Essential Paediatrics

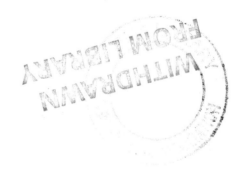

For Churchill Livingstone:

Commissioning editor: Ellen Green
Project development manager: Barbara Simmons
Project manager: Frances Affleck
Designers: Sarah Cape, Judith Wright

Essential Paediatrics

Edited by

David Hull

BSc MB FRCP FRCPCH DObstRCOG DCH
Formerly Professor of Child Health,
Medical School,
University of Nottingham,
Nottingham, UK

Derek I. Johnston

MA MD FRCP FRCPCH DCH
Consultant Paediatrician,
University Hospital,
Queen's Medical Centre,
Nottingham, UK

FOURTH EDITION

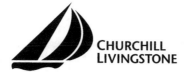

CHURCHILL LIVINGSTONE

EDINBURGH LONDON NEW YORK OXFORD PHILADELPHIA ST LOUIS SYDNEY TORONTO
1999

CHURCHILL LIVINGSTONE
An imprint of Elsevier Limited

Fourth Edition 2000
  Reprinted 2001, 2003, 2005, 2006 (twice), 2008 (twice)

ISBN 978 0 443 05958 2

International Student Edition ISBN 978 0 443 05959 9

British Library Cataloguing in Publication Data
A catalogue record for this book is available from the British Library.

Library of Congress Cataloging in Publication Data
A catalog record for this book is available from the Library of Congress.

Medical knowledge is constantly changing. As new information becomes
available, changes in treatment, procedures, equipment and the use of drugs
become necessary. The author and publisher have, as far as it is possible,
taken care to ensure that the information given in this text is accurate and up
to date. However, readers are strongly advised to confirm that the information,
especially with regard to drug usage, complies with current legislation and
standards of practice.

 your source for books,
journals and multimedia
in the health sciences

www.elsevierhealth.com

Working together to grow
libraries in developing countries

www.elsevier.com | www.bookaid.org | www.sabre.org

ELSEVIER   BOOK AID International   Sabre Foundation

The
publisher's
policy is to use
**paper manufactured
from sustainable forests**

Printed and bound in the United Kingdom

Transferred to Digital Print 2010

Preface

The main objective of *Essential Paediatrics* is to provide medical students with an introduction to the care of children that stimulates interest and then satisfies a growing appetite for more in-depth information. The challenge has been to balance an introduction to normal health in children and young persons with the increasing complexity and specialisation that is a feature of contemporary paediatric medicine and surgery. Despite society's increasing realisation that health in early life determines the pattern of adult life and death, most trainee health professionals have to absorb their core paediatric knowledge over a matter of weeks. It was with this pressure in mind that *Essential Paediatrics* emerged as a teaching tool in the then newly established Nottingham University Medical School. The text has been and continues to be tested by successive groups of Nottingham students and teachers, and we are also grateful to those readers from further afield who have made valid criticism and valuable suggestions. In this era of clinical governance and evidence-based medicine, our readers have the right to expect that core information can justify its inclusion!

This new edition of *Essential Paediatrics* benefits from a new infusion of contributors and ideas. All chapters have been revised and several have been radically restructured. Many sources have been tapped to ensure that contemporary research and epidemiological data enhance the core information. We hope that liberal use of lists, tables and figures enriches the text and helps readers to maintain perspective and priority when encountering potentially complex topics.

The illustrations frequently highlight the doctor-child relationship, and it remains a paramount objective of *Essential Paediatrics* that students are encouraged to practise their newly acquired skills in all the settings in which they are privileged to meet children.

Nottingham 1999   D.H.
                                                                                                          D.I.J.

Acknowledgment

Many of the colour illustrations in the Skin chapter were reproduced by kind permission from Churchill Livingstone's Colour Guide series: Thomas R & Harvey D *Neonatology*; Thomas R & Harvey D *Paediatrics*; Wilkinson JD, Shaw S, Fenton DS *Dermatology*.

Contributors

Charles P. J. Charlton
B Med Sci (Hons) MB ChB MRCP FRCPCH
Consultant Paediatric Gastroenterologist, University Hospital,
Queens Medical Centre, Nottingham, UK
Chapter 10 Gut

David A. Curnock
MA MB BChir FRCP FRCPCH DCH
Consultant Paediatrician, City Hospital, Nottingham, UK
Chapter 4 Newborn

Martin Hewitt
BSc MD FRCP FRCPCH
Consultant Paediatrician/Oncologist, University Hospital,
Nottingham, UK
Chapter 12 Blood
Chapter 13 Malignancy

Neil Marlow
MA DM FRCP FRCPCH
Professor of Neonatal Medicine, University of Nottingham,
Nottingham, UK
Chapter 4 Newborn

David H. Mellor
MD FRCP FRCPCH DCH
Consultant Paediatric Neurologist, University Hospital,
Nottingham, UK
Chapter 19 Brain, cord, nerve, muscle
Chapter 20 Seeing, hearing, speaking and learning

John B. Pearce
MB BS MPhil MRCP FRCPsych
Professor of Child and Adolescent Psychiatry,
University of Nottingham, Nottingham, UK
Chapter 21 Emotions and behaviour

Leon Polnay
FRCPCH FRCP DCH
Professor of Community Paediatrics, University of Nottingham,
Nottingham, UK
Appendix C Child health promotion programme

Nicholas Rutter
MD FRCP FRCPCH
Professor of Paediatric Medicine and Honorary Consultant
Paediatrician, University of Nottingham, Nottingham, UK
Chapter 9 Heart

Stephanie A. Smith
BM BS FRCPCH
Consultant Emergency Paediatrician, University Hospital,
Nottingham, UK
Chapter 7 Hazards

Alan Smyth
MD FRCPCH
Consultant in Paediatric Respiratory Medicine,
Nottingham City Hospital, Nottingham, UK
Chapter 8 Airways and lungs

Terence Stephenson
BSc DM FRCP FRCPCH
Professor of Child Health, University of Nottingham,
Nottingham, UK
Chapter 3 Fetus

Helen Venning
BMedSci BM BS FRCP FRCPCH
Consultant Paediatric Rheumatologist, University Hospital,
Nottingham, UK
Chapter 18 Bone and joint

David A. Walker
BMedSci BM BS FRCP FRCPCH
Consultant Paediatric Oncologist and Senior Lecturer,
University of Nottingham, Nottingham, UK
Chapter 12 Blood
Chapter 13 Malignancy

Alan R. Watson
BMedSci MB ChB FRCP FRCPCH
Consultant Paediatric Nephrologist, City Hospital, Nottingham, UK
Chapter 11 Urinary tract and testes

Hywel C. Williams
MSc PhD FRCP
Professor of Dermato-Epidemiology, Queen's Medical Centre,
Nottingham, UK
Chapter 17 Skin

I.D. Young
MD FRCP MSc DCH
Professor of Paediatric Genetics, City Hospital, Nottingham, UK
Chapter 2 Genes

Contents

1. The ill child 1
2. Genes 12
3. Fetus 31
4. Newborn 43
5. Nutrition 74
6. Infection 90
7. Hazards 110
8. Airways and lungs 121
9. Heart 136
10. Gut 159
11. Urinary tract and testes 183
12. Blood 202
13. Malignancy 213
14. Growth 230
15. Endocrine 243
16. Metabolism 260
17. Skin 269
18. Bone and joint 280
19. Brain, cord, nerve, muscle 293
20. Seeing, hearing, speaking and learning 314
21. Emotions and behaviour 326

Appendices
A. Normal values 355
B. National immunisation schedule 360
C. Child health promotion programme 361

Index 367

Editor's note

For ease of reading, the masculine gender is used throughout this book, except where obviously inappropriate, but the feminine is intended to be equally applicable.

The ill child

THE INTERVIEW
THE PROBLEMS
MORTALITY

In paediatric practice it is not possible to make a full diagnosis or draw up an appropriate care programme without some knowledge of the child's age, size, abilities and personality. Furthermore, children are part of a family; to understand them one must know something of their family; of their parents' life styles, family life and capacity to look after their children and in particular their relationships to our patient and their attitudes towards the illness. As children grow older and become more independent they relate more directly to the community, to their school and their peers. Thus, it is helpful to know the main features of that community and the child's and family's relationship to it. The mode of presentation, the symptoms and even the signs of disease may be influenced by the nature of the child, his family and their surroundings and experiences. Likewise, treatment will depend on the reserves and resources of the family and community.

THE INTERVIEW

First impressions are important. Even very young children are quick to sense an atmosphere and the reactions of their parents to it. As they grow older they become expert at masking their feelings. In uncertain situations they are more likely to demonstrate what they think by actions rather than words. They will look to and reach for those they trust. Children, not unlike adults, warm to those who like and admire them, and they are less suspicious than adults of ulterior motives. A relaxed, friendly beginning to the interview not only eases its passage, but is essential for its success.

Establishing trust

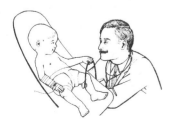

It is a matter of sensitivity and judgement to know how to make the first introductions. In the UK shaking hands is probably right for most parents but not for most children. It is impolite not to know the child's name and what he or she would like to be called. All Susans do not like to be called 'Suzie'. The sex of the child is not always evident from appearances. Sometimes the dress and the hair style may be very misleading and you may wonder why. Even under such circumstances, to call a boy 'she' is a mistake. His mother will not like it and neither will he if he is old enough to understand. Never refer to the baby as 'it'.

The interview

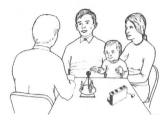

Next ascertain the names and the relationship to the child of the adults who accompany him. Children belong to their parents, parents are responsible for their children so it is the parents' point of view that, in the first instance, you want to know. Not infrequently parents differ in their interpretation of their child's symptoms and signs. Neither parent has a monopoly on objectivity. Sometimes an unaccompanied mother will say, referring to her husband, that 'he disagrees with me and says I fuss too much', or alternatively that 'he told me to bring her along because she is not right'. Some grandparents are a tremendous support to their children when they start their own families but others tend to be interfering busy bodies. The latter, if they are present at the interview, should be encouraged not to interrupt or enlarge upon the history given by the parents, though their attempts to do so may help in understanding the total situation.

The ability and willingness of children to describe their own symptoms varies widely. If in doubt always ask. It is instructive, for example, to find out why the child thinks he has been brought to see you. The answers are often revealing if not too helpful with the diagnosis. Another very important question, possibly best asked at the end of the interview, is what does the child and what do the parents think is the cause of the child's illness? In particular, what do they fear it might be?

In the main, children are not interested in adult talk so as the interview gets underway the majority of the younger ones will become restless and seek ways of entertaining themselves; but never make the mistake of thinking that they are not listening to what is being said. Toys for every age group should be scattered on the desk, shelves and floor.

Suggested types of toys to have on hand

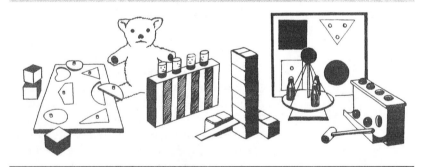

Play will not only occupy the youngster, it will also give valuable clues to his motor skills, mental abilities, interests and personality. So while taking the history you can often learn a lot by watching the child. In particular, the way he moves, how he uses his eyes and ears and hands and feet. Does he follow up a challenge? Is he constructive? Is he relaxed? Watch the interplay between the child and parents, and the child and yourself. It will not only help interpret the history but also give some indication of how best to examine the child later to get the most information. For example, if a 4 year old stays on his mother's knee and demands that the toys be brought to him, he is obviously feeling very threatened or is limited either by his illness or in his abilities. In these circumstances it is probably wisest to make the preliminary examination at least while the child is on his mother's knee. Know something about the toys in the room; for example, at what stage can a child be expected to put a square block in a square hole, or to lift it out to find pictures underneath, or to name what they see. If he does not do it you have not learnt much—it might be simply because of the situation—but if he does, you may have learnt a great deal.

History

Every doctor develops his own way of collecting information. It is best to start by noting the main complaint or complaints. If there are a number, then a simple opening problem list helps. Then enlarge and define each problem and enquire about associated problems. An obsessional enquiry about all the bodily functions is not usually necessary, it wastes time and may interrupt the flow of the interview. However for most medical problems, and always for any child admitted to hospital, certain background information is essential.

Firstly, it is important to collect information about the child's own life. Was the pregnancy, labour and birth normal? What was the birth weight? How was the child in the first days of life? It may be important to note whether the baby was breast or bottle fed and when he was weaned. Has he had the common childhood infections? Has he been immunised? Has the child been treated in hospital and, if so, when and where and for what?

Secondly, an assessment should be made as to how the child is progressing. Full assessment of motor and language achievement and mental and social responses demands considerable skill and experience. For most purposes a simple enquiry about the principal stages of development is all that is required and should be within the competence of anyone presuming to advise parents about the care of their children. Plot on the charts of normal development what his parents say they can do—and parents are usually right—and what you observed the child does in clinic. For the older child, ask about progress at school. It is not acceptable to make a note that the child is slow or retarded without indicating the basis for that conclusion. Indeed, labels of that nature are best avoided altogether. If a child is not speaking at 3 years of age, write that he has delayed speech, but do not

Steps in development

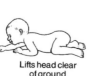

Lifts head clear
of ground

Sits with
support

Sits on
own

Crawling

Stages in development

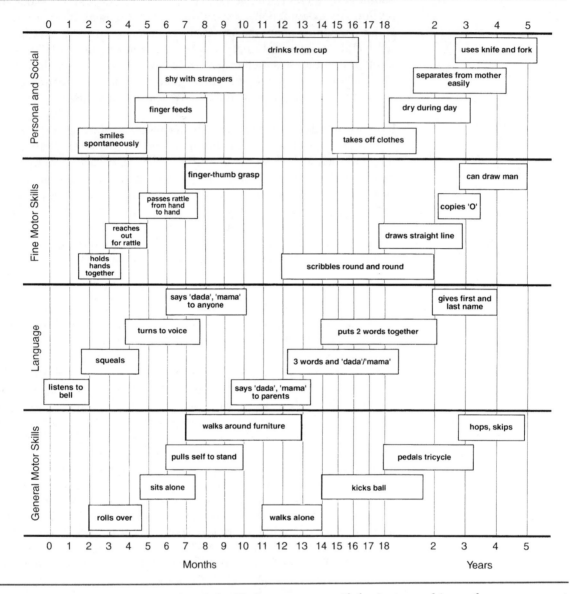

guess at the likely cause, even if, for instance, his mother appears not to understand even your simplest questions.

Always ask about the health of the rest of the family. This is important for a variety of reasons. The first, and perhaps the most obvious, is that the child might have an inherited disorder. Collect the information carefully and record it using accepted symbols and notation (see Ch. 2). Secondly, if environmental factors are important, then other members of the family may also be affected. This might include anything from respiratory infections to the inhalation of lead. Thirdly, the presence of chronic illness in other members of the family may be the reason why the parents are concerned about the child before you. It may be that the family's stress has helped precipitate the child's problems. The fourth, though not the most important, is probably the most interesting reason. There are often family complaints, headaches, stomach aches, weariness, which determine the family language of disease and colour the way the child and his parents interpret his symptoms and signs. This will be particularly so if there is a strong behavioural component to his problem.

Examination

Examining children can be fun, but it may involve games when you do not want to play, and occasionally it can be singularly frustrating. Children, even the smallest infants, will try and work out your intentions by looking into your eyes. People with kind eyes do not mean to hurt! The parents may be more nervous about what you might do than the child himself, so they need reassurance as well. Some parents attempt to comfort their children by telling them not to worry 'the doctor won't hurt you'. Up until that time it may not have entered their heads that you might, so be prepared for the protests. Some mothers may say such things in an attempt to put you off any examination which might be uncomfortable or embarrassing. Always encourage the parents to help you with the examination by holding or distracting the child, unless, of course, the youngster is approaching puberty when his independence is to be respected.

Clinicians have different practices about clothes. Undressing disturbs babies and they do not like it. Older infants hold onto their clothes as a protection, so they may object to their removal. From 3 years onwards there is usually no problem until puberty. Then the youngster must be handled with all the care and sensitivity you would extend to royalty! So it can be very useful to make observations while the child is clothed and undisturbed. Palpation and auscultation can easily be performed through vest and pants. On the other hand, some babies and children will remain undisturbed and, indeed, may expect you to undress them, and you can learn a great deal by the handling involved. It is a form of palpation which children understand and further palpation afterwards is usually acceptable. If the child shows uncertainty ask the parents to undress him. Even the most defensive child is usually happy for you to observe him naked from a distance.

Although the collection of the information may be disorderly, its recording in the notes must not be. In most situations it is important to record aspects of the child's size. Weight and length or height must be measured accurately. In certain situations, skull circumference and very occasionally skin fold thicknesses may also be measured. The data is recorded in the notes and on the appropriate charts (see Ch. 14). Note the child's general behaviour and awareness. You may wish to make you own evaluation of the child's capabilities and record them with the parents' reports of his achievements. Next, observe the child. Much of the information you seek may be obtained by careful observation. In general terms, is the appearance at all unusual? If so, try to define why: is it the shape of the head, the mould of the ears, the position of the eyes, bodily proportions or the posture? Does the child look like his parents? Has he got any of the recognised major or minor anomalies?

Then specifically assess the child's general size, proportions and nutritional state. Note the nature and distribution of any skin lesions or rashes. Then examine the system or systems that are the source of the complaint.

Respiratory disorders are often most easily observed. Avoid percussion or auscultation until you have noted the respiratory rate and the movement of the diaphragm and chest wall with quiet breathing and the effect of a stronger respiratory effort performed on request in an older child, or with a cry in a baby. Determine whether or not the lung is overinflated by percussion of the upper edge of the liver.

Listen to the heart

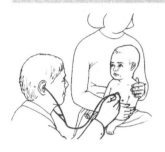

Interpretation of breath sounds and additional noises can be difficult in the very young. Fine crackling noises on inspiration (crepitations) may be heard on careful auscultation in apparently normal babies. If they are persistent and bilateral in a distressed toddler they usually indicate bronchiolitis or, very rarely, left heart failure. Coarse intermittent noises during both inspiration and expiration (rales) usually signify liquid debris in the larger airways. They may be transmitted from the back of the throat. Harsh and more persistent noises superadded on to the breath sounds (rhonchi), indicating a more persistent obstruction, are less frequently heard in children. Continuous noises, hardening and extending the breath sounds (bronchial breathing) may be heard in babies over most of the upper back, and usually are transmitted sounds from the main airway. When the airway is partially obstructed the noise becomes harsher and more vibrant and is called a stridor. This term covers a wide range of sounds, some fine and high pitched, some low and coarse. The character depends on the site, the nature of the obstruction and the narrowness of the aperture. Wheezing is heard when the mid airways are narrowed; always check if it is bilateral.

Examination of the cardiovascular system begins by recording the rate, rhythm, strength and character of the peripheral pulses. Palpate and percuss the anterior chest wall to determine the heart size, the site and nature of the apex beat and to detect the presence, if any, of a thrill. Then listen to the first heart sound, then the second, then the sounds in between and then the murmurs between the heart sounds. For each murmur you will wish to know its timing, character, loudness, site and distribution. Check if it is transmitted into the neck.

Percuss the liver

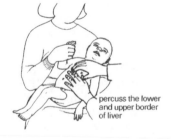

percuss the lower and upper border of liver

Always observe the abdomen before you palpate. Look for swellings and movements. Ask if anywhere is tender, and if you can, watch the child's face and not his abdomen while you palpate. After general palpation in the four quadrants, systematically determine the position and size of the liver, spleen, kidneys and bladder. If an organ is enlarged, note its position, size, surface and texture, the character of the edge if it has one, and whether or not it is tender. When examining the back of the chest, look at the spine, particularly the lower end.

Again, examination of the locomotor and nervous systems is more by observation than manipulation. In babies and infants always palpate the anterior fontanelle or head 'soft spot'. It usually closes in

Palpate the fontanelle

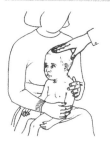

Look at the ear drum

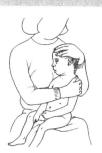

the middle of the second year. Note if it is pulsating: it usually does. You can record the heart rate from it. The fontanelle may be full or flat. Ask yourself the following questions: Can the child see? Hear? Move his eyes and head well and in all directions? Move all limbs, and is the movement normal and full? Is the contour and position of each limb normal? Is the power good? When you handle the infant, note the tone on passive movement of the limb. Is there any limitation in the movement at any joint? Are the joints unduly lax and hyperextendable? Again, watch the child's face while you move their limbs. Eliciting the reflex responses rarely adds useful information in children but it is as well to keep up the habit for the odd occasion when it does. In the infant the percussing finger can be used as the hammer.

Finally, examine with a light. If necessary, check the eyes and then the ear drums and finally the throat. Never force yourself upon the child. Never force their mouth open against their will: be patient. Ask yourself, is the information you wish to gather as important as all that? Do not use a dry stick to depress the tongue when a smooth teaspoon handle will do just as well. Spoons are meant to go into mouths. Before you finish, should you bother to record the blood pressure? If disease of the kidney or heart is suspected, the answer is yes.

This completes the general examination. During it you may have included specific observations or examinations, for example, to see if the testes are in the scrotum, the femoral pulses are present, the hips in joint, the characteristic of unusual lumps, the presence of the signs of puberty, etc.

Once the clinical enquiry is complete the next step is to re-examine the initial list of problems; some may be easily dealt with by appropriate advice, on the other hand new problems may have arisen. Draw up a new list and indicate what steps you propose to follow through further enquiry, investigation or treatment. Discuss these steps with the parents and, in a form that he may understand, with your patient.

THE PROBLEMS

Every week practising paediatricians see a condition, anomaly, or a sign that they have never seen before and in such a situation their actions depend on their basic scientific knowledge. Every month they will treat a condition which is known but rare, then they rely on colleagues who have reported their observations in the medical literature. However, the substance of doctors' practice is with diseases they have seen before, and their management of these problems will be influenced as much by their own previous experience and by their knowledge of their own patients and their community as it is by therapies recommended in textbooks. What are these common problems? Obviously, these will vary from place to place and from community to community, and on whether the doctor works in a family practice, a child health clinic or a district hospital.

Family practice

Work in General Practice	
Problem	Number*
Cystic fibrosis	10
Diabetes	30
Epilepsy	110
Asthma	4020
Eye disorders	5120
Skin disorders	9400
Ear disorders	9560

*Numbers of children (0–15 years) consulting family doctors in a resident population of 250 000 per year

Each group of four family doctors in the UK has about 8000 people registered in the practice. The birth rate runs at around 12.0 births per 1000 population, thus there will be, on average, 96 births in their practice each year and 1440 child patients spread between 0 and 15 years of age. Between 15 and 20% of the family doctor's work is with children. Disorders of the respiratory system are by far the commonest, followed by skin conditions, infectious diseases, gastrointestinal disorders, problems with eyes, ears and teeth. Social and administrative problems form the bulk of the remainder. Only 10% of children's disorders are judged to be serious and in need of specific therapy, though it is likely that medicine will be prescribed in over half the cases.

Only occasionally will an individual family doctor have to care for a child with some of the conditions which are often seen in hospital. Thus, on average, a family doctor will see a child presenting with mental retardation, diabetes or epilepsy every 5 years or so, a child with Down syndrome every 20 years, cystic fibrosis every 40 years and muscular dystrophy every 480 years!

Hospital service

One in five children visit the accident and emergency department of the local hospital each year. Ninety per cent are taken directly to hospital. The common reasons are home and road accidents, accidental poisoning, acute respiratory illness, fevers, convulsions and acute bowel upsets. Between 70 and 75% of attendances are for cuts, bruises, fractures, dislocations and head injuries.

Patients referred to the paediatric consultancy service usually have less acute conditions. The commoner problems include recurrent respiratory infections, asthma, failure to thrive, small size, suspected developmental delay, convulsions or suspected convulsions, nocturnal enuresis and constipation. There are usually special clinics for children with chronic illnesses, for example for children with diabetes, leukaemia, neurology, short stature, cystic fibrosis and renal disorders. Children with physical and mental handicaps are assessed in a special developmental assessment unit by a team which includes physiotherapists, occupational therapists, psychologists, teachers and audiometricians, as well as doctors from various disciplines.

Admission to hospital is avoided if it is at all possible. Half of the admissions are for medical conditions, and half for surgery—general, ENT, orthopaedics, etc. It is now usual for parents to stay with their children and share in their care (see Hospital Paediatrics).

Reasons for admission to a medical ward: 1996–97			
Asthma	15.8%	Bronchiolitis	4.9%
Febrile convulsion	9.2%	URTI	4.3%
Ingestion	7.1%	Convulsions	3.6%
Gastroenteritis	6.6%	Croup	2.8%
Vomiting	5.9%	Others	34.3%
Fever	5.5%		

*Note: 60% stayed for less than a day

Child health service

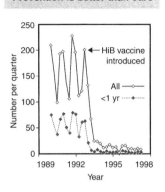

Prevention is better than cure

Many family doctors work in group practices in health centres. Working with them in the primary care team are health visitors. In some centres one doctor in the group, with the health visitors, holds regular child health clinics in order to examine routinely every child and provides a preventive health service. In others, a consultant paediatrician or clinical medical officer from the community child health service attends the clinic. Healthy babies are examined routinely at 6 weeks of age and then at regular intervals afterwards. The predominant problems in the early months are related to feeding, nutrition, bowels and general growth and development. Hearing is assessed at 6–9 months of age. The infants are examined for vision abnormalities and the development of squints. The clinics also have responsibilities for the immunisation programme and health education. After the age of 5 years surveillance is continued by the school health services. See Appendix C.

Child health promotion programme: see Appendix C for details		
0–3 days	anomalies, defects	2$\frac{1}{2}$–3 years development, behaviour, vision
6 weeks	review mother and child, feeding and sleeping	4$\frac{1}{2}$–5 years readiness for school
6–8 months	mobility, skills, language, behaviour	

Social paediatrics

The distribution of health problems differs across the town. Certain inner city areas, deprived by most material and social standards, have a higher incidence of most medical problems and the children who live there are, in general, less physically, mentally and socially able. At a disadvantage from birth, these children 'born to fail' are less able to form secure relationships and thus are themselves less likely to establish a strong family environment for their own children. Breaking this circle of events is one of the major tasks of community paediatric care (see Community Paediatrics). It is a challenge that the health service staff share with social workers and teachers.

Social class and health disasters

Health disaster	Social class					
	I	II	IIIN	IIIM	IV	V
Perinatal death (per 1000 births)	6.6	6.0	7.1	7.6	9.5	9.6
Infant death (per 1000 births)	5.6	5.3	6.4	6.5	8.3	11.2
Childhood death (per 100 000 pop.)	23	21	24	28	33	51

MORTALITY

Happily, infant and child mortality rates continue to fall. The rates are highest for the very young.

Neonatal mortality. Around 30% of neonatal deaths are due to congenital abnormalities incompatible with independent life, and over 40% are very immature and even with artificial respiratory and nutritional support do not survive the first few days after birth. With the continuing improvements in general health, antenatal care and appropriate genetic counselling, it is likely that the perinatal mortality will continue to fall. (Note that the definition for the perinatal mortality rate (MR) changed in 1993.)

Post-neonatal mortality. Older infants rarely die in hospital. The majority of children dying between 4 weeks and 1 year, post-neonatal infant deaths, die suddenly at home (SUDI—sudden unexpected death in infancy). Often nothing abnormal is found at post mortem and there are no suspicious curcumstances (SIDS—sudden infant death syndrome). Despite much research, the cause of SIDS is still not clear. Some consider that it might be due to a confusion in respiratory control precipitated by a respiratory infection or unexpected regurgitation. Another possibility is that the infants over-react to a fever, or are unable to lose heat and that hyperpyrexia is the cause of death. SIDS was found to be less common in cultures which traditionally place their infants on their backs to sleep. This practice has now been adopted around the world. Rates of post-neonatal death in the UK fell sharply between 1988 and 1991 and have continued to fall but more slowly since.

The incidence of SIDS is higher in families living in poor housing, when the parents are inexperienced or of limited ability, or when there is domestic stress. Early infant death occurs more often in babies born prematurely or experiencing problems in the newborn period. These characteristics can be identified at birth and if the families are given extra advice and support during the early months, the number of post-neonatal infant deaths will fall further.

Some of the infants who die unexpectedly do have evidence of known disease, or non-specific signs of illness at autopsy. A small percentage (under 2%?) have been found to be due to an inherited metabolic disorder. Some studies suggest that as many as 10% are due to 'gentle smothering', that the parents had acted against their infant. There are also a small number of infants with severe abnormalities, persisting problems due to immaturity or fulminating infections who die in the 1–12-month period.

Deaths over 1 year of age. An unexpected death of a child over the age of 1 year is rare. Many are due to accidents; others are due to previously diagnosed malignancies. The remainder include children with inherited diseases, for example, cystic fibrosis, muscular dystrophies and progressive encephalopathies. Acute infections, which

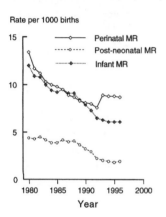

Deaths in the first year of life

Rate per 1000 births

Perinatal MR
Post-neonatal MR
Infant MR

used to be a major cause of death, are usually controllable; but occasionally the onset can be so sudden and death follows so quickly that therapeutic measures cannot be introduced in time, for example in meningitis with septicaemia or an intravascular coagulopathy, severe gastroenteritis and fulminating respiratory infections.

Causes of death in childhood (England & Wales 1991: population 49 million)

Cause of death	Age group			
	4 wk–1 yr	1–4 yr	5–9 yr	10–14 yr
Congenital abnormalities (%)	17	20	12	9
Sudden unexpected death (%)	41	4	0	0
Respiratory illness (%)	10	8	3	7
Cancer (%)	1	13	27	19
Injuries and poisoning (%)	4	22	31	35
Others (%)	27	32	27	30
Boys total numbers	1243	554	431	354
Girls total numbers	863	439	248	222

BIBLIOGRAPHY

Botting B (ed) 1995 The health of our children. OPCS, London
Committee on Child Health Services 1976 Fit for the future. Report Cmnd 6684, Chairman Court S D M. HMSO, London
Forfar J O (ed) 1988 Child health in a changing society. Oxford University Press, Oxford
House of Commons, Health Committee 1997 Child and adolescent mental health services. HMSO, London
House of Commons, Health Committee 1997 Health services for children and young people in the community: home and school. HMSO, London
House of Commons, Health Committee 1997 Hospital services for children and young people. HMSO, London
House of Commons, Health Committee 1997 The specific health needs of children and young people. HMSO, London
Inequalities in health 1988 (includes the Black Report and the Health Divide). Penguin Books, Harmonsworth
Milner A D, Hull D 1998 Hospital paediatrics, 3rd edn. Churchill Livingstone, Edinburgh
On the State of Public Health The Annual Report of the Chief Medical Officer of the Department of Health for the years 1996/7. HMSO, London
Polnay L, Hull D (eds) 1993 Community paediatrics, 2nd edn. Churchill Livingstone, Edinburgh
Report of the Chief Medical Officer's Expert Group 1993 The sleeping position of infants and cot death HMSO, London
Smith R (ed) 1991 The health of the nation. BMJ, London
Spencer N 1996 Poverty and child health. Radcliffe Medical Press, Oxford

2 Genes

CHROMOSOMES AND
  CHROMOSOMAL
  ABNORMALITIES
COMMON AUTOSOMAL
  ABNORMALITIES
COMMON SEX CHROMOSOME
  ABNORMALITIES
SINGLE GENE (MENDELIAN)
  INHERITANCE
MULTIFACTORIAL (POLYGENIC)
  INHERITANCE
RECENT ADVANCES IN
  MOLECULAR GENETICS
GENETIC COUNSELLING

Genetic disorders can become apparent at any age from conception to senescence, but it is in childhood that they make their greatest impact. Approximately 1 in 40 of all babies has a major malformation identifiable at birth and in over half of these infants genetic factors can be implicated. Inherited disorders also account for 50% of all cases of childhood blindness and deafness, and together with congenital malformations are responsible for 25–30% of all hospital admissions and deaths occurring in the paediatric age group.

As a result of continuing progress in obstetrics, community paediatrics and the treatment of both infection and cancer, it is likely that the relative contribution of genetic disease to childhood morbidity and mortality will increase, in parallel with the general public's knowledge of genetics and expectations of good health. Recognition of the importance of genetic disorders in childhood has coincided with a scientific explosion in molecular biology, which has revolutionised understanding of the mechanisms of inheritance and opened up new avenues for the prevention and sometimes the treatment of inherited disease.

CHROMOSOMES AND CHROMOSOMAL ABNORMALITIES

Genes consist of DNA and are tightly packaged in chromosomes which are present in all nucleated cells. Electron microscopy reveals that the DNA is coiled around histone proteins, the precise function of which is unclear. Normally, each cell contains 46 chromosomes comprising 22 pairs of autosomes and a single pair of sex chromosomes, XY in the male and XX in the female. During meiosis I each pair separates so that each gamete receives a single 'haploid' set consisting of 23 chromosomes. Successful fertilisation results in restitution of the normal 'diploid' complement of 46 chromosomes.

Whereas genes cannot be directly visualised, it is possible to detect alterations in both the number and structure of human chromosomes using a high powered light microscope. Peripheral blood lymphocytes or skin fibroblasts can be cultured in the laboratory. Cell division is arrested during metaphase, the stage of maximum

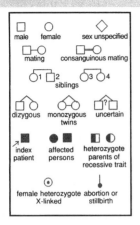
chromosome condensation. The cell nuclei are then swollen by adding a hypotonic solution which separates the individual chromosomes and renders them readily visible by light microscopy. The chromosomes are then stained to facilitate their individual identification and subsequent analysis. The overall chromosome constitution is known as a karyotype and can be illustrated by photographing the metaphase spread down the microscope and then arranging the chromosomes in matching pairs in descending order of size. Normally it takes at least 3 days to obtain a satisfactory chromosome analysis using circulating lymphocytes.

The karyotype of a female infant with Down syndrome resulting from the presence of an additional number 21 chromosome (trisomy 21)

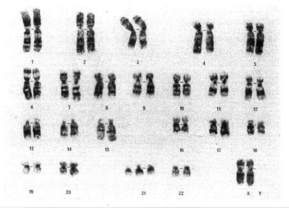

The majority of chromosomal abnormalities arise as de novo events due to an error in gametogenesis in one of the parents. Many individuals with an autosomal imbalance are unable to reproduce so that the issue of risks to their offspring is largely unimportant. However, autosomal rearrangements may exist in a balanced form such as a translocation or inversion, and carriers of these rearrangements may be at high risk of transmitting the rearrangement in an unbalanced form and therefore of having a handicapped child. This is discussed in the section on Down syndrome below.

Any loss or gain (imbalance) of autosomal material is likely to have adverse effects on both mental and physical development. Generally, alterations in the number or structure of the sex chromosomes have a much milder effect than autosomal imbalance, although certain sex chromosome abnormalities such as Turner syndrome and Klinefelter syndrome are associated with a high incidence of infertility.

Spontaneous abortions. At least 15% of all recognised pregnancies end in spontaneous miscarriage. In 40% of these there is a chromosomal abnormality consisting most commonly of autosomal trisomy, monosomy X (i.e. 45, X), triploidy or tetraploidy.

Perinatal mortality surveys. In most developed nations, the perinatal mortality rate is around 1%. Approximately 25% of these babies die as a direct consequence of a serious malformation: 5% have a chromosomal abnormality such as trisomy 13 or trisomy 18.

Newborn surveys. The pooled results of several surveys show that a chromosomal abnormality is present in 0.6% of all newborn infants. In one-third of cases this is present in a balanced form.

Mental retardation. Surveys in the community show that chromosomal abnormalities account for at least 30% of all cases of moderate and severe mental retardation. Trisomy 21 and the fragile X syndrome are the most common causes.

COMMON AUTOSOMAL ABNORMALITIES

Down syndrome (T21)

Incidence. This condition affects approximately 1 in 700 babies and is found in all ethnic communities. There is a well recognised association with advancing maternal age, with the incidence rising to 1% when a mother reaches the age of 40 years. Advanced paternal age has very little effect.

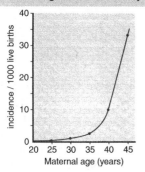

Incidence of Down syndrome vs maternal age at time of delivery

incidence / 1000 live births vs Maternal age (years)

Clinical features. The most striking feature in the neonate is hypotonia, and although the diagnosis is usually evident at this time, it may sometimes be missed if the baby is very premature or his facial features are concealed by ventilatory apparatus. In infants and older children the most characteristic features are upward sloping palpebral fissures and protruding tongue, single palmar creases, mild short stature and mild to moderate developmental delay. IQ scores range from 25 to 70 and social skills often exceed other intellectual parameters. Children with Down syndrome are usually happy and sociable.

Clinical features in Down syndrome	
General	**Limbs**
Neonatal hypotonia	Fifth finger clinodactyly
Mild–moderate mental retardation	Single palmar crease
Short stature	Wide gap between first and second toes
Cranio-facial	**Other**
Brachycephaly	Congenital heart disease (40%)
Epicanthic folds	e.g. common atrio-ventricular canal,
Protruding tongue	ASD, PDA, VSD, Fallot tetralogy
Small ears	Anal atresia
Upward sloping palpebral fissures	Duodenal atresia
Strabismus and/or nystagmus	
Increased incidence of leukaemia (1%)	

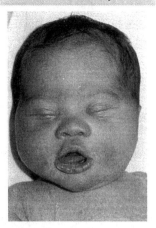

Typical facial appearance of an infant with Down syndrome

Note the upward sloping palpebral fissures and protruding tongue

Life expectancy in Down syndrome has improved dramatically as a result of the widespread availability of antibiotics and advances in cardiac surgery. Approximately 15–20% of Down syndrome children die before the age of 5 years, usually as a result of severe inoperable congenital heart disease. Life expectancy for the remainder is well into adult life. By the age of 40 years almost all individuals with Down syndrome will have developed Alzheimer disease, probably as a direct result of a gene dosage effect, because the gene which codes for the amyloid protein which is associated with Alzheimer disease is located on chromosome 21.

Cytogenetic aspects. Chromosomal abnormalities in Down syndrome are listed below. By far the most common finding is straightforward trisomy 21. Molecular studies have revealed that the additional number 21 chromosome is derived from the mother in 95% of cases. The recurrence risk in these families is approximately 1%. If a female with Down syndrome due to trisomy 21 conceives, then there is a risk of 50% that the baby will also have trisomy 21. Males with Down syndrome have rarely if ever reproduced.

Chromosome findings in Down syndrome	
Trisomy 21, e.g. 47,XY,+21	95%
Mosaicism, e.g. 46,XX,/47,XX,+21	2%
Unbalanced Robertsonian translocation, e.g. 46XX,–15,+t(15q21q)*	3%

* This karyotope can be interpreted as showing that the patient is a female (46,XX) with Down syndrome due to the replacement of a normal number 15 chromosome (–15), by a translocation chromosome consisting of the fused long arms of one number 15 chromosome and one number 21 chromosome (+t(15q21q)).

Children with mosaic Down syndrome are usually less severely affected than in the full-blown syndrome, and if only a small proportion of cells are trisomic then these individuals may lead normal lives. In the event of reproduction, there is a relatively high risk that the baby will have full trisomy 21, with the precise risk equalling the proportion of gametes which carry an additional number 21 chromosome.

When a child has Down syndrome as a result of an unbalanced Robertsonian translocation, there is a probability of around 25% that one of the parents will carry this in a balanced form. The remaining 75% of cases arise as de novo events and convey a low recurrence risk of approximately 1%. If, however, a parent is shown to be a carrier then there will be a significant risk that a future child will be affected, usually of the order of 2–5% for a carrier male and 10–15% for a carrier female. In the very rare event that a parent carries a balanced 21q21q Robertsonian translocation, the risk of Down syndrome in liveborn offspring will be 100%.

Edwards syndrome

Incidence. Trisomy 18 affects approximately 1 in 3000 neonates with a male to female ratio of 1 : 3. There is a weak association with advanced maternal age: 25% of all cases are conceived by mothers aged 35 years or over.

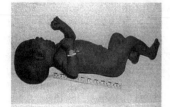

Lateral view of a baby with trisomy 18 showing prominent occiput and overlapping fingers

Clinical features. Intrauterine growth retardation is common and the mean birth weight is under 2.0 kg. Characteristic features are listed below; 90% of affected babies have congenital heart disease and 50% die during the first week of life. Almost all cases have died by the age of 1 year. Surviving infants and children show severe retardation of growth and development.

Clinical features in trisomy 18

General	Limbs
Intrauterine growth retardation	Clenched hands with second and fifth fingers
Severe failure to thrive	overlapping third and fourth fingers
Mental retardation	Small nails especially on fifth finger
	Short dorsiflexed big toes
	Rocker-bottom feet
Cranio-facial	**Other**
Prominent occiput	Cardiac abnormalities
Low-set dysplastic ears	Oesophageal atresia
Short narrow palpebral fissures	Tracheo-oesophageal fistula
Small mouth and small jaw	Spina bifida

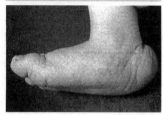

'Rocker-bottom' foot in a baby with trisomy 18

Cytogenetic aspects. Most cases show straightforward trisomy 18. Molecular studies indicate that the additional number 18 chromosome has been inherited from the mother in over 90% of cases. Rarely an unbalanced translocation is found, in which case parental chromosome studies must be initiated. Mosaicism with a normal cell line sometimes occurs and probably accounts for most long-term survivors.

Patau syndrome (T13)

Incidence. This disorder is found in approximately 1 in 5000 newborn babies, and, as with the other autosomal trisomies (18 and 21), there is an association with advanced maternal age.

Clinical features. Almost all babies with trisomy 13 have marked dysmorphic features and major internal abnormalities. Survival beyond a few weeks is very unusual with 50% of affected babies dying within 3 days of birth. Long-term survivors show severe handicap.

Clinical features in trisomy 13

General		Limbs
Hypertonicity in neonatal period		Polydactyly (post-axial, i.e. on ulnar side)
Severe failure to thrive with early death in most cases		Single palmar creases
		Talipes
Cranio-facial		**Other**
Facies type I	Holoprosencephaly, e.g.:	Cardiac abnormalities
	absent nose (premaxillary agenesis)	Exomphalos
	single nostril (cebocephaly)	Cryptorchidism/hypospadias
	proboscis (ethmocephaly)	Polycystic kidneys
	single eye (cyclops)	
Facies type II	Microphthalmia	
	Large bulbous nose	
	Cleft lip/palate	
	Small ears/scalp defects	

Cytogenetic aspects. In 80% of cases there is regular trisomy 13. Most of the remaining 20% have an unbalanced translocation and occasionally one of the parents is found to carry this in a balanced form. Mosaicism with a normal cell line results in less severe features.

Cri-du-chat syndrome (5p-)

Incidence. This is a very rare condition with an incidence of 1 in 50 000.

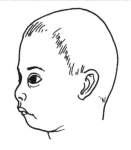

Facial features of cri-du-chat

Clinical features. Usually there is a high pitched cat-like cry in the newborn period and early infancy. External anomalies are minimal and may consist of microcephaly only with a round face and abnormal palmar creases. Severe internal abnormalities are very unusual so that most affected children show long-term survival. Intellect is severely impaired.

Cytogenetic aspects. Usually there is loss (deletion) of a small portion of material from the end of the short arm (p for 'petit') of one number 5 chromosome. Because this may have resulted from malsegregation of a balanced rearrangement, it is important that parental chromosome studies are undertaken.

Microdeletion syndromes

Loss of a small number of contiguous genes constitutes a 'microdeletion'. Microdeletions are usually not visible under the microscope but can be detected instead using the technique known as fluorescence in-situ hybridisation (FISH). This involves hybridising a DNA probe from the critical region to the patient's chromosomes. Failure of the probe to hybridise to one of the relevant chromosomes indicates that there is a microdeletion in that particular chromosome.

It is now known that several previously unexplained syndromes are caused by microdeletions. For example Williams syndrome is caused by a microdeletion in the long arm of chromosome 7. The deleted region includes the locus for elastin which almost certainly explains why most children with Williams syndrome have supravalvular aortic stenosis.

Syndromes associated with microdeletions

Syndrome	Chromosome location
Williams	7q11
WAGR	11p13
Angelman	15q11 (mat)
Prader–Willi	15q11 (pat)
Smith–Magenis	17p11
Di George/Shprintzen	22q11

COMMON SEX CHROMOSOME ABNORMALITIES

Klinefelter syndrome (47, XXY)

Incidence. Chromosome surveys of large numbers of consecutive newborn infants have shown that this condition affects approximately 1 in 1000 males. Many cases are not diagnosed until adult life.

Clinical features. Male infants with Klinefelter syndrome are entirely normal and there is no increase in the incidence of congenital malformations. Intellectual development in childhood may be mildly impaired with average verbal IQ being 10–20 points below that of unaffected siblings and controls. Adults with Klinefelter syndrome tend

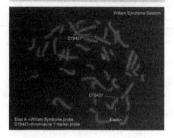

FISH showing failure of the elastin probe to hybridise to one number 7 chromosome in a child with Williams syndrome

to be slightly taller than average with long lower limbs. Thirty per cent show mild to moderate gynaecomastia, and all are infertile with small soft testes; otherwise sexual performance in adult life is usually satisfactory. Testosterone replacement therapy should be commenced at adolescence and appears to have a beneficial effect both on psychosexual development and the long-term prevention of osteoporosis.

Cytogenetic aspects. In 80–90% of cases there is a 47,XXY karyotype. Molecular studies have shown that the additional X chromosome is as likely to have come from the father as the mother. The remaining 10–20% of cases show either mosaicism with a normal cell line resulting in only minor problems or the presence of additional X chromosomes (e.g. 48,XXXY or 49,XXXXY) which are usually associated with more marked hypogonadism and mental retardation.

Turner syndrome (45,X)

Incidence. Loss of a sex chromosome (i.e. 45,X) is a common finding in abortus material and only around 3–5% of Turner syndrome conceptions survive to the third trimester. The incidence in liveborn female infants is 1 in 2500.

Clinical features. During pregnancy Turner syndrome may present with generalised hydrops or localised nuchal swelling which may be mistaken on ultrasonography for an encephalocele. This excess of tissue fluid is due to delayed maturation of the lymphatic drainage system. In surviving babies the vestiges of this intrauterine oedema manifest as residual neck webbing, puffy hands and feet and small hyperconvex nails. Fifteen per cent of cases have coarctation of the aorta.

Short stature is the most common presenting feature in childhood, when examination may also reveal a low posterior hairline, increased carrying angles, widely spaced nipples (shield chest) and Madelung deformity at the wrists.

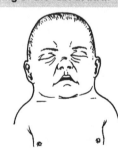

Webbing of the neck and swelling of the feet at birth

Presentation in adult life is with primary amenorrhoea and infertility. In Turner syndrome the ovaries develop normally during the first half of intrauterine life. Thereafter, they regress ('ovarian dysgenesis'), leaving only small strands of ovarian tissue ('streak gonads'). Treatment with genetically engineered growth hormone is beneficial for the short stature seen in Turner syndrome, and oestrogen replacement therapy should be commenced around the time of the onset of puberty. It is important to stress that the majority of girls cope with normal schooling, although they have increased difficulty with abstract concepts such as mathematics.

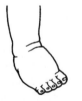

Cytogenetic aspects. In 50% of cases there is only one sex chromosome, i.e. 45,X. Molecular studies have revealed that this is usually maternal in origin with loss of the X or Y chromosome having occurred in spermatogenesis. In the remaining cases there may be either a deletion of the short arm of one X chromosome, or an isochromosome consisting of two long arms with no short arm. Very rarely there may be mosaicism with one cell line showing the presence of a Y chromosome, i.e. 45,X/46,XY. In these cases there is a small risk of malignant change in the streak gonads, which should therefore be removed prophylactically.

Fragile X syndrome

Incidence. This affects approximately 1 in 2000 males and is the commonest inherited cause of mental retardation.

Clinical features. Affected males usually have a long face with large ears and a prominent jaw. Large testes (macro-orchidism) develop after puberty. In childhood autistic behaviour and convulsions may be noted and most affected males are moderately to severely retarded.

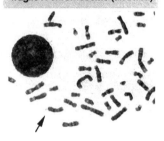

Part of a 'metaphase spread' showing the presence of a fragile X chromosome (arrowed)

Genetic aspects. The diagnosis used to be made by demonstrating the presence of a gap ('fragile site') at the end of the long arm (q) of an X chromosome. Technically this is difficult and special cultures are needed so that the laboratory should always be informed if this diagnosis is suspected. The diagnosis is now made by DNA analysis of the fragile X locus known as *FRAXA*. The *FRAXA* mutation consists of an increase in the number of CGG trinucleotide repeat sequences. Normally the *FRAXA* locus contains between 10 and 50 copies of this triplet repeat. An increase to between 60 and 200 is known as a premutation. When a female carrier of a premutation transmits this to a child there is a high probability that it will increase in size ('expand') to cause the full syndrome in a male infant and mild retardation in a female infant.

SINGLE GENE (MENDELIAN) INHERITANCE

A condition or trait resulting from a germ-line mutation in DNA is said to show single gene inheritance. Over 8000 human characteristics or diseases have been attributed to single gene defects. As an alternative, the term Mendelian is sometimes used in recognition of the fact that Gregor Mendel, an Austrian monk, was the first to recognise the underlying principles of single gene inheritance. Ironically the significance of Mendel's work was only recognised long after his death, so that he could have had no idea that his observations would ultimately prove to be of such major importance.

Autosomal dominant

A condition occurring in someone with only a single copy of an abnormal gene located on one of the autosomes is said to show autosomal dominant inheritance. Over 5000 conditions or traits showing this pattern of inheritance have been identified. Some of these disorders, such as polydactyly, may be very mild, whereas others, such as the lethal forms of osteogenesis imperfecta, are very severe.

Autosomal dominant inheritance

affected   unaffected

both affected   both unaffected

Example

The fundamental principles of autosomal dominant inheritance are:

1. Each time an individual with an autosomal dominant disorder has a child there is 1 chance in 2 that the child will inherit the disorder. Thus these conditions tend to be transmitted from generation to generation, giving rise to the appearance of 'vertical' transmission in a pedigree.
2. Generally males and females are equally affected and each can transmit the disorder to individuals of either sex. This contrasts with sex-linked inheritance in which male to male transmission cannot occur.
3. When two parents, both with the same autosomal dominant disorder, have a child, risks to the child are:
   1 in 4 for inheriting both copies of the mutant gene;
   1 in 2 for inheriting one copy of the mutant gene;
   1 in 4 for inheriting neither copy of the mutant gene.
   Usually individuals with two copies of the mutant gene (homozygotes) are very severely affected, e.g. early lethality in achondroplasia and ischaemic heart disease by early adult life in familial hypercholesterolaemia.

Genetic counselling is complicated by the fact that many autosomal dominant disorders show quite marked variation in their degree of severity, even among affected individuals within a family. For example, some individuals with neurofibromatosis show only *café au lait* patches and have no clinical problems, others may be quite severely retarded or have serious illness as a result of tumour formation. This is known as 'variable expressivity'. Occasionally an autosomal dominant disorder may appear to completely skip a generation, with the individual who must have transmitted the condition from grandparent to grandchild showing absolutely no clinical abnormality. Such an event represents an example of 'non-penetrance'.

Common examples of autosomal dominant inheritance

Disorder	Chromosomal location
Achondroplasia	4
Apert syndrome	10
Familial hypercholesterolaemia	19
Holt–Oram syndrome	12
Huntington disease	4
Marfan syndrome	15
Myotonic dystrophy	19
Neurofibromatosis1	17
Osteogenesis imperfecta	7/17*
Polycystic kidney disease (adult onset form)	4/16*
Polyposis coli	5
Spherocytosis	8
Tuberose sclerosis	9/16*

*These disorders show genetic heterogeneity, i.e. the same phenotype can be produced by mutations at different loci.

The individual in a family who is the first to be affected is said to represent a 'new mutation'. The recurrence risk to his or her siblings will be very low, whereas the risk to each of his or her offspring will be 1 in 2. For many conditions, such as achondroplasia and Apert syndrome, it has been noted that the mean age of the fathers of children who represent new mutations is greater than average.

As a general rule, autosomal dominant disorders tend to be associated with structural abnormalities, in contrast to autosomal recessive disorders which are often due to defective enzyme activity. There are however, a few notable exceptions, such as several forms of porphyria, which show autosomal dominant inheritance and are caused by a 50% reduction in enzyme activity.

Autosomal recessive

An autosomal recessive disorder is one which occurs only in individuals who inherit two copies of an abnormal autosomal gene, one from each parent. Affected individuals are said to be homozygous; carriers are heterozygous. Over 2000 disorders or traits showing autosomal recessive inheritance have been described.

Autosomal recessive inheritance

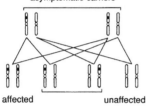

asymptomatic carriers

affected   unaffected

asymptomatic carriers

The basic principles of autosomal recessive inheritance are:

1. When parents have had one affected child, the risk to each subsequent offspring is 1 in 4. This risk applies equally to males and females.
2. Usually an autosomal recessive disorder affects only members of a single sibship in a family—'horizontal' transmission. This is because an affected individual can transmit only one of his or her abnormal genes to each child, who in order to be affected would have to inherit another abnormal gene from the other parent.
3. Autosomal recessive disorders, particularly those which are rare, show an increased incidence in the offspring of consanguineous parents. It has been estimated that most humans carry at least one deleterious autosomal recessive gene. Therefore when close relatives marry, there is a risk (usually small) that they may both carry a common ancestor's abnormal gene and transmit it in double dose to a child.

Example

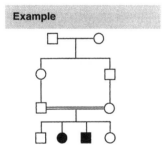

Some autosomal recessive disorders show a particularly high incidence in certain ethnic groups or communities One possible explanation is a 'founder effect' in a population which is restricted in its choice of marital partners by geographical or religious factors. Thus if one of the founders of a genetic 'isolate' carried a harmful autosomal recessive gene, it is possible that this could by chance have become widely established in the relevant community. This may be the explanation for the high incidence of Tay–Sachs disease in the Ashkenazi Jewish population in the Eastern United States.

Another possible explanation is heterozygote advantage. Carriers of some autosomal recessive disorders may be biologically fitter than non-carriers. By far the best known example is sickle cell disease, carriers of which are relatively immune to infection by malaria. Consequently in areas where malaria is endemic, carriers of the sickle cell gene are at a distinct biological and hence reproductive advantage. This concept may also apply to cystic fibrosis, although no underlying mechanism for carrier advantage has been identified.

Autosomal recessive disorders which have a high incidence in particular ethnic groups	
Disorder	Ethinic group
α_1-antitrypsin deficiency	Scandinavians
Congenital adrenal hyperplasia (21-hydroxylase deficiency)	Eskimos
Cystic fibrosis	Western Europeans
Sickle cell disease	Afro-Caribbeans
Tay–Sachs disease	Ashkenazi Jews
Alpha-thalassaemia	Orientals
Beta-thalassaemia	Mediterranean races and orientals

Sex-linked (X-linked)

Sex-linked disorders are those which are caused by abnormal genes on the X chromosome. If the disease is not manifest in women who have only a single copy of the abnormal gene, then the disorder is said to show X-linked recessive inheritance. Over 500 X-linked recessive disorders or traits have been recognised.

The essential features of X-linked recessive inheritance are:

X-linked recessive inheritance

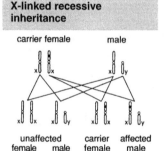

1. Each time a carrier has a child, there is 1 chance in 2 that she will transmit the abnormal gene, so that for each daughter there is 1 chance in 2 of being a carrier and for each son, 1 chance in 2 of being affected. This is sometimes referred to as a vertical or 'knight's move' pattern of inheritance.
2. When an affected male has children, he will transmit the abnormal gene to all of his daughters who will be carriers and to none of his sons who will therefore not be affected, i.e. male to male transmission cannot occur.

Rarely a woman may be affected with a sex-linked recessive disorder. This may be because she has inherited two copies of the abnormal gene, one from her carrier mother and one from her affected father; or she has Turner syndrome (45,X) or testicular feminisation, a very rare condition in which affected 'women' have a 46,XY karyotype with female habitus and external genitalia because of insensitivity to testosterone during embryogenesis; or because Lyonisation (X chromosome inactivation) has not occurred in a random fashion, either by chance or because of an abnormality or rearrangement involving one of her X chromosomes. Most commonly this takes the form of a balanced X-autosome translocation.

One of the greatest problems posed by sex-linked recessive disorders is carrier detection. By definition carriers are usually entirely healthy. Sometimes it is possible to show that a woman is likely to be a carrier using appropriate biochemical tests. For example, serum creatine kinase levels are raised in approximately two-thirds of all carriers of Duchenne muscular dystrophy. Generally, however, these indirect measurements of gene activity are not very reliable and this is one of the reasons why the recent isolation of many of the important X-linked genes has proved to be so valuable.

Molecular techniques have also revealed that occasionally a woman may transmit a sex-linked recessive disorder to more than one child, even though tests indicate that the woman does not have the mutation in DNA extracted from her circulating lymphocytes. It is believed that this is due to the presence of a mutant gene bearing cell line in one of her ovaries (gonadal mosaicism). This phenomenon has also been observed in males, who, though unaffected, may transmit the disorder to more than one daughter.

Sex-linked disorders	
Sex-linked recessive	**Sex-linked dominant**
Bruton agammaglobulinaemia	Incontinentia pigmenti
Duchenne muscular dystrophy	Vitamin D resistant rickets
Factor VIII deficiency (haemophilia A)	
Factor IX deficiency (haemophilia B = Christmas dis.)	
Glucose-6-phosphate dehydrogenase deficiency	
Lesch–Nyhan syndrome	
Red–green colour blindness	

Sex-linked dominant

A small number of X-linked disorders are manifest in both the heterozygous female and the hemizygous male. An affected female will transmit the disorder on average to half of her daughters and to half of her sons. An affected male will transmit the disorder to all of his daughters and to none of his sons.

Mitochondrial inheritance

Each mitochondrion carries a small amount of DNA which codes for 13 proteins involved in the mitochondrial respiratory chain. Disorders which result from mutations in mitochondrial DNA include very rare forms of encephalopathy and myopathy. Mitochondria are transmitted only by ova and not by sperm, so that mitochondrial inheritance is characterised by transmission exclusively through females.

Genomic imprinting

Studies in mice have shown that apparently identical genes inherited from each parent may sometimes differ in their expression in offspring. This memory or 'imprint' of parental origin is probably due to different patterns of DNA methylation during meiosis and gametogenesis. The effect of this imprint persists throughout life but is altered during gametogenesis in the offspring depending on whether transmission is occurring in the ova or the sperm. It is not yet known how extensively imprinting occurs in humans, nor is it clear how important this mechanism is in causing disease. One observation which can be explained by imprinting is that if a de novo deletion occurs on the long arm of the number 15 chromosome inherited from the father, this results in the Prader–Willi syndrome (hypotonia in infancy, mild mental retardation and obesity), whereas if a similar deletion occurs on the maternally inherited number 15 chromosome this results in Angelman syndrome (convulsions, ataxia, severe mental retardation and inappropriate laughter). Thus, lack of paternally imprinted genes causes Prader–Willi syndrome whereas lack of maternally imprinted genes causes Angelman syndrome.

MULTIFACTORIAL (POLYGENIC) INHERITANCE

This is the term used to describe the pattern of inheritance observed for several relatively common conditions which appear to result from the interaction of a genetic predisposition with adverse environmental factors. The genetic susceptibility is determined by the additive effects of many genes and hence is known as polygenic. Conditions believed to show multifactorial inheritance include many of the more common congenital malformations along with acquired disorders of childhood and adult life.

Various mathematical models have been formulated to explain multifactorial inheritance. The simplest is based on the assumption that there is an underlying 'liability', made up of both genetic and environmental factors, which shows a normal distribution in the general population. Those individuals whose liability falls beyond an arbitrary threshold superimposed on the normal curve develop the disorder.

Hypothetical curves of liability for the general population and for close relatives of affected individuals

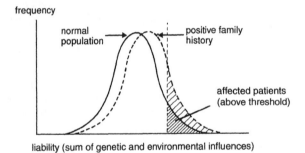

Because of shared genes the liability curve for close relatives of an affected individual will be shifted to the right, so that they will therefore show an increased incidence of the disorder.

The characteristic features of multifactorial inheritance are:

1. Risks to close relatives are generally less than in single gene disorders.
2. Risks to siblings and offspring of an affected individual are roughly comparable.
3. Risks decline sharply as the relationship with the affected individual becomes more distant. For example, the risk to the first degree relatives (siblings and offspring) of someone with a neural tube defect is 4–5%, whereas for second degree relatives (nephews, nieces, grandchildren) the risk is 1–2%. For third degree relatives such as first cousins, the risk is close to the general population incidence.
4. Risks to close relatives are greater if more than one family member is affected. For parents who have had two children with a neural tube defect, the risk that a third child will be affected rises to 10–12%.
5. If the index case is very severely affected then the risks to close relatives are greater. This is most noticeable for cleft lip/palate, for which the risk rises from 2% for the sibling of someone with cleft lip to 6% if the index case has bilateral cleft lip and palate.

The concept of multifactorial inheritance is not entirely satisfactory because the underlying mechanisms are not well understood and parameters such as liability cannot be measured. Ultimately it may emerge that at least some of the conditions for which multifactorial inheritance has been proposed are actually caused by mutations at a single major locus interacting with a polygenic background and/or environmental factors. Research using molecular techniques suggests that this may be the case for asthma, diabetes mellitus and schizophrenia.

Multifactorial disorders

Congenital malformations/disorders of infancy	Acquired disorders of childhood and adult life
Cleft lip/palate	Asthma
Congenital dislocation of the hip	Depression
Congenital heart disease	Diabetes mellitus
Neural tube defects	Epilepsy
Pyloric stenosis	Glaucoma
	Hypertension
	Schizophrenia

Neural tube defects

Clinically and embryologically these can be divided into disorders resulting from a defect in neurulation (anencephaly and craniorachischisis) and those resulting from defective canalisation of the neural tube (lumbosacral lesions). There is some evidence that genetically these are distinct and different entities, although both forms have been observed to occur within the same family. Clinical aspects of neural tube defects are described in Chapter 4. Factors known to contribute to the aetiology of neural tube defects include poor socioeconomic circumstances, diet and a Celtic ancestry. Prenatal diagnosis programmes have been established in the United Kingdom and elsewhere based on assay of maternal serum α-fetoprotein at 16 weeks' gestation. This is elevated in 60–70% of mothers carrying a fetus with an open lesion. More specific prenatal diagnosis is based on ultrasonography or amniocentesis.

Accumulating evidence indicates that folic acid taken by the mother around the time of conception prevents the development of a neural tube defect in a genetically susceptible embryo. This is a universally acceptable means of primary prevention, which emphasises the importance of focusing on the search for potentially treatable or avoidable environmental trigger factors.

RECENT ADVANCES IN MOLECULAR GENETICS

During the last decade new and exciting developments in molecular biology have greatly enhanced understanding of the molecular basis of disease. These have proved particularly valuable for the investigation and diagnosis of inherited disorders both in affected individuals and in their relatives. The following are areas of special relevance for paediatrics.

Gene tracking

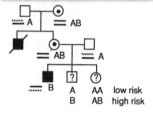

The principles underlying the use of linked DNA markers in gene tracking

A   AA   low risk
B   AB   high risk

This technique can be used to determine whether an individual, who could be an unborn baby, a child or an adult, is likely to have inherited a single gene disorder known to be running in the family. The underlying principle is relatively complex and relies on study of the cosegregation of the disease with DNA markers known to be linked to the disease locus. These DNA markers are usually identified using the technique known as the polymerase chain reaction (PCR) to identify randomly occurring DNA polymorphisms such as microsatellites. These are scattered throughout the genome and show a high degree of variation from person to person. By study of the linkage pattern in the family, it may be possible to determine which DNA marker is cosegregating with the disease gene.

Applications

Prenatal diagnosis. Some parents who are known to be at high risk of having a child with a serious genetic disease may request prenatal diagnosis followed by termination of the pregnancy if the baby is found to be affected. Examples of diseases in which gene tracking has been used for this purpose include beta-thalassaemia, cystic fibrosis and Duchenne muscular dystrophy.

There are a few situations in which prenatal diagnosis may facilitate early treatment. In congenital adrenal hyperplasia due to 21-hydroxylase deficiency, impaired synthesis of cortisol results in increased secretion of adrenocorticotrophic hormone (ACTH), which in turn stimulates the fetal adrenal glands to produce excess androgens. This usually leads to virilisation of an affected female fetus. However, if the diagnosis can be made early in pregnancy by analysis of DNA obtained at chorion biopsy, then administration of dexamethasone to the mother may suppress the fetal pituitary–adrenal axis thereby preventing virilisation.

Preclinical diagnosis. Approximately 25–40% of cases of retinoblastoma are hereditary. The risk that a child of someone with hereditary retinoblastoma will develop the condition is close to 50%. It is strongly recommended that regular ophthalmoscopy should be carried out in these children during at least the first 5 years of life. This is not easy in young children and may involve general anaesthesia. If DNA analysis indicates that a child has inherited his or her parent's retinoblastoma gene, then obviously very frequent ophthalmoscopy is mandatory. If, however, it is shown that a child has almost certainly not inherited the retinoblastoma gene, then it would be reasonable to omit some or all of the ophthalmological assessments.

The same principle applies to disease of adolescent or adult onset such as polyposis coli and polycystic kidney disease, in both of which it could be argued that early diagnosis might be beneficial to the child's long-term prognosis. However at the present time the full ethical aspects of this so-called 'predictive testing' in children have not been clarified. The general feeling at present is that the medical benefits of early diagnosis and treatment should outweigh any possible psychological disadvantages of alerting a child to the certainty of a potentially serious adult-onset disease.

Carrier detection. Women who have male relatives with a sex-linked recessive disorder may wish to know whether they are carriers and therefore at risk of having affected sons. Until recently for conditions such as Duchenne muscular dystrophy and haemophilia, carrier detection was based upon biochemical assays (creatine kinase and factor VIII levels respectively) which were not always reliable in distinguishing carriers from non-carriers. The availability of DNA markers closely linked to these disease loci has now enabled most female relatives of affected males to be given a very accurate estimate of their carrier status.

Direct mutation analysis

Indirect mutation analysis as outlined in the previous section enables disease status to be predicted based on the study of the cosegregation of DNA markers linked to the disease locus. This method has the disadvantages that DNA has to be obtained from several members of the family, at least one family member has to be heterozygous at the marker locus, and there is a small risk that disease status will be predicted incorrectly due to recombination (crossing-over) occurring between the disease locus and the marker locus during prophase of meiosis I.

Direct mutation analysis, by contrast conveys none of these disadvantages and can be used as a precise diagnostic test for conditions such as cystic fibrosis, which can be difficult to diagnose in neonates using conventional methods. Many techniques for direct mutation analysis have been devised. Some of the simpler approaches are:

Change in a restriction site. A point mutation can be detected easily if it alters a restriction enzyme cleavage site. For example, in the sickle cell gene a thymine to adenine mutation in the sixth codon/residue of the β-globin gene results in loss of an *MstII* cleavage site, so that the fragments normally produced by the Southern blotting technique are altered in size. This permits very precise diagnosis of heterozygotes (carriers of the trait) and homozygotes (patients with sickle cell disease) by molecular studies.

Use of an oligonucleotide probe. A very short probe will only hybridise to a patient's gene if it is an exact copy. A single base mismatch resulting from a point mutation will prevent hybridisation. Oligonucleotide probes of around 20 bases can be used for diagnosing several diseases such as α_1-antitrypsin deficiency and beta-thalassaemia.

Chemical cleavage mismatch. In this technique a probe, which is an exact match for the normal gene, is hybridised to the patient's DNA. The resulting hybrid molecule is then exposed to an agent which will only cleave the probe if there is a mismatch resulting from a point mutation

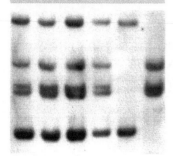

Deletion analysis of the Duchenne muscular dystrophy gene in six affected boys

In the right hand lanes, several bands are missing indicating deletion of a portion of their dystrophin gene

in the patient's gene. Cleavage can be detected by the presence of two bands on a gel instead of one.

Deletion analysis: Southern blotting. It is now known that deletions in the dystrophin gene on the short arm of the X chromosome account for approximately two-thirds of all cases of Duchenne muscular dystrophy. These deletions can be demonstrated in a Southern blot by hybridising the patient's DNA, which has been cleaved into lots of tiny fragments, with a suitable probe. A deletion mutation can be deduced by the absence of several bands on the blot.

Deletion analysis: polymerase chain reaction (PCR). The PCR technique enables a specific sequence or portion of a gene to be amplified up to 1 million fold. If a deletion is present in the sequence which is amplified, this will result in production of a smaller fragment than that found in unaffected individuals. This approach has proved particularly useful for diagnosing carriers of cystic fibrosis. Approximately 75% of all cystic fibrosis genes in western Europeans show a deletion of codon number 508 (the so-called ΔF508 mutation). Thus if 98 base pairs of the cystic fibrosis gene including codon 508 are amplified, then in an affected patient who is homozygous for the deletion, two fragments, each 95 pairs long, will be generated. Carriers of the deletion will be identified by the presence of one normal 98 base pair band and one truncated 95 base pair band.

Deletion analysis. Shows separation of the normal (N) and deleted (Δ F) cystic fibrosis genes by polymerase chain reaction followed by electrophoresis. HD represents a heteroduplex band which forms in samples from heterozygotes. The individuals shown in lanes 2 and 8 are homozygous affected, those in lanes 5 and 7 are homozygous normal, and those in lanes 1, 3, 6, 9 and 10 are heterozygous

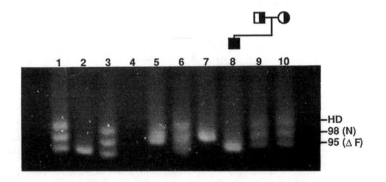

Oncogenes

These are genes which are normally involved in basic cell functions such as division, proliferation and differentiation, by the production of proteins such as growth factors and growth factor receptors. Overactivity therefore results in uncontrolled cell proliferation with possible induction of malignant transformation.

Mechanisms which can disturb the function of an oncogene include: a point mutation in a coding exon, a translocation resulting in loss of normal gene suppression or synthesis of an altered gene product (e.g. Burkitt lymphoma) and gene amplification which may be the result of a mutation in a gene controlling DNA synthesis (e.g. neuroblastoma).

Anti-oncogenes are genes which normally control cell turnover and therefore act as tumour suppressors. Loss of an anti-oncogene in a cell which is already primed by a mutation involving the homologous anti-oncogene results in malignant transformation. The dominantly inherited genes which account for retinoblastoma and polyposis coli are examples of tumour suppressor genes.

Gene therapy

No effective means of gene therapy exists at present, but recent advances in molecular biology have raised hope that direct replacement of an abnormal gene by its normal counterpart may soon be possible. Public unease at the prospect of 'tinkering' with genes has been alleviated by a universal consensus that gene therapy should be used exclusively to cure an illness rather than for eugenic purposes such as increasing intelligence or athletic prowess, and that treatment should be directed primarily at altering a body tissue (somatic therapy) rather than altering the heritable underlying genetic constitution (germ-line therapy).

Gene insertion: physical methods. Various strategies have been applied with only limited success. These include microinjection of DNA, exposure of recipient cells to high voltage electric current, and the formation of cell permeable DNA–liposome complexes.

Gene insertion: viral agents. Several types of viruses have been used to try to transport 'foreign' DNA into cells. These include retroviruses and adenoviruses. Retroviruses can incorporate up to 7 kb of DNA and can be rendered incapable of replication before being allowed to infect host cells in vitro. However animal trials of retrovirus mediated gene therapy have not been very successful. Adenoviruses can incorporate larger quantities of foreign DNA and can be targeted to specific tissues such as the respiratory tract. Unfortunately they tend to induce a host immune response and clinical trials have shown only transitory benefit.

Disorders suitable for gene therapy. In order to be a candidate for gene therapy a disorder has to have a well defined genetic or biochemical defect, the relevant gene must have been isolated along with its control sequences, and the target organ has to be easily accessible for manipulation either in vivo (e.g. respiratory tract mucosa) or in vitro (e.g. bone-marrow, liver, tumour infiltrating lymphocytes). Examples of disorders which might be treatable by gene therapy in the foreseeable future are indicated below. No consistently effective gene therapy exists at present for any disorder in children or adults.

Disorders which might be suitable for gene therapy	
Haematopoietic	— haemoglobinopathies
	— immunodeficiencies
Hepatic	— α_1-antitrypsin deficiency
Metabolic	— hypercholesterolaemia
	— phenylketonuria
Oncogenic	— solid tumours by insertion of tumour necrosis factor gene into tumour-infiltrating lymphocytes
Endocrine	— diabetes mellitus, growth hormone deficiency
Respiratory	— α_1-antitrypsin deficiency
	— cystic fibrosis

GENETIC COUNSELLING

This can be defined as the process whereby an individual is alerted to the possibility of developing and/or transmitting an inherited illness and how this might be avoided. The key underlying principle is that individuals seeking help should be provided with information rather than advice, thereby enabling them to make their own informed decisions about future child-bearing. It is universally agreed that genetic counselling should be non-coercive, non-directive and non-judgemental, with no attempt being made to direct the patient along a particular course of action.

Much genetic counselling can be and is undertaken by general practitioners and paediatricians. Patients with relatively complex problems can be referred to specialist genetic clinics held at most large hospitals and teaching centres. These are usually located at or close to one of the regional genetics centres which have been established throughout the United Kingdom. These centres are responsible for several tasks, including the maintenance of registers of families in which individuals may be at risk of developing or transmitting a genetic disease. The role of these 'genetic' registers is to ensure that a rapid means of two-way communication exists, so that members of these families can seek information at short notice and in turn be alerted to new developments and technical innovations.

BIBLIOGRAPHY

Connor J M, Ferguson-Smith M A 1997 Essential medical genetics, 5th edn. Blackwell Science Publications, Oxford
Harper P S 1998 Practical genetic counselling, 5th edn. Butterworth Heinemann, Oxford
Jones K L 1997 Smith's recognizable patterns of human malformation, 5th edn. Saunders, Philadelphia
McKusick V A 1998 Mendelian inheritance in man, 12th edn. Johns Hopkins University Press, Baltimore
Mueller R F, Young I D 1998 Emery's elements of medical genetics, 10th edn. Churchill Livingstone, Edinburgh

3 Fetus

PERICONCEPTIONAL MEDICINE
THE PLACENTA
EXAMINATION OF THE FETUS
DRUGS WHICH CROSS THE
    PLACENTA
FETAL TRANSPLACENTAL
    INFECTIONS
INFECTIONS ACQUIRED DURING
    VAGINAL DELIVERY
MATERNAL IMMUNOGLOBULINS

In the main, the fetus is protected against diseases which attack the mother. However, because the fetus lies hidden, unobserved within the uterus, he can become ill without the mother being aware of what is happening. There are also situations, fortunately rare, when the fetus is seriously harmed by agents which either have little effect on the mother, for example rubella virus, or which might even benefit her, for example various drugs. Despite advances in obstetric and perinatal care, fetal life carries a greater risk of morbidity or mortality than any other period in childhood. Thus in England and Wales each year of the 700 000 births, around 3000 are stillborn and 48 000 are born at a disadvantage with a low birth weight due to either growth restraint or premature birth.

PERICONCEPTIONAL MEDICINE

This is the actual size of an 8-week fetus

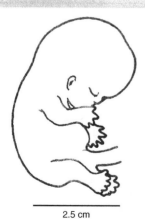

2.5 cm

Life begins not only before birth but, in a sense, before conception. The health and diet of the parents, especially the mother, can affect the early development and future wellbeing of their child. For example, folic acid reduces the risk of neural tube defects whereas large doses of vitamin A may be teratogenic. Certain foods are associated with listeriosis; uncooked eggs, soft or blue-veined cheeses, unpasteurised milk, and pâté. Poor diet, along with maternal infection and substance abuse, may contribute to the higher fetal loss rates in areas of social deprivation. Risks are also higher if the mother is very young or very old, already has a large family, or if there is a multiple pregnancy. Less common environmental risks to gametes and the fetus are radiation and certain chemicals.

Because many of these agents carry the greatest risk around the time of conception, before the mother is certain that she is pregnant, there have been calls for preconceptual clinics to promote healthy diet and behaviour in prospective parents. As a minimum, obesity, smoking, alcohol intake, sexually transmitted diseases, diabetes and hypertension could be screened for and a history of inherited diseases sought. Ensuring parental health before pregnancy is one way of preventing ill health in the next generation of children.

THE PLACENTA

The tissues of the mature human placenta, unlike many other mammalian species, are derived entirely from the fetus. The placenta starts to develop shortly after the blastocyst implants in the uterine wall. It is situated outside the body of the fetus, and is connected to it by an umbilical cord of blood vessels. Despite being antigenically different from the maternal tissues, the placenta is immunologically privileged and is not rejected.

The placenta, in a single structure, combines many functions which are performed by separate organs after birth. It acts as a fetal lung and a fetal kidney. It transfers nutrients and substrates essential for growth and metabolism, a role the gut later fulfils. The placenta allows heat loss, a function of the skin postnatally. It is a barrier to the transfer of cells from mother to fetus, and vice versa, which would be damaging and allow the cell-mediated immunity of the maternal 'host' to reject the fetal 'graft'. It prevents uptake of large molecules, such as hormones which would interfere with fetal homeostasis, and yet selectively transfers IgG to reduce the risk of infection. It is an important site of hormone production. It grows rapidly early in gestation, the placental to fetal weight ratio changing from 4 : 1 at 10 weeks to 1 : 5 at term. Finally it is a disposable organ with a finite life span which naturally separates from the fetus at birth and is safely expelled despite its very vascular structure. The loss of this low-resistance vascular bed triggers the circulatory changes which occur after birth. Towards the end of pregnancy fetal demands for oxygen and nutrients reach a point where they may challenge the capacity of the utero-placental unit to supply them. At this stage, any disturbance of that supply line may interfere with fetal growth or development.

The blood supply to the fetus

Uterine artery   Umbilical vein

Placenta   liver   brain   carcass

Uterine vein   Umbilical artery

Mother   **Fetus**

EXAMINATION OF THE FETUS

In the past, the assessment of fetal growth depended on a knowledge of the date of the last menstrual period and an estimation of fetal size by palpation of the mother's abdomen. Now ultrasound techniques provide a more accurate means of measuring growth.

Most women in the United Kingdom have a 'dating scan' in the first half of pregnancy to confirm that fetal size corresponds to the period of amenorrhoea. Serial scanning of the fetus allows detection of problems such as structural abnormality (e.g. hydrocephaly, diaphragmatic hernia, abnormal limbs) or abnormal intrauterine growth. Symmetrical growth retardation from early pregnancy suggests an intrauterine infection or dysmorphic syndrome, whereas asymmetrical growth retardation in the final trimester, with relative preservation of head growth, is usually the result of fetal 'starvation' due to utero-placental dysfunction.

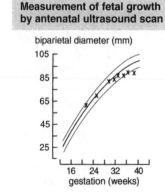

Measurement of fetal growth by antenatal ultrasound scan

biparietal diameter (mm)

105

85

65

45

25

16   24   32   40
gestation (weeks)

Fetal health

Amniocentesis

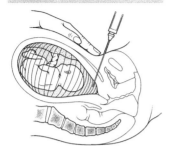

Some abnormalities which may cause a rise in α-fetoprotein in maternal blood

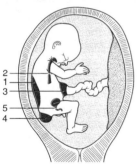

1 open neural tube defect
2 oesophageal atresia
3 exomphalos
4 sacrococcygeal teratoma
5 bladder neck obstruction
6 fetal-maternal heamorrhage

Evaluation of fetal health is more difficult than fetal growth. Soon after implantation, the detection of human chorionic gonadotrophin (hCG) in maternal urine is the basis of biochemical pregnancy testing. Early in pregnancy, before detailed visualisation of the fetus is possible (see below), we remain dependent on the measurement of proteins and hormones of fetal, maternal and placental origin to monitor the health of the conceptus. The production of oestradiol and progesterone is transferred from the corpus luteum to the fetoplacental unit in the middle of the first trimester. The synthesis of fetal proteins such as α-fetoprotein (AFP) increases throughout the first trimester.

In certain fetal abnormalities, AFP leaks from the fetus into amniotic fluid and thence into the maternal circulation. Amniotic fluid and maternal blood AFP levels are increased if the fetus has an open neural tube lesion (spina bifida or anencephaly), an anterior abdominal wall defect (gastroschisis or exomphalos) or a germ cell tumour (e.g. sacrococcygeal teratoma). Maternal serum AFP levels are used for screening at around 16 weeks of pregnancy, but because the elevated maternal blood levels overlap with the upper end of the normal range, the definitive diagnosis of fetal anomalies depends on detailed ultrasound scanning.

Down syndrome can also be screened for using maternal serum. The principal early second trimester markers are AFP, unconjugated oestriol (both of which are reduced in Down syndrome) and hCG (which is elevated). These form the basis of the 'triple test' at 19 weeks' gestation and, taken with the maternal age, can be used to compute a modified risk of an affected pregnancy. Again, this is only a screening test.

Confirmation of Down syndrome depends on examination of the chromosomes in fetal cells obtained either by amniocentesis (transabdominal needle aspiration of the amniotic fluid around the fetus) or by chorionic villus sampling (transabdominal or transcervical placental biopsy).

In the second half of pregnancy, ultrasound characteristics such as the 'biophysical profile' have largely superseded the previous biochemical and hormonal tests used to monitor feto-placental wellbeing.

The 'biophysical profile' comprises:
- fetal heart rate variability
- fetal breathing movements
- fetal body movements
- fetal tone
- amniotic fluid volume.

Although the placenta functions as the fetal kidney in terms of excretion of waste products, the fetal kidney itself produces urine from early in gestation which contributes to amniotic fluid volume and is swallowed and reabsorbed from the gut of the fetus. Hence, fetal renal disease (absence of the kidneys, obstructive uropathy) is associated with oligohydramnios, as is premature rupture of the fetal membranes, whereas atresia of the gastrointestinal tract and large diaphragmatic hernias are associated with hydramnios. Amniotic fluid volume can be estimated using ultrasound scans.

Ultrasound: normal head

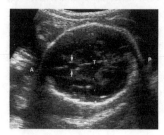

In fetal life, the respiratory tract is also filled with amniotic fluid and it appears that fetal 'breathing' activity, an important determinant of fetal lung development, is affected by the absence of amniotic fluid. As a result, pulmonary hypoplasia is a serious complication of oligohydramnios. Limb and facial deformities can also occur leading to the appearances described as fetal inertia syndrome, because the fetus is squashed rather than floating within a fluid-filled container. Attempts to assess amniotic fluid volume, fetal 'breathing' activity and lung volume by ultrasound scan have been used to estimate the likelihood of lung hypoplasia, but this is not reliable. Most fetal medicine specialists will combine the biophysical profile with Doppler studies of the blood flow velocity in the umbilical artery. If the Doppler studies show decreased forward flow (i.e. from fetus to placenta) in the umbilical artery, this suggests increased placental resistance due to placental vascular disease. This is often associated with an increased risk of adverse outcome pre- and postnatally (poor fetal growth, intrauterine asphyxia or death, necrotising enterocolitis in the neonatal period). Hence, these detailed fetal assessments help guide the optimum gestation at which to deliver the baby. If born too early, the complications of prematurity may be fatal; if the obstetrician waits too long, the fetus may die in utero.

Fetal diagnosis

Ultrasound: normal spine

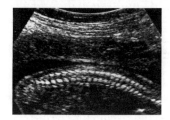

A detailed ultrasound scan is offered to all women at 20 weeks' gestation but especially if there is a previous history of congenital abnormality or fetal loss. A scan at this stage can reliably detect structural abnormalities such as spina bifida, exomphalos and renal abnormalities and the presence of abnormal collections of fluid. Early dysmorphic features can sometimes be seen, for example in Down or Turner syndrome, and a four-chamberr view of the fetal heart can detect half of the 8/1000 incidence of congenital heart disease. Fetal arrhythmias can also be diagnosed.

Ultrasound is also used to direct amniocentesis, cordocentesis and chorionic villus biopsy. Amniocentesis and chorionic villus sampling carry an approximately 1% risk of abortion in the second trimester. Cell-free amniotic fluid can be used for biochemical measurements (e.g. α-fetoprotein in neural tube defects and metabolic markers of a number of organic acid and mucopolysaccharide disorders). The fetal cells within amniotic fluid obtained at 16 weeks can be cultured for subsequent karyotyping, molecular biological techniques or assay of enzyme activity in suspected inborn errors of metabolism.

As the human placenta is derived entirely from fetal tissue, chorionic villus biopsy, either by the transabdominal or transcervical route, provides a source of fetal cells as early as 10 weeks which can be subjected to the same enquiry as amniotic cells but with more rapid results. Early sexing of the fetus enables the parents to choose selective termination of male fetuses if there is a history of sex-linked disorders. Cordocentesis is used to obtain fetal red cells to diagnose haematological disease, such as thalassaemia, to monitor the severity of rhesus haemolytic disease, or to obtain fetal white cells for rapid karyotype or

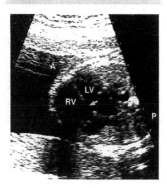

Ultrasound: arrow points to ventricular septal defect

Fetal therapy

enzyme assay. Some inborn errors of metabolism can only be diagnosed antenatally from fetal tissue and fetal liver biopsy may then be necessary.

Early detection of fetal abnormalities may allow the parents to opt for termination or enable the paediatric staff to anticipate problems at delivery and ensure correct follow up. Occasionally, fetal therapy is recommended (see below).

Once labour starts, some indication of the likelihood of fetal hypoxia can be gained by analysis of the fetal heart rate, recorded either by transabdominal ultrasound or, once the presenting part can be reached, by a fetal ECG electrode applied to the fetal scalp. Normally, the fetal heart rate shows variability due to sympathetic and parasympathetic innervation, chemoreceptor activity, sleep patterns and circulating catecholamines. Loss of variability, prolonged decelerations or sustained bradycardia are all sinister changes but a normal trace does not exclude serious fetal compromise. A more direct estimate of fetal hypoxia and acidosis is measurement of fetal pH, or lactate, from capillary blood samples obtained from the presenting head or breech.

Medicine. Fetal medicine is based on the premise that certain drugs, if given to the mother, may cross the placenta and exert desirable pharmacological effects on the fetus. In families with a child previously affected by congenital adrenal hyperplasia, maternal administration of dexamethasone in a subsequent affected pregnancy will suppress fetal ACTH release by negative feedback, and hence limit the accumulation of the adrenal steroids which masculinise the female fetus. Digoxin has been given to treat fetal supraventricular tachycardia which, if untreated, may result in fetal heart failure, hydrops (oedema, ascites, pericardial and pleural effusions and hepatomegaly) and intrauterine death. Glucocorticoids given to the mother in the latter half of pregnancy mature the fetal lungs and induce surfactant production and should be used whenever premature labour threatens with the risk of respiratory distress syndrome. Immunoglobulin infusion to the mother may ameliorate fetal alloimmune thrombocytopenia. Maternal intrapartum ampicillin reduces the risk of neonatal Group B streptococcal infection in at-risk women.

In theory, intra-amniotic administration of drugs is feasible and absorption could occur across fetal skin, lung or gut. Amnio-infusion of saline has been tried in an effort to combat the pulmonary hypoplasia resulting from oligohydramnios.

Non-pharmacological fetal interventions have also been attempted, the intrauterine treatment of severe rhesus haemolytic disease being the most successful. The fetus can be given rhesus negative red cell transfusions either intraperitoneally or by cordocentesis. Such therapy allows the pregnancy to continue to a safe gestation without the development of hydrops, although the fetal bone marrow is suppressed for some months and postnatal anaemia may require further transfusions. Platelet transfusions can be given to correct fetal thrombocytopenia in iso- or alloimmune thrombocytopenia but obviously the risks of an invasive procedure are greater.

Surgery. Needle aspiration of cysts, bladder, hydrothorax or ascites may be performed for diagnostic or therapeutic purposes, and vesico-amniotic or pleuro-amniotic shunts can be inserted to prevent reaccumulation of fluid. Fetal renal function can be assessed by quantification of urine flow and urine biochemistry and these complement estimation of liquor volume and the gross appearances of the kidneys on ultrasound scan. However, the long-term benefits of these intervention strategies remain controversial. 'Open' fetal surgery for diaphragmatic hernia has been undertaken following hysterotomy and the fetus then returned to the uterine cavity to continue the pregnancy. Theoretically, fetal bone marrow transplantation may one day be feasible to cure severe thalassaemia and storage disorders in utero. The last decade has seen great advances in the technology available to undertake fetal diagnosis and therapy. Hopefully, the next decade will shed more light on when these techniques should be used and whether they confer real, long-term benefits.

DRUGS WHICH CROSS THE PLACENTA

Drugs affecting the embryo

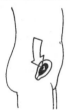

thalidomide
antimitotic
alchol
anticonvulsants
ethisterone
warfarin

Drugs which cross the placenta and affect the newborn infant

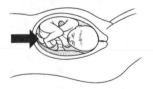

anaesthetics
sedatives
opioid analgesics
narcotics
anticonvulsants
antihypertensives
prostaglandin-synthetase inhibitors

There is no doubt that some drugs cause embryopathy. There is some suspicion that others may have harmful effects. Difficulty in establishing causality is due in part to the fact that the drug may only occasionally have this harmful effect, and in part to the fact that the end pathology may not be specific.

Maternal smoking in pregnancy increases the risk of miscarriage, stillbirth, premature birth and cot death. As little as 10 cigarettes a day will lower birth weight. Cytotoxic agents can kill the fetus, but if the pregnancy continues the fetus may survive with deformities. Progesterone preparations will masculinise the female fetus. Alcohol can cause facial abnormalities, growth retardation and mental handicap and the risk starts to increase once more than 7 units of alcohol per week are consumed, i.e. one drink per day. Some anticonvulsant drugs (e.g. phenytoin) and the anticoagulant warfarin have been associated with dysmorphic features and a variety of abnormalities. Certainly there is sufficient evidence to recommend that they are not given during pregnancy unless there is evidence that the maternal benefit outweighs the fetal risk.

Drugs administered to the mother prior to delivery may affect the baby's behaviour immediately after birth. Sedatives and anaesthetics which cross the placenta will make the newborn sleepy and inactive. The babies of mothers receiving anticonvulsant therapy may have withdrawal symptoms. These babies become hyperactive and difficult to feed and some have 'jittery' episodes. Infants of drug addicts (heroin, methadone, codeine, cocaine) may show severe withdrawal symptoms and require careful management over the first few weeks of life. Maternal analgesia with inhibitors of prostaglandin synthesis (e.g. non-steroidal anti-inflammatory drugs) may induce premature closure of the fetal ductus arteriosus. Large volumes of intravenous dextrose given to the mother in labour can cause dangerous neonatal hyponatraemia.

FETAL TRANSPLACENTAL INFECTIONS

Organisms that have been proven to cross the placenta and affect the fetus are few.

Rubella

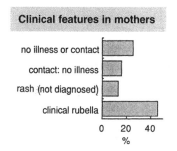

Clinical features in mothers

Women who have their first attack of German measles during early pregnancy may or may not have a suggestive rash. The risks to the fetus are considerable, particularly if viraemia occurs in the first trimester. A large percentage of pregnancies abort or the surviving fetus can suffer serious organ damage. The viraemia may persist throughout pregnancy and the infant may continue to excrete virus for many years afterwards. During this time the disease process continues. It is because of the terrible consequences of this otherwise trivial infection that rubella immunisation was offered previously to all teenage girls. Nevertheless, fetal damage due to rubella continued to occur because some girls missed or declined immunisation. Therefore, in an effort to eradicate all rubella from the community, rubella immunisation is now recommended for all children, boys and girls, at 15 months and the incidence of congenital rubella has fallen dramatically.

Clinical features. A surviving fetus may be left with congenital heart defects, deafness and eye disorders, particularly cataracts. A small percentage present at birth with purpura, thrombocytopenia and hepatosplenomegaly and have X-ray evidence of bony lesions. Many have an associated encephalopathy and are subsequently mentally handicapped. Eighty-five per cent of infants infected during the first 8 weeks of pregnancy will have detectable defects, usually multiple, in contrast to only 15% of infants infected at 16–20 weeks (usually sensorineural deafness only). There appears to be little risk from exposure after 22 weeks.

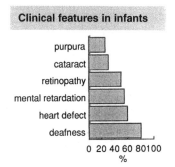

Clinical features in infants

If a pregnant woman has contact with suspected rubella it is essential to determine whether she is vulnerable to primary infection or whether she has protection from previous exposure. If the diagnosis is suspected, blood is taken and tested for serum haemagglutinin inhibition antibodies (HI) for rubella. If antibodies are high within the incubation period, the patient can be considered to be protected by a previous infection. If they are low, further samples should be taken. A rise in titre confirms primary infection and the risk of fetal damage and many consider this grounds for a therapeutic abortion. Diagnosis in a newborn is confirmed by the presence of a specific rubella IgM antibody.

Cytomegalovirus disease

Cytomegalovirus (CMV) is the commonest congenital infection in the United Kingdom (3 per 1000 live births). In common with rubella virus, CMV produces a mild disease in adults. It is also widespread in the community; 50% of pregnant women in the United Kingdom have antibodies to CMV. It has been estimated that between 1 and 5% of pregnant women contract CMV infections and that the fetus is affected in around 50%. Infection in early pregnancy may cause abortion or a spectrum of malformations including growth failure, microcephaly, mental retardation and deafness. CMV infection in late pregnancy may produce a systemic illness in the fetus causing purpura, hepatosplenomegaly, pneumonia and encephalitis in the newborn.

Overall, about 5% of infected infants will have clinical signs at birth, and this group invariably has long-term sequelae. Another 5% develop severe handicaps later (particularly sensorineural deafness) despite an asymptomatic neonatal period.

Due to the absence of clinical illness in the adult, the infection in the mother often passes undetected. However, the presence of virus in the urine of the newborn with raised CMV-specific IgM antibody confirms the diagnosis. At present there is no reliable vaccine available for protection against CMV infections.

Unlike rubella, routine serological screening for CMV in pregnancy and the option of termination cannot be justified because fetal infection can occur following primary or recurrent CMV infection in pregnancy, damage can occur following infection at any time in pregnancy, and 90% of infants will be unaffected.

Human immunodeficiency virus

HIV may be transmitted from mother to child before, during or after birth, but because transplacental maternal antibodies persist until up to 18 months of age, neonatal diagnosis is difficult in asymptomatic infants. Tests to detect viral antigen are not yet widely available. Postnatal infection via breast milk may occur and breastfeeding should be avoided if a safe alternative is available.

Approximately one-third of infants born to HIV-positive mothers will ultimately be shown to be infected. The prognosis for this group is variable but many develop full-blown AIDS. Clinically, there may be serious opportunistic infections in the first year of life or a spectrum of non-specific features such as lymphadenopathy, hepatosplenomegaly, chronic diarrhoea, failure to thrive and encephalopathy.

Maternal treatment with anti-retroviral agents such as zidovudine reduce transmission to infants. Sadly the cost of these drugs prohibits their use in areas of the world such as Africa where the disease is most devastating.

Parvovirus B19 infection

Seventy per cent of adults are seropositive for this virus which causes slapped cheek syndrome and erythema infectiosum (5th disease) in children. Infection is often subclinical. In pregnancy, the risk of transplacental transmission is estimated at 33%, with an increased incidence of abortion and hydrops fetalis. However, there is no evidence of damage in the 85% of infants who survive maternal infection and therefore termination of pregnancy is not indicated.

Herpes varicella zoster infection

Eighty-five per cent of women have antibodies to HZV and therefore, while they may develop shingles in pregnancy, the fetus will not be at risk from maternal chickenpox. In seronegative mothers who are first infected early in pregnancy, chickenpox rarely affects the fetus, although if it does the complications are severe (the 'varicella syndrome'—scarring skin lesions, chorioretinitis, cataracts and CNS damage). The greatest risk to the infant is if the mother first develops the rash between 4 days before delivery and 4 days after delivery, in which case there is no time for protective transplacental maternal antibodies to be acquired and neonatal mortality is high. The transplacental transmission rate to the fetus of this late-onset maternal HZV is 25% and these infants should be given passive immunisation with zoster immune globulin as soon after birth as possible. Acyclovir is usually reserved for those infants who show clinical features of neonatal HZV. In view of the high mortality rate, a mother developing the rash perinatally should be isolated and should barrier nurse her infant and not breastfeed until all the skin lesions have crusted over.

Listeria monocytogenes

Maternal infection with these Gram-positive bacteria may result in abortion or preterm labour. Fetal infection is acquired predominantly transplacentally, although other routes are by inhalation of infected liquor or by ascending infection from the genital tract. The organism has been isolated from under-cooked chicken, unpasteurised milk and soft cheeses, and gives rise to a mild 'flu-like' systemic illness in the mother. Infants infected prenatally present soon after birth with a generalised septicaemic illness which may include pneumonia, meningitis and a rash. The liquor may be offensive and discoloured. There is a 30% mortality. Those infected during vaginal delivery present after 1–8 weeks, usually with meningitis, and have a better prognosis. Ampicillin and gentamicin are synergistic and maternal treatment may improve the prognosis for the fetus.

Toxoplasmosis

Toxoplasma gondii, a protozoon parasite, affects animals as well as man. In the United Kingdom, only 20% of women are protected by antibodies. Maternal infection may not produce any clinical symptoms. Only a small percentage of women contract the infection in the first part of pregnancy but when they do so the organism may invade the placenta and spread to the fetus. Infection occurs from ingestion of undercooked meat or of oocysts excreted in cat faeces. Pregnant women should not empty cat litters and should wear gloves for gardening.

The risk of transplacental transmission is about 40% but only 10% of these show clinical features at birth. Toxoplasmosis has widespread effects on the developing brain, causing hydrocephalus or microcephaly with cerebral calcification and a chorioretinitis. There is usually resultant mental handicap with other neurological abnormalities. The major late risk to the 90% who show no features at birth appears to be chorioretinitis, which may only appear in adulthood. In the newborn, diagnosis is confirmed by the presence of toxoplasma-specific IgM antibody. If infection is confirmed in the first trimester, when the risk to the fetus is greatest, termination may be

Fetal infections

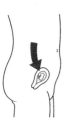

Treponema pallidum (syphillis)

rubella virus

Herpes varicella and zoster

cytomegalovirus

plasmodia (malaria)

Toxoplasma gondii

human immuno-deficiency virus

parvovirus

considered or the mother treated with spiramycin which reduces the risk of fetal infection.

Others

Syphilis is now very rare in the United Kingdom. The same is true for congenital tuberculosis. Worldwide, malaria commonly affects the placenta and may interfere with fetal growth. Occasionally the parasites cause fetal disease.

INFECTIONS ACQUIRED DURING VAGINAL DELIVERY

A sterile infant passing through the vagina is at risk of contracting a wide range of infections, particularly from pathogenic organisms in the maternal bowel. If the membranes have ruptured prematurely, the infant may be infected 2 or 3 days prior to birth by organisms entering the uterus via the vagina. There has been some concern that, even without rupture of the membranes, infection can ascend to the placenta and the fetus.

Gonococcal ophthalmia

Infection due to *Neisseria gonorrhoea* acquired during birth can lead to a purulent conjunctivitis, which if not treated promptly results in corneal ulceration and perforation. Treatment is with topical and systemic penicillin.

Chlamydia

The endocervix is the site most frequently infected by *Chlamydia trachomatis* in women and chlamydia is a cause of conjunctivitis in the newborn in the first month of life. Chlamydial pneumonia is rarer and difficult to diagnose, as symptoms appear 4–6 weeks after birth. Chest X-ray shows widespread pneumonitis.

Pneumonia and meningitis

Listeria or group B streptococcal organisms in the vagina can be drawn into the respiratory tract and produce a bacterial pneumonia in the first few days of life. The possibility needs to be recognised and vigorous antibiotic therapy given for septicaemia as meningitis may quickly follow. All infants with respiratory distress should be given penicillin because of the very high mortality from group B streptococcal infection.

Herpes simplex infections

Herpes virus type 2 infection (HSV) is a sexually transmitted disease. The cervicitis is frequently asymptomatic but it creates a major risk for the fetus. Ascending infection may result in abortion or, in later pregnancy, premature birth. There is a high (40%) risk of direct infection during vaginal delivery. Neonatal herpes infection is frequently fatal and obstetricians regard active genital herpes as an indication for elective caesarean section. The risk to the fetus is less if the lesions represent reactivation rather than primary infection. The risk of post-natal spread to a baby from a parent with a 'cold sore' is very low but topical treatment with acyclovir should be given to the mother.

Neonatal disease usually presents in the first week with localised, vesicular skin lesions or with a generalised viraemia with hepatosplenomegaly, jaundice, petechiae, encephalopathy and seizures. There may be chorioretinitis or cataract and increased white cells in the cerebrospinal fluid (CSF). Rapid diagnosis is by electron microscopy or antigen detection of fluid from blisters. All neonatal HSV should be treated with intravenous acyclovir.

Hepatitis B virus

Hepatitis B is a major health problem in developing countries. It contributes to a high mortality from cirrhosis and hepatocellular carcinoma. The pool of chronic carriers is perpetuated by maternal–child transfer at birth. Screening for HBs, a surface antigen, is carried out in all non-Caucasian women in the United Kingdom and Caucasian women with previous hepatitis, drug abuse or with a sexual or occupational life style suggestive of increased exposure to HBV. If the mother is also positive for the E antigen of HBV, her blood is highly infective, whereas if the anti-HBe antibody is present, the infectivity is much lower. Although HBV can be transferred to the fetus at any time during pregnancy or delivery, or to the baby post-natally, the combination of active immunisation (with HBV vaccine) and passive immunisation (with anti-HBs immunoglobulin) shortly after birth followed by active immunisation again at 1 and 6 months appears to reduce the risk of subsequent HBV carriage, cirrhosis and hepatoma.

MATERNAL IMMUNOGLOBULINS

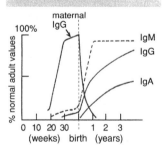

Immunoglobulin levels before and after birth

The immune defence mechanisms develop early in fetal life, but in the absence of exposure to antigens, specific antibodies are not produced. The human fetus gains some specific protection by the transfer of maternal IgG across the placenta. In general the maternal immunoglobulins confer benefit but they can also cause problems. The commonest example is the transfer of maternal antibodies against the fetal blood cells as in rhesus and ABO incompatibility.

Less commonly, mothers suffering from autoimmune diseases may transfer damaging antibodies to the fetus. Thus, the infants of mothers with platelet antibodies may develop purpura in the first 2–3 days of life due to the transfer of platelet antibodies across the placenta. Similarly, the infants of mothers with systemic lupus erythematosis may develop either systemic disease, heart block or a transient lupus rash on the face. Likewise, babies of mothers with myasthenia gravis may have transient but severe hypotonia. Infants of women with circulating thyroid stimulating antibodies, irrespective of the mother's own biochemical thyroid status, may develop all the signs of thyrotoxicosis after birth including exophthalmos.

Fetal determinants of adult disease

Evidence is accumulating that some of the risk of disease in adulthood is attributable to events during fetal life. Systolic blood pressure in men

Transient disorders in the newborn caused by maternal immunoglobulin

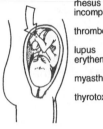

rhesus incompatibility

thrombocytopenia

lupus erythematosis

myasthenia gravis

thyrotoxicosis

at retirement is inversely related to birth weight and the risk of ischaemic heart disease is greater the lower the fetal/placental weight ratio. It appears that fetal life may represent a 'critical window' of time when insults, such as poor fetal growth, may result in that individual being programmmed to be at greater risk of degenerative diseases many decades later.

Programming for longevity: experience in early life has long lasting effects (Barker 1994)					
Trimester	Effects	Birth weight and shape	Weight at 1 yr	Adult life	Death
First	Down regulation of growth	Reduced *proportional*	Reduced	▲ BP	Haemorrhagic stroke
Second	Disturbed feto-placental unit	Reduced *thin*	Normal	▲ BP Non-insulin dependent diabetes	Coronary heart disease
Third	Brain growth sustained at expense of trunk	Normal *short*	Reduced	▲ BP ▲ LDL and cholesterol ▲ Fibrinogen	Coronary heart disease Thrombotic stroke

REFERENCE

Barker D J P 1994 Mothers, babies and disease in later life. BMJ Publishing Group, London

Barker D J P, Bull A R, Osmond C, Simmonds S J 1990 Fetal and placental size and risk of hypertension in adult life. British Medical Journal 301: 259–262

Broughton Pipkin F, Hull D, Stephenson T J 1994 Fetal physiology. In: Lamming G E (ed) Marshall's physiology of reproduction, 4th edn. Chapman and Hall, London

Chamberlain G 1995 Turnbull's obstetrics, 2nd edn. Churchill Livingstone, Edinburgh

Cleary M A, Wraith J E 1991 Antenatal diagnosis of inborn errors of metabolism. Archives of Diseases in Childhood 66: 816–822

Gluckman P D, Heymann M A 1993 Perinatal and pediatric pathophysiology. Edward Arnold, London

James D K, Stephenson T J Fetal nutrition and growth. In: Broughton Pipkin F, Chamberlain G (eds) Clinical physiology in obstetrics, 3rd edn. Blackwell Science, Oxford (in press)

Polin R A, Fox W W 1992 Fetal and neonatal physiology. WB Saunders, Philadelphia

Van Wijngaarden W, Stephenson T J Counselling about paediatric problems. In: James D K, Steer P J, Weiner C P, Gonik B (eds) High risk pregnancy, 2nd edn. W B Saunders, Philadelphia (in press)

4 Newborn

ROUTINE EXAMINATION OF THE
  NEWBORN
BIRTH INJURIES
TRANSITION TO INDEPENDENT
  LIFE
SIZE AT BIRTH
RESPIRATORY PROBLEMS IN THE
  NEWBORN
JAUNDICE IN THE NEWBORN
GASTROINTESTINAL PROBLEMS
NEURAL TUBE ABNORMALITIES
CLEFT LIP AND PALATE
NEONATAL INFECTIONS
NEONATAL CONVULSIONS

In our concern to provide every mother and her child with a safe birth we must not overlook the importance of their first meeting face to face. They have a deep basic need to 'recognise' and respond to each other. Fascinating research has demonstrated how very aware and responsive human newborns are to their new environment and how natural and robust this developing relationship is. If the mother is ill, the delivery difficult, or the newborn infant is sick or weak, it is even more important for the caring staff to encourage the establishment and the strengthening of this key relationship between mother and child. Problems with bonding have been shown to lead to poor feeding patterns, failure to thrive, and the longer-term consequences of maternal neglect, including an increased risk of child abuse and post-neonatal infant death.

ROUTINE EXAMINATION OF THE NEWBORN

The average newborn!

body weight	3.5 kg
body length	50 cm
head circumference	35 cm
HB	18 g/dl
blood volume	300 ml

'Is my baby all right?' is often the first question that mothers ask after delivery and it is so difficult to answer if he is not! As soon as the baby is born a quick but careful scrutiny of the face, eyes, mouth, chest, abdomen, spine and limbs should exclude major abnormalities; a lusty cry and the development of a suffuse pink blush over the face and body denote satisfactory immediate adjustment to independent existence. Together they are sufficient to answer the mother's pressing question.

If there is difficulty establishing adequate breathing, then the appropriate steps in resuscitation should be taken. If the baby is small, immature or injured, he must be given extra support and protection. If you are not sure of the sex of the infant do not make a guess. Explain to the parents that occasionally it can be difficult to tell immediately and that tests will be necessary. If the mother has had hydramnios then a firm tube must be passed into the stomach to exclude oesophageal atresia, a congenital abnormality which is usually associated with a trachea-oesophageal fistula. At some point over the next 48 hours all infants should be examined thoroughly and at leisure, preferably in the mother's presence, ideally with both parents, and only after the details

Incidence of the commoner malformations in Great Britain (these figures are approximate)	
Malformation per 1000 live births	
Anencephaly and spina bifida	<1.0
Cleft lip/cleft palate	1.4
Club foot	1.2
Congenital hip dislocation	1.5
Congenital heart malformation	7.5
Down Syndrome	1.4

of the medical history of the family, the pregnancy and labour are known. This first medical examination is a screening procedure, and its aim is to discover disorders which are open to early management. The baby should be naked in a warm room, and the mother should be able to see clearly what you are doing. The examination needs to be thorough and in a logical sequence; first assess overall size, proportions and maturity, then look for structural abnormalities, starting with the head and eyes and then the ears, mouth, chest, abdomen and limbs, hands and feet. Note any accessory tags, digits and dimples. Many abnormalities follow failure of complete union in the midline, and so a quick check along the midline is worthwhile, and this should include a close look at the palate and anus. Respiratory disorders are more easily seen than heard. Palpating the peripheral pulses may suggest, if full, a ductus arteriosus, or, if weak, a major defect causing poor systemic cardiac output. The presence or absence of femoral pulsations must always be noted. Abnormal heart sounds and murmurs are more difficult to interpret; if there is doubt, it is better to find an opportunity to re-examine the baby later. If the murmur persists but the baby is otherwise well, then the parents are told of the finding and a follow-up examination is arranged. Two other conditions are specifically sought; congenital dislocation of the hips, and in boys, the presence of testes in the scrotum.

The third stage of this examination is to assess the baby's behaviour and responsiveness. The mother and the midwife will usually be quick to tell you about the baby's feeding, behaviour, crying and sleeping patterns. An unduly floppy or sleepy baby, an irritable or restless baby, or a poor 'suckler' all call for more careful evaluation, particularly in relation to the establishment or otherwise of satisfactory breastfeeding. Parents should be reassured about minor anomalies. Finally give the parents an opportunity to ask any other questions.

Minor anomalies

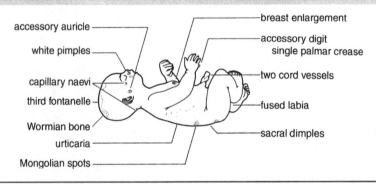

Capillary or macular haemangioma (stork bites, salmon patch) around the eyes and at the nape of the neck are seen in 30–50% of babies. Those around the eyes usually disappear in the first year. Those at the nape may persist.

Blue-black pigmented areas (mongolian blue spots) at the base of the back and on the buttocks are unimportant and are common in infants of dark-skinned parents but can also occur in Caucasian infants. They usually fade over the first year or so.

Urticaria of the newborn is a fluctuating, widespread, erythematous rash with a raised white or cream dot at the centre of the red flare. It is usually most marked on the trunk and is most evident on the second day. It disappears spontaneously, requiring no treatment.

Heat rash (miliaria) is seen in mature infants nursed in warm humid atmospheres. Both red, macular patches and superficial, clear vesicles may be seen, most evident on the forehead and around the neck. The lesions clear in a cool environment.

Breast enlargement is seen in both girl and boy infants and the breasts may even secrete small amounts of milk ('witch's milk'). As a parallel endocrine-mediated event girls may discharge a mucous plug from the vagina and there may be scanty vaginal bleeding on about the fourth day.

White pimples (milia) on the nose and cheeks are very common and are found in about 40% of infants. They are blocked sebaceous glands and clear spontaneously.

Cysts in the mouth occur on the palate near the midline (Epstein pearls) and larger ones on the gums (epulis) and on the floor of the mouth. Epstein pearls and most of the others resolve spontaneously. Teeth may be present at birth: some are loose and have to be removed.

Accessory skin tags on the face, anterior to the ears (accessory auricles) or loosely attached, vestigial, extra digits can usually be dealt with easily but this should preferably be done by the surgical team.

Sacral dimples should be explored gently to exclude underlying sinuses.

The skull

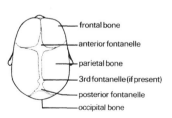

- frontal bone
- anterior fontanelle
- parietal bone
- 3rd fontanelle (if present)
- posterior fontanelle
- occipital bone

Some anomalies, although relatively unimportant in themselves, may be associated with more important underlying abnormalities. The fontanelles (head 'soft spots') are occasionally wide and extra bones may float in the space, wormian bones. If skin defects overlie the posterior fontanelle chromosomal abnormalities should be considered. A third fontanelle is occasionally found between the anterior and posterior fontanelles and is common in trisomy 21.

Oddly shaped ears and two cord vessels may be associated with renal abnormalities. A single palmar crease, instead of the usual two, may sometimes be associated with other abnormalities, including Down syndrome. Abnormalities of the face, jaws and ears, including accessory auricles, may be associated with varying degrees of deafness, and a newborn hearing test should be arranged.

Congenital postural deformities

The posture of the infant after birth often reflects his position in utero. However, with more freedom, the infant soon chooses to curl into a compact shape with arms and legs flexed. If there is a reduced amount of amniotic fluid to cushion the fetus, then towards the end of gestation the infant may be so tightly packed within the uterus that deformations of the musculoskeletal system develop. These congenital postural deformities may mould the head into odd shapes (dolichocephaly, plagiocephaly), suppress or distort the chin, resulting in it being unduly small (micrognathia), or cause mandibular asymmetry or neck muscle contractures and torticollis. The shoulders may be dislocated, the chest wall compressed, the hands and feet distorted (club hand, club foot). These effects are usually multiple and are seen in their extreme form in renal agenesis, and very little amniotic fluid is present (oligohydramnios). The presenting part is often the most deformed. One special example of postural deformity associated with intrauterine position is dislocation of the hip, which is more common in breech presentation.

Intrauterine postures

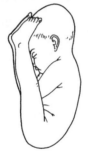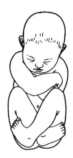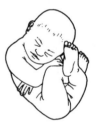

Biochemical screening

The number of inherited biochemical disorders or variations which can be recognised by relatively simple and cheap biochemical tests increases yearly. It is the simplicity and cheapness of the test which makes it feasible to test the blood of every newborn infant. The tests are primarily intended to screen for phenylketonuria, hypothyroidism and cystic fibrosis, but other conditions including galactosaemia, maple syrup urine disease and homocystinuria may be identified. The blood test (often called the Guthrie test) is performed when milk feeding has been established, between the sixth and eighth day after birth.

BIRTH INJURIES

The short journey down the birth canal is not without potential hazards for the infant but fortunately the risks are becoming less as the techniques for recognising fetal distress improve. Infants who are

Caput succedaneum (common)

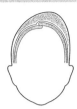

Cephalhaematoma (occasional)

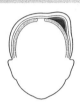

Subaponeurotic haemorrhage (rare)

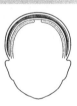

judged to be too big for the birth canal or who fail to advance during labour and become distressed are delivered by caesarean section, making heroic obstetric manipulations to achieve vaginal birth rarely necessary. The risk of birth trauma is greater in breech deliveries, premature births, precipitate deliveries and when the baby is unexpectedly large.

Some of the damage caused by the birth is unsightly but quickly resolves. Inevitably, the presenting part becomes oedematous and bruised. This caput succedaneum is commonly found on the back of the head and happily it clears spontaneously in a few days. However, the swelling looks uncomfortable when it involves the breech and scrotum and may be very unpleasant in a face presentation. The face also looks bloated, blue and bruised when the cord is pulled tightly around the neck (an appearance called 'traumatic cyanosis'), and there may also be retinal and conjunctival haemorrhages. As the fetal head is pushed down the birth canal it rotates and the apex of the parietal bones may catch the ischial spines and be dented like a ping pong ball or the outer shelf may be cracked and crepitus may be felt, or a cephalhaematoma may form beneath the separated periosteum, producing a lump the size of a small hen's egg. Again, these injuries are of little import although the cephalhaematoma may take many months before it finally disappears. Rarely a bleed may occur under the aponeurosis (subaponeurotic haemorrhage). In this case the bleeding is not confined to a single cranial bone like a cephalhaematoma but spreads rapidly over the head and down towards the eyes. A significant fraction of the blood volume may be lost into this haematoma.

Severe compression with extreme moulding of the skull can tear the tentorium cerebelli and its accompanying vein. The resulting haemorrhage is likely to cause permanent damage or death. The baby may be born in a state of shock and may not respond to resuscitative procedures.

Birth injuries

Fractures	Nervous tissue damage
	brain bleed (tentorial tear)
clavicle	spinal cord
	upper brachial plexus
humerus	
ribs	**Dislocations**
	shoulder
	hip

Manipulation of the spine and arms, which is most likely to be required for breech deliveries, may damage the cervical spinal cord with residual palsies in arms and legs, or lead to stretching and damage of the upper part of the brachial plexus causing weakness or paralysis of abduction at the shoulder, flexion at the elbow and extension and supination of the wrist (Erb palsy). The arm is dropped into the position a waiter adopts in the expectation of a tip. The weakness usually resolves spontaneously in a few weeks.

Rough handling may lead not only to fracture of the skull but also of the clavicle, humerus or ribs. These injuries may pass undetected immediately after birth, but can be recognised when a lump appears due to callus formation around the fracture. During labour, pressure from the ischial spines or from forceps blades may compress the facial nerve as it leaves the parotid gland. Usually the resultant facial palsy is transient, but occasionally the pressure causes overlying fat necrosis with permanent scarring and a residual palsy.

TRANSITION TO INDEPENDENT LIFE

The fetus, floating in the amniotic fluid, 'breathes', 'feeds' and 'excretes' through the placenta. The fetal lungs are filled with fluid secreted by the alveolar cells to a volume close to the functional residual capacity found after birth. Following delivery, the placenta is discarded and 'dies' while the independent infant activates his own system for obtaining oxygen and nutrients and discarding waste.

The most urgent requirement is to breathe. To do this lung liquid must be displaced by air. During a vaginal birth the thorax is squeezed in the birth canal and lung liquid can sometimes be seen pouring out of the baby's nose when his head is just emerging from the birth canal. Once the infant gasps, air is drawn into the lung and lung liquid disappears to the periphery of the respiratory tree. From there it is cleared by the pulmonary circulation and lymphatics. Failure to complete this process satisfactorily is one factor leading to transient tachypnoea.

As the infant passes down the birth canal his head is squeezed, then released and exposed to the cooling air. His limbs are pushed, pulled and finally allowed to drop into positions they have never occupied before. His umbilical cord is intermittently obstructed, stretched and finally clamped. His arterial oxygen concentration falls and that of carbon dioxide rises. Many of these stimuli provoke a gasp. On average, newborn infants gasp after 6 seconds and the majority have done so by 20 seconds. With these efforts the lungs rapidly fill with air and a residual lung volume is formed. Once this is achieved, tidal breathing begins, commencing on average after 30 seconds, and the majority of infants are breathing regularly by 90 seconds.

As the lungs expand and fill with gas, the pulmonary vascular resistance falls, the pulmonary blood flow increases and the pressure in the left atrium rises closing the foramen ovale. As a consequence of these changes, oxygenated blood passes through the ductus arteriosus;

Onset of breathing

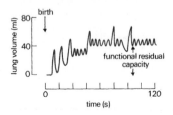

oxygen has a direct effect on the muscle of the ductus causing contraction and physiological closure, anatomical closure proceeds more slowly over the following weeks.

Circulatory adjustments after birth

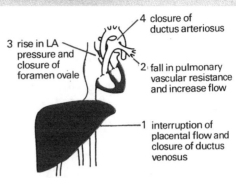

3 rise in LA pressure and closure of foramen ovale

4 closure of ductus arteriosus

2 fall in pulmonary vascular resistance and increase flow

1 interruption of placental flow and closure of ductus venosus

Occasionally, in hypoxaemic infants, the ductus may remain open, or the physiologically closed ductus may reopen, and so add to the infant's problems sometimes to the point of precipitating heart failure.

Hypoxaemia, hypoxia and perinatal compromise

The fetus normally has a low arterial oxygen concentration in utero, i.e. is hypoxaemic, but perfusion is normal, acidosis does not develop and there is no fetal compromise. Where oxygen delivery to the tissues is compromised because of profound hypoxaemia or poor circulation, acidosis develops and the fetus is described as hypoxic.

Infants may become hypoxic in utero for a variety of reasons. If the disorder is not reversed they will be in poor condition at birth and they must be resuscitated immediately. Many of the babies who appear all but dead at birth, but who respond promptly to active resuscitation, may make a full recovery. More commonly, infants are reasonably oxygenated at birth but due to previous hypoxia or sedative drugs given to the mother they fail to begin adequate ventilation, and then become compromised and require resuscitation. Many factors are associated with perinatal hypoxia, including the general wellbeing of the mother and the maturity and nutrition of the infant.

Causes of intrauterine hypoxia

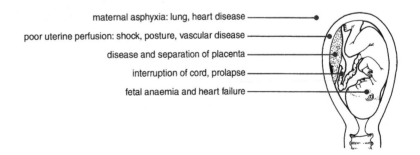

maternal asphyxia: lung, heart disease

poor uterine perfusion: shock, posture, vascular disease

disease and separation of placenta

interruption of cord, prolapse

fetal anaemia and heart failure

With increasing hypoxia the infant becomes blue and then white, hypotonic, unresponsive, and the heart rate begins to fall. Five features: colour, tone, response to stimulation, respiration and heart rate were arranged into a scoring system by an American anaesthetist, Dr Virginia Apgar; scores of 0 representing apparent stillbirth and scores of 8–10 the normally adapted infant. The most important features to watch are the infant's attempts to breathe and the rate and strength of the pulse. Those who fail to breathe should be actively resuscitated when the heart rate begins to fall.

Assessment of neonatal condition at birth—the Apgar Score			
	0	1	2
Response to stimulation	None	Facial grimace	Cry
Respiration	Absent	Gasping	Regular
Heart rate/minute	0	< 100	> 100
Colour of trunk	White	Blue	Pink
Muscle tone	Flaccid	Some flexion	Normal with movement

Resuscitation

The newly born baby is gently dried and wrapped in a warm towel. The time of birth is noted. Resuscitation then proceeds as 'ABCD'— **A**irway, **B**reathing, **C**irculation, **D**rugs. The upper airway is cleared by gentle suction of excess fluid and any inhaled vernix, blood or meconium. If during this procedure the infant fails to make any respiratory effort then a gasp may be provoked with gentle stimulation. If this is not effective then the other bizarre methods used in the past, for example pinching, slapping, injecting respiratory stimulants, or putting champagne or pepper on the nasal mucosa, are not likely to work!

The next step is to expand and ventilate the lungs. Often simple inflation of the lungs will initiate a gasp with spontaneous breathing. If it does not, the lung should be ventilated at a rate between 20 and 30 inflations per minute with pressures limited to 30 cmH$_2$O. The majority of infants will quickly become pink and begin breathing within 2 or 5 minutes.

Steps in resuscitation: watch the clock

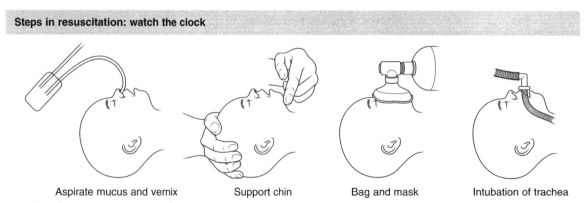

Aspirate mucus and vernix   Support chin   Bag and mask   Intubation of trachea

The most effective method of inflating the lungs is via an endotracheal tube. If the lungs do not expand then either there is a rare abnormality of the airways or lungs, or the endotracheal tube is not in the trachea. Clumsy insertion of the tube can damage the upper airways; energetic and faulty inflation may damage the lungs. If either the skill or the equipment is not available for intubation then the infant can be resuscitated nearly as well with a face mask, which fits snugly over his mouth and nose, and a bag which delivers small volumes of gas. It is essential to hold the lower jaw forward to ensure a clear airway.

If the infant fails to become pink with good expansion of the lungs, he is probably in a state of shock. If the apex rate is less than 60 and falling, start cardiac massage, encircling the chest with both hands, thumbs to the fore and using both thumbs to exert pressure on the lower half of the sternum at 100–120 beats per minute 3–5 compressions to one inflation of the lungs. Rarely adrenaline 10 µg/kg (0.1 ml/kg of 1 : 10 000 solution) may be required to re-establish the heart beat. Poor perfusion may be corrected by giving 10–20 ml/kg albumin into the umbilical vein. Further adrenaline at the higher dose of 1.0 ml/kg is then given if there is no response. Hypoglycaemia may be treated with 5 ml/kg 10% dextrose.

Occasionally, the difficult decision of whether or not to resuscitate has to be made, especially when babies are born at the limits of viability (22–24 weeks' gestation). An experienced neonatologist should be called to these deliveries and the baby's gestation, birth weight and degree of bruising are taken into account together with the baby's condition at birth, the presence or absence of a heart beat and efforts to breathe.

Reasons for failure to respond to resuscitation

Brain damage
  haemorrhage: ischaemia
Upper airway obstruction
  laryngeal spasm
  laryngeal stenosis
Lung pathology
  pneumothorax
  hypoplasia
  effusion
  diaphragmatic hernia
Small chest cage
Shock due to ruptured viscera

Neonatal effects of perinatal hypoxia

Fetal hypoxia during delivery may have both immediate and long-term effects. Hypoxia may be acute and total, for example when cord pulsation ceases following cord prolapse, or more commonly occurs intermittently or partially ('chronic partial'). These may be difficult to distinguish at birth. The results of hypoxia may be observed in many body systems. In the term baby, poor condition at birth may lead to neurological compromise, with general hypoxic changes throughout the brain but mainly affecting the basal ganglia and cortex. Clinically this may be manifest as initial irritability and poor feeding, followed in more severe cases by lethargy and seizures which develop after the first few hours. This encephalopathy is related to the development of cerebral oedema and tends to improve as tissue healing occurs after a few days. Hypoxic renal, pulmonary and gastrointestinal changes may occur. In preterm infants, perinatal hypoxia increases the risk of respiratory distress syndrome and two specific brain lesions: intraventricular haemorrhage and periventricular leucomalacia (softening of the white matter around the lateral ventricles). Where chronic hypoxia occurs before labour intrauterine growth may be restricted producing a small-for-gestational-age baby. Such babies are at increased risk of acute hypoxia in labour and must be monitored carefully.

Severe perinatal hypoxia is responsible for some disabling brain

Effects of hypoxia

Brain	Fits, irritability, abnormal tone, hypo- and hyper-ventilation
Heart	Hypotension
Lungs	RDS, haemorrhage, aspiration
Kidneys	Oliguria (tubular necrosis), vein thrombosis
Bowels	Ileus, perforation, necrotising enterocolitis
Liver	Raised enzymes
Metabolic	Hypoglycaemia, coagulopathy

injuries in term children, manifest as cerebral palsy and learning difficulties, the extent of which become apparent as the child develops. Milder hypoxic insults are popularly thought to cause problems such as hyperactivity, fits and learning problems, but there is little good evidence for this. Some babies make remarkable recoveries after perinatal hypoxia, so parents can often be encouraged to be reasonably optimistic. Poor prognostic signs include the severity of encephalopathy, a prolonged period before suckling feeds are established (over 7 days) or brain injuries visible on CT or MR imaging.

In very preterm babies, outcome is less predictable after the development of intraventricular haemorrhage or periventricular leucomalacia. There is value in serial cerebral ultrasound scanning—in the presence of a normal scan, major disability is unlikely, but where cystic changes have developed cerebral palsy will develop in about half the babies.

SIZE AT BIRTH

Plotting birth weight on charts of body weight against gestational age helps to define particular groups of babies. Babies with birth weights between the 10th and 90th centile lines are considered 'normal weight for dates', those with birth weights over the 90th centile are termed 'large for dates', and those under the 10th centile 'small for dates'. Small-for-dates babies are also described as 'small for gestational age', 'light for dates' or dysmature. It is important to determine whether a baby is large for dates or small for dates or preterm or post-term, for each has special problems which can be anticipated and treated.

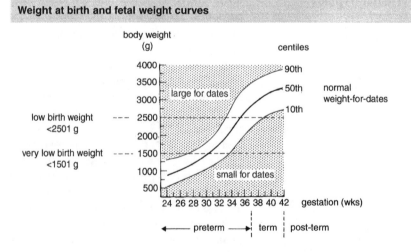

Weight at birth and fetal weight curves

Large-for-dates infants

By definition 10% of normal babies will be large for dates. The most important pathological cause is maternal diabetes mellitus. These babies may be large and obese, due to fetal hyperinsulinism which occurs as a result of fluctuations in maternal glucose concentrations. In the past many were stillborn; with improved antenatal care this is now unusual, but they are still at an increased risk of having a congenital abnormality or problems during birth (their broad shoulders causing shoulder dystocia) and after birth they are more likely to develop hypoglycaemia, respiratory distress and jaundice. Their hyperexcitability, jitteriness and immaturity may initially cause feeding difficulties. With meticulous control of the diabetic state during the whole of pregnancy, many if not all these problems can be avoided. There is increasing evidence that tight diabetic control in very early pregnancy will reduce the incidence of congenital abnormalities.

Low birth weight

Small-for-dates infants: characteristics

Wasted
White or pale pink
Length > 50 cm
Head circumference > c.35 cm
Thick, dark hair
Skin: dry, loose, thick
Ears, breast tissues, genitalia –
  all mature
Good muscle tone

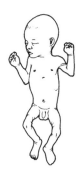

Small-for-dates infants: problems

Respiratory:
  birth asphyxia
  meconium aspiration
  pulmonary haemorrhage
Hypothermia:
  large surface area
Infections in utero:
  toxoplasma, rubella, CMV,
  herpes virus
Metabolic:
  symptomatic hypoglycaemia
Congenital anomalies

About 7% of births in the United Kingdom are of low birth weight, defined as all those weighing 2500 g or less. The incidence is lower in Scandinavian countries and higher in Third World countries. The low-birth-weight group includes a disproportionate number of the babies with problems. In the United Kingdom about 60% of stillbirths and 70% of first week deaths are of low birth weight. Low birth weight is associated among other things with poor socioeconomic conditions, congenital abnormalities, intrauterine infections, multiple pregnancies, poor placental function, and maternal starvation, illness, smoking, drug and alcohol abuse. Low birth weight may be due to premature or preterm birth, before 37 weeks, or poor fetal growth (small-for-dates infant). Although they may be of the same weight, preterm and small-for-dates infants look different and have different problems. Some babies are both preterm and small for dates and are at risk of the problems of both groups.

Small-for-dates infants. Although many small babies will have birth weights below the 10th centile, others fail to grow normally during pregnancy and are at particular perinatal risk. It is preferable to recognise these infants before birth as they are at greater risk from perinatal hypoxia and may be in need of prompt and skilful resuscitation. Small-for-dates infants are particularly susceptible to hypoglycaemia in the first days after birth. Early feeding is commenced at 50% more than normal requirements and the blood glucose is monitored as appropriate. Should the blood glucose concentration fall below 2.6 mmol/l, it should be rechecked after a feed; intravenous glucose therapy is required if a low blood sugar persists or if the child has signs of neurological dysfunction, such as seizures or drowsiness.

Small-for-dates babies have a lower perinatal mortality rate than babies of similar birth weight who are appropriately grown but preterm, but their eventual outlook may not be so good. Those who are small but perfectly proportioned, suggesting intrauterine growth restriction early in the pregnancy, may remain small, and their learning abilities are more likely to fall below the average. The situation is complex because of the association with poor socioeconomic status.

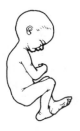

Preterm infants. The survival rates of preterm babies have improved over the years. Much of this progress is due to better management. Neonatal care is provided at two levels. Special care is for well preterm infants who need to be carefully watched and monitored in a relatively stable environment and where special expertise is available to help them establish and maintain adequate nutrition. This is all that is usually required for the more mature preterm infant (33–36 weeks). Intensive care is for sick and very immature infants who require a strictly controlled environment and respiratory support with a ventilator, or as high dependency care which involves more monitoring and support, often with parenteral nutrition.

Survival for infants without malformation decreases with decreasing gestational age from over 95% at 30–32 weeks to about 40% at 25–26 weeks. Most babies who are born before 32 weeks now survive without major disabilities, the risk rising as gestation falls. About 10% of babies born before 29 weeks (birth weight below 1.0 kg) are left with a significant disability. Premature birth brings with it a number of immediate problems:

Nutrition. As the ability of the weak preterm infant to suckle is limited they often require to be fed for some weeks after birth using a nasogastric tube. Recent work suggests that breast milk, which may be fortified with commercial calorie and mineral supplements, and milks formulated specially for very low birth weight infants (under 1.5 kg), result in better growth and development. The immature bowel adjusts surprisingly well, although there may be a functional ileus for the first few days after birth.

Thermal stability. Premature babies have a high surface area to body weight ratio and little subcutaneous fat—over the first few days they lose water rapidly through their skin (transepidermal water loss). These physical characteristics make it difficult for them to maintain thermal stability. As cold exposure increases energy expenditure and jeopardises their survival, great attention must be paid to keeping them warm. To provide a controlled ambient temperature the smaller premature infants are nursed in incubators with high humidity.

Respiratory difficulties. Because of their immaturity many preterm babies have difficulty expanding their lungs and the work of breathing is greatly increased due to the idiopathic respiratory distress syndrome. Also their respiratory drive varies, and this is apparent in their periodic breathing pattern which becomes troublesome when it leads to long apnoeic spells.

Liver immaturity. Physiological jaundice is more frequent and more prolonged in immature infants but with careful nursing, early establishment of feeding and the use of phototherapy, exchange transfusions should rarely be necessary. It is thought that the preterm brain is more at risk from damage due to high bilirubin levels.

Infections. Because of their delicate surfaces and limited immunological competence, premature babies are more susceptible to infections. Because of their weak defence systems, they do not show the symptoms and signs that are seen in older infants. Their clinical state changes rapidly from bacteraemia, to septicaemia, to death. Associated meningitis can easily pass undetected. Therefore in any infant suspected of having an infection, it is necessary to perform a 'septic screen' including culture of urine, blood and cerebrospinal fluid and to commence therapy with broad spectrum antibiotics before the results come back.

Intraventricular haemorrhage (IVH). Small haemorrhages into the germinal layer lining the lateral ventricles in the brain are commonly seen on cerebral ultrasound scanning of preterm babies, especially those who have experienced hypoxia or severe respiratory problems. These may extend into the ventricular system and a few infants subsequently develop hydrocephalus. However, the majority seem to recover without serious long-term effects.

Ultrasound: hydrocephalus

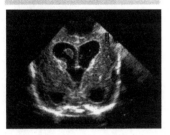

Periventricular leucomalacia (PVL). Ischaemia or infarction of the brain parenchyma may lead to changes recognised initially as 'flare' on cranial ultrasound examination. Sometimes this resolves, but in other babies these damaged areas of brain break down to form cysts. Cystic periventricular leucomalacia has a much poorer outlook than haemorrhage confined to the ventricles. Where these changes extend beyond the frontal lobes of the brain about 9 out of 10 children develop spastic cerebral palsy.

Ultrasound: periventricular leucomalacia

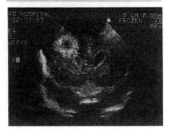

Necrotising enterocolitis (NEC). This is a serious condition affecting the bowel during the first 3 weeks. It is much commoner in the smallest preterm infants. The cause is not known but hypoxic damage to the bowel wall possibly associated with umbilical catheterisation, apnoeic spells and septicaemia, and the colonization of the bowel with certain organisms are probably precipitating events. Isolated cases occur but so do worrying outbreaks within neonatal units. The baby vomits bile-stained fluid, the abdomen distends and blood and mucus appear in the stools. The diagnosis is confirmed by abdominal X-ray which shows thickened bowel wall containing intramural gas. Perforation may occur. Oral feeds are stopped for at least a week, and intravenous feeding is used. Broad spectrum antibiotics and metronidazole are given intravenously. Surgical resection of perforated and necrotic bowel may be needed.

Retinopathy of prematurity (ROP). In the 1950s it was found that preterm infants who inhaled gas mixtures with high oxygen concentrations were at risk of developing abnormal vascularisation at the back of the eye (retrolental fibroplasia or retinopathy of prematurity). Some of these babies became blind. Oxygen excess is not the only cause of ROP and it is the tiniest, most immature infants (under 30 weeks or 1250 g birth weight) who are most at risk. It is important to measure the percentage of oxygen in the inspired gas (FiO_2) and the partial pressure of oxygen in arterial blood (PaO_2), so that oxygen is not given in excess. Newer monitors allow the continuous non-invasive monitoring of oxygen saturation or transcutaneous oxygen levels. However, even with strictly controlled oxygen levels some very immature infants develop retinopathy of prematurity and, untreated, a few go on to partial or complete blindness. Associated disorders include intraventricular haemorrhage, apnoeic attacks, patent ductus arteriosus, septicaemia and metabolic acidosis and any or all may play a part in its causation. All babies under 31 weeks or 1500 g should be screened by an ophthalmologist and more severe disease treated before severe visual impairment ensues.

Nutritional deficiencies. Once they have adjusted to extra-uterine life and feeding has been established, preterm babies can grow at a rate similar to that which they would have achieved in utero. This high growth rate can lead to vitamin deficiency, so vitamin supplements are given. Significant iron transfer takes place across the placenta during the third trimester of pregnancy. Preterm infants are commonly given iron supplements from the fourth week. Calcium, phosphate and vitamin D supplementation all appear to be necessary to avoid osteopenia of prematurity, a condition that develops in some preterm infants in the first months and is characterised by an elevated alkaline phosphatase level and occasionally fractures.

Other hazards. Premature babies are often born unexpectedly and are therefore more likely to experience hypoxia during birth and their delicate tissues are more likely to be damaged. They are susceptible to hypoglycaemia, metabolic acidosis, and peripheral oedema. The delicate preterm infant is also more easily damaged by nursing and medical procedures. For example, if hypertonic solutions like 10% glucose, calcium or amino acid preparations leak out of a peripheral vein they quickly cause necrosis which can result in a permanent scar.

Prognosis. The outlook of prematurely born infants, particularly those with only moderate problems adjusting to extra-uterine life, is good. The majority reach their expected size and ability level. Until recently infants born before 26 weeks were thought not to be viable. It was exceedingly rare for infants weighing less than 750 g to survive. Now, with intensive care, including if necessary artificial ventilation and intravenous nutrition, more and more are surviving and it is important to assess the quality of survival. Between 5 and 10% of babies with birth weights below 1500 g are found to have a major handicap such as cerebral palsy, developmental delay, blindness or deafness. Very preterm children are also at greater risk of sudden infant death syndrome. Most children without major disability will attend normal school and grow up normally. A proportion may have educational, attentional or behavioural problems which may be attributable to prematurity or to the socio-environmental situations associated with preterm birth.

Chemical burn

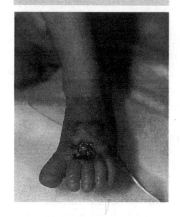

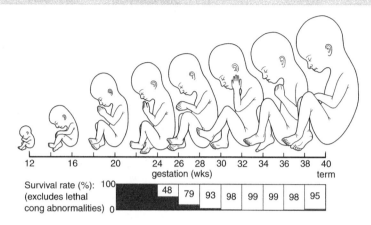

Survival rates in preterm infants admitted for neonatal intensive care (Nottingham 1996)

gestation (wks)

Survival rate (%): (excludes lethal cong abnormalities)

| 48 | 79 | 93 | 98 | 99 | 99 | 98 | 95 |

RESPIRATORY PROBLEMS IN THE NEWBORN

Respiratory distress is recognised by tachypnoea (a respiratory rate of more than 60 per minute); recession of the intercostal spaces, sternum and subcostal areas; flaring of the ala nasae; expiratory grunting, and cyanosis or the need for oxygen to remain pink. Respiratory failure may be due to a wide variety of both pulmonary and extrapulmonary causes.

Lung disorders due to aspiration

An infant may aspirate foreign material before, during and after birth.

Intrauterine pneumonia. Occasionally babies are born with lung consolidation due to material aspirated from the amniotic fluid. This 'congenital pneumonia' is associated with prolonged rupture of the fetal membranes, amnionitis and fetal hypoxia. If organisms are present they are usually *E. coli*, other gram-negative bacteria or the beta-haemolytic streptococcus group B. All can produce an aggressive infection leading to septicaemia and meningitis. The babies develop respiratory distress in the first few hours after birth. A chest X-ray shows patchy shadowing. A septic screen is performed and broad spectrum antibiotics started without delay. Group B streptococcus can also cause a fulminating septicaemia and meningitis 2–6 weeks after birth. Less common but important lung infections are caused by *Listeria monocytogenes* and by chlamydia.

Meconium aspiration. Hypoxia during labour may provoke mature infants to gasp. If there is meconium in the amniotic fluid, or if the

Lung disorders

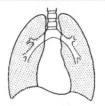

ground-glass appearance + air bronchogram: idiopathic respiratory distress syndrome

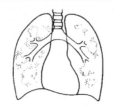

patchy collapse with overinflation meconium aspiration

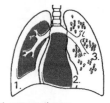

1. pneumothorax
2. pneumomediastinum
3. interstitial emphysema

baby's head is in the birth canal surrounded by vernix, meconium and blood, these tenacious materials may be drawn into the upper airway and then into the respiratory tree. This may result in patchy lung collapse, and other areas of overinflation, due to a ball valve effect of the meconium plug allowing air in but not out. The infants may have severe respiratory difficulties for some days, and complications like pneumothorax and pneumomediastinum are common and may be fatal. Oxygen will be needed, and any tension pneumothorax must be drained. Supportive ventilation is difficult. Several new techniques can help the most severely affected babies, including extracorporeal membrane oxygenation (ECMO) in which an oxygenator takes over the function of the baby's lungs until spontaneous recovery of the aspiration occurs. It is better to try to prevent the meconium reaching the lungs by clearing the airways promptly at birth. If meconium is seen around the larynx, the baby is intubated and suction applied directly to the endotracheal tube as it is withdrawn. In skilled hands this can be repeated several times in the first few minutes before the baby is ventilated for resuscitation.

Milk aspiration. It is quite a challenge for the newborn infant to separate in the pharynx the air breathed in through the nose and milk sucked in through the mouth. Often air is swallowed; and occasionally milk may be inhaled. Obviously the latter is the more dangerous and every effort must be made to anticipate and avoid it. Aspiration of feeds is quite a common occurrence in preterm babies and in full-term babies with a neurological or cardiorespiratory problem. Those with structural anomalies of the nose, mouth and oesophagus are particularly at risk, for example cleft palate, choanal atresia and oesophageal atresia. Management of these babies requires considerable nursing skill and judgement. A nasogastric or nasojejunal feeding tube may be needed, or even total parenteral nutrition for a while.

Transient tachypnoea of the newborn. This is not so much an aspiration as a delay in the clearance of lung fluid which is naturally present in utero. The rapid breathing usually settles within a few hours of birth, and chest X-ray shows the fluid as streaky shadows spreading out from the mediastinum and in the horizontal fissure on the right.

Disorders due to lung immaturity

Respiratory distress syndrome (RDS). The more immature the infant the greater is the risk of respiratory distress and the lower the survival rate. In the adult, alveolar spaces are clustered around the terminal bronchioles; in the infant at term a single, simple sac is found at the end of each bronchiole. The alveolar epithelium has two types of cells. The type II pneumocytes secrete a complex of lipoproteins, surfactant, which has the property of lowering surface tension. In some preterm infants these cells seem unable to release or produce enough surfactant, with the result that the air sacs collapse each time the infant breathes out, and the work of breathing is greatly increased. The pulmonary capillaries ooze liquid and red cells into the interstitial space causing oedema and haemorrhage. The protein leaked into the alveolar sacs form 'hyaline' membranes which can be clearly seen on light microscopy. This finding led to the disorder being called hyaline membrane disease, but in early severe forms membranes may not have had sufficient time to form.

The ability of the type II cells to release surfactant can be assessed before birth by measuring the ratio in the amniotic fluid of two of the lipoproteins which make up surfactant, lecithin and sphingomyelin, although this is not now commonly used. Certain stimuli, including maternal ill health, uterine contractions and drugs may induce the cells to begin secreting earlier in gestation. Steroids given to the mother at least 24–48 hours before a very preterm delivery have been shown to reduce both the incidence of RDS by 40% and the severity of the illness. They have proved to be a very important factor in the improvements in survival that have been seen over the past few years. Perinatal hypoxia, acidosis and hypothermia have the opposite effect and inhibit surfactant synthesis. Within a few days of birth, whatever the gestation, the cells begin to function and produce adequate surfactant.

As the affected infants have difficulty forming and maintaining a functional residual capacity, they are recognised clinically by their struggle to draw in air and to hold it. Each diaphragmatic tug pulls in the lower rib cage and soft tissues of the neck. An expiratory grunt accompanies each effort. The signs appear at birth or soon after, with apparent increasing severity. If the infant survives then improvement is usually seen after the second or third day and the lungs appear to recover fully. It might be deduced from the pathogenesis that the disorder will vary in severity and this is true; at one extreme it produces an unimportant transient disturbance in the respiratory pattern, at the other it leads to increasing cyanosis, acidosis and death in the first hours after birth.

The diagnosis is confirmed by the chest X-ray which shows a diffuse ground glass appearance with an air bronchogram. The management requires considerable medical and nursing skill and involves continuous

Radiograph: RDS

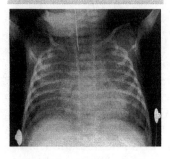

Radiograph: BPD

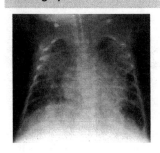

Radiograph: pneumothorax

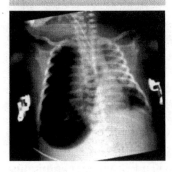

monitoring of many features of the baby, (heart rate (HR), respiratory rate (RR) (PaO_2) and of his environment (temperature (T), FiO_2) as guides for respiratory support, nutrition programmes, and intravenous therapy. Initially oxygen can be given in a headbox, and then as additional support is needed, by a nasal tube delivering a continuous positive airways pressure (CPAP) and finally by intermittent positive pressure ventilation (IPPV) or high frequency oscillatory ventilation (HFOV) via an endotracheal tube. Surfactant replacement therapy, either as artificial or bovine- or porcine-derived product, can now be given and large trials have shown benefit in terms of reduction of disease severity, and survival may be improved by up to 40%.

Chronic lung disease (bronchopulmonary dysplasia, BPD). Forcing the lungs open when they are not ready by using high inflation pressures from a mechanical ventilator together with raised inspired oxygen concentrations can result in the development of chronic lung disease in some preterm infants with respiratory distress. The X-ray reveals areas of patchy collapse and fibrosis interspersed with areas of cystic change and overdistension. The infants may remain dependent on IPPV for many days, but it has now been shown that giving dexamethasone can significantly reduce the duration of assisted ventilation. The babies can be weaned down onto CPAP and then onto added oxygen alone over a period of weeks. Most recover well but others continue to need respiratory support and some die of chronic respiratory failure, cor pulmonale or added infections.

Pulmonary haemorrhage may complicate hypoxia and atelectasis, or occasionally appear to be a primary problem. It also occurs during recovery from hypothermia and may be a complication of surfactant therapy.

Apnoeic attacks are a common problem in sick and preterm newborn infants. The respiration of infants at risk must be continually monitored and stimulation may be required to restart breathing. Occasionally CPAP or intubation and supportive ventilation may be required. Respiratory stimulants like caffeine may help in preterm infants.

Pneumothorax may occur spontaneously but is also a common complication of respiratory distress syndrome and of meconium aspiration, especially when CPAP or IPPV are being used. The air leak can be confirmed by transilluminating the affected side with a powerful fibreoptic light or by X-ray. The air can be aspirated with a syringe and needle, but it will usually require placement of a chest drain.

Extrapulmonary causes of respiratory distress. Three non-lung diseases may present with respiratory symptoms. *Cerebral hypoxia* can produce bizarre respiratory patterns mimicking dyspnoea, though more commonly it leads to hypoventilation. If lung expansion matches respiratory effort this possibility should be considered. *Metabolic* *acidosis*, frequently an outcome of disorders of amino acid metabolism, presents with hyperventilation, deep and effective breaths. *Congenital heart disease* is perhaps the most difficult to exclude. Auscultation may not help or be positively misleading; assessment of peripheral perfusion, an ECG, chest X-ray and echocardiography are often more helpful. Babies with cyanotic heart disease will not improve on breathing 100% oxygen, whereas babies with a respiratory cause for cyanosis will respond with a clear rise in PaO_2 ('the nitrogen washout test'). Sometimes there is no structural heart defect but the baby's circulation continues in the fetal pattern, bypassing the lungs and causing cyanosis ('persistent fetal circulation'). Although associated with other lung disease, it may occur by itself. It is characterised by pulmonary vasoconstriction and can be treated with a variety of vasodilator drugs, including inhaled nitric oxide and tolazoline. Babies who fail to respond can be treated with extra-corporeal membrane oxygenation (ECMO).

JAUNDICE IN THE NEWBORN

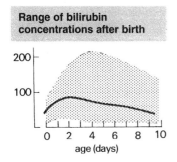

Range of bilirubin concentrations after birth

Many healthy normal newborn infants develop jaundice after birth. In utero, bilirubin crosses the placenta and is excreted by the mother. After birth, the infant must activate his own excretory systems but there is usually some delay and blood bilirubin concentrations rise. This 'physiological' jaundice appears at 2–3 days of age and begins disappearing towards the end of the first week; the bilirubin is largely unconjugated and the baby remains generally well. There is considerable variation from one infant to another. The condition is more severe and prolonged in preterm infants; if hypoxia and hypoglycaemia further limit bilirubin conjugation; and if the infant has an ileus or bowel obstruction then there may be increased enteric reabsorption of bilirubin. The diagnosis of physiological jaundice is made by the typical presentation, and by excluding other more serious causes.

Kernicterus

Unconjugated bilirubin is lipid soluble and travels in the circulation largely bound to albumin. It is the small fraction of free bilirubin which escapes from the vascular compartment and enters the cellular lipid fractions of brain cells, which may cause transient or permanent damage, kernicterus. When this happens the infant behaves abnormally, feeds badly and may fit and develop opisthotonus when the back is arched and the head thrown back. This is now a very rare problem but it can result in death or residual brain damage, often with severe choreoathetosis and mental handicap. High-tone deafness is common after hyperbilirubinaemia, and hearing should be tested carefully in early life.

In healthy full-term infants unconjugated bilirubin concentrations above 450 µmol/l are considered dangerous, but much lower thresholds apply to preterm babies and those who are sick. The risks are greater when albumin levels are low or when there is competition for albumin binding by, for example, free fatty acids and drugs like

Causes of neonatal jaundice, by time of appearance

First 24 hours of life	2nd–5th day	End of 2nd week onwards
Haemolytic diseases	Physiological	Breast milk jaundice
Rhesus incompatibility	Infection	Hypothyroidism
ABO incompatibility	Bruising	Hepatitis
G6PD deficiency	Galactosaemia and other	Biliary atresia and other
Spherocytosis	metabolic diseases	biliary tract problems
Congenital infections	Familial non-haemolytic jaundices	Pyloric stenosis
	Infants of diabetic mothers	

sulphonamides. Various diseases can cause unconjugated bilirubin to rise to dangerous levels, and these are best considered chronologically.

Jaundice: first 24 hours

A few babies who are jaundiced at birth are suffering from one of the congenital infections which can cross the placenta and may severely damage the fetus: toxoplasmosis, rubella, cytomegalovirus, herpes virus and syphilis. The jaundice is usually mixed conjugated and unconjugated, and the babies have other signs of the infection. Most early jaundice, including that due to congenital infection or early bacterial sepsis, is however due to excess haemolysis.

Haemolytic diseases of the newborn. Haemolysis of the newborn red cells may be caused by antibody from the mother, which can only happen if the maternal and fetal blood are incompatible. Some of the most severe problems are due to rhesus incompatibility. The problems occur after the mother has been sensitised by either a mismatched blood transfusion, or from fetal blood entering her circulation during a miscarriage or, more commonly, at the end of a previous pregnancy during labour and delivery. She reacts to the fetal blood by producing antibodies. The concentration of the antibodies is measured serially during pregnancy in affected mothers. It is these IgG class antibodies which cross the placenta in increasing concentrations during the pregnancy, and which cause haemolysis in the fetal circulation. When the condition is mild, the fetus and newborn tolerate the small increase in haemolysis rate, although after birth the baby may become moderately jaundiced and have mild anaemia. With higher rates of haemolysis, the bilirubin levels in the fetus may still stay low because the unconjugated bilirubin passes back across the placenta and the fetus can tolerate moderate anaemia, but after birth the bilirubin concentrations rise rapidly and dangerous bilirubin levels may be reached within 24 hours. In the severe forms with high rates of haemolysis the fetus is unable to maintain his haemoglobin and becomes severely anaemic, and this with an associated general disturbance in fetal metabolism leads to severe oedema (hydrops fetalis), a condition which is usually fatal.

The aim of obstetric management is to deliver the baby before the anaemia becomes critical. A measure of the state of the fetus can be gained by serial analysis of amniotic fluid, taken by amniocentesis for bilirubin products, or by cordocentesis and measurement of fetal haemoglobin. If the fetus is very severely affected and too immature to be delivered, fetal blood transfusions can be given in utero to correct the anaemia. Rhesus incompatibility is now far less common, following the discovery that administration of anti-D antibodies to the mother immediately after birth destroys any red cells which might have leaked into the maternal circulation and so reduces the risk of the mother producing antibodies.

Incompatibility of the ABO system is more common, and produces a similar but usually milder clinical picture. The mother is usually group O and the baby A or B. There is a marked rise in the titres of the naturally occurring anti-A or anti-B haemolysins, but these drop back to normal levels after the pregnancy, and the next pregnancy is not at greater risk, unlike rhesus disease.

Haemolysis due to a deficiency of one of the red cell enzymes. Many Mediterranean, Afro-Caribbean and Oriental babies have relative lack of glucose-6-phosphate dehydrogenase. A screening test is available. Those affected have to avoid a number of drugs which precipitate haemolysis. Finally abnormalities of the red cell shape, such as spherocytosis, can result in increased osmotic fragility and haemolysis.

Jaundice: 2–5 days

Before jaundice at this age can be labelled 'physiological', the baby has to be examined carefully to exclude any infection. Bruising, especially in forceps or breech deliveries, may be exacerbating the jaundice. Investigation for metabolic abnormality and infection is necessary if the baby is acidotic and ill.

Jaundice: 2 weeks onwards

Many babies who are being breastfed have a prolongation of their jaundice. This does not rise to harmful levels, and the mother is encouraged to continue breastfeeding, but the diagnosis can only be made by exclusion. Thyroid function tests are needed to exclude hypothyroidism. Persistent jaundice accompanied by pale stools and dark urine points to a conjugated or obstructive jaundice, and the urgent task of differentiating between neonatal hepatitis and an anatomical obliteration of the biliary tree, most commonly extrahepatic biliary atresia.

Management

Having established the cause of the jaundice, bilirubin levels can be measured serially. This is especially important in haemolytic disease because the bilirubin level may rise rapidly. Good hydration and an adequate calorie intake help the liver to conjugate the bilirubin efficiently. The hyperbilirubinaemia can be treated by using phototherapy. Light of wavelength 450 nm from the blue band of the visible spectrum (*not* ultraviolet) converts unconjugated bilirubin by photodegradation to a biliverdin-like pigment which is water soluble and harmless. Light of the correct wavelength is produced by fluorescent tubes or more specialised blue lamps. Care is needed with temperature control and fluid balance. If there is a risk of the bilirubin

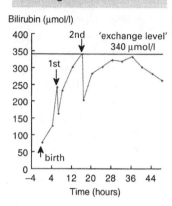

Exchange transfusion

Bilirubin (μmol/l)

rising to dangerous levels in spite of phototherapy and the measures above, then an exchange transfusion is performed. During this procedure blood is alternately withdrawn and transfused in 10–20 ml aliquots via a catheter in the umbilical vein, until 60–70% of the infant's red blood cells have been replaced. In rhesus incompatibility an exchange transfusion is often needed shortly after birth, even before bilirubin levels have had time to rise, in order to remove from the baby's circulation the antibodies which are causing the haemolysis.

This coagulation disturbance arises from vitamin K deficiency and the resulting impairment of hepatic production of factors II, VII, IX and X. Early onset disease develops between the 2nd and 4th days after birth and presents with gastrointestinal bleeding. Late onset, 2–8 weeks after birth, is rarer but commonly presents with intracranial bleeding. The risk is highest in babies who are breastfed, premature or who have been hypoxic. The occasional tragedy due to this readily preventable condition merits the prophylactic administration of vitamin K to all newborn infants shortly after birth.

GASTROINTESTINAL PROBLEMS

Oesophageal atresia

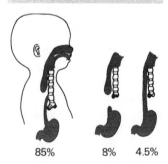

Tracheo-oesophageal fistula

85%   8%   4.5%

Oesophageal atresia (incidence 1 : 2500) is usually associated with a tracheo-oesophageal fistula. In every infant born to a mother with hydramnios, it should be excluded by passing a firm, large-bore (12G) tube through the mouth into the stomach. After birth, the affected infant is unable to swallow his own saliva and bubbles fluid from the mouth, another sign requiring investigation. It is always a sad event when the diagnosis is made only after the child has choked over his first feed. It is the condition of the lungs as well as the extent of the abnormality which dictates the success of surgical correction.

The diagnosis is confirmed radiologically by passing a firm, radio-opaque tube into the upper pouch and taking a lateral film of the chest, and an anteroposterior film of the chest and abdomen. Air in the stomach confirms the presence of a fistula. Associated anomalies may include ano-rectal agenesis and cardiac defects, particularly Fallot tetralogy.

Congenital diaphragmatic hernia

Congenital diaphragmatic hernia (incidence 1 : 2200) is due to a defect of the haemidiaphragm, usually the left. Fetal ultrasound can make the diagnosis before birth, and allows for delivery and management in a unit experienced in neonatal surgery. Where the diaphragmatic defect is the only anomaly, the baby may appear well at birth, but observation will show a deep chest and a scaphoid abdomen. Respiratory distress develops as the child swallows air, which passes into the small bowel within the chest cavity. The resulting mediastinal shift leads to

Diaphragmatic hernia

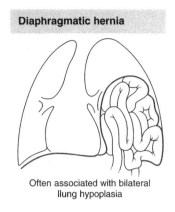

Often associated with bilateral
llung hypoplasia

Small bowel obstruction

Duodenal atresia

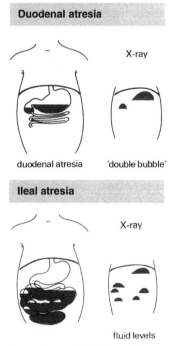

duodenal atresia   'double bubble'

Ileal atresia

fluid levels

Large bowel obstruction

compression of the previously unaffected lung. The diagnosis is confirmed by X-rays of the chest and abdomen. A nasogastric tube should be passed to empty the stomach and small bowel. Endotracheal intubation and ventilation may be necessary pre-operatively.

Babies with diaphragmatic hernias commonly have severe pulmonary hypoplasia which may prevent initial resuscitation or complicate preparation for surgery. Persistant fetal circulation (q.v.) may complicate the course and children with this condition are among the sickest infants treated by a neonatal service. Ventilation, often using HFOV, pulmonary vasodilators and occasionally ECMO may be required, but mortality may be as high as 20–40%. Other associations include heart defects and gut malrotation.

The most common form of organic obstruction of the small bowel is meconium ileus. Other causes of small bowel obstruction in the neonatal period include atresia, stenosis and diaphragms of the duodenum, jejunum or ileum, midgut volvulus, Ladd's band associated with failure of caecal descent, enterogenous cyst and milk curd obstruction. Meconium ileus and atretic lesions will present very early with distension and vomiting within hours of birth. The other lesions may not produce symptoms for some days or even a week or two after birth.

Vomiting of green rather than yellow bile-stained material suggests organic obstruction. Meconium may or may not have been passed in the early hours after birth. The area of distension will depend on the level of the obstruction; in duodenal obstruction it is confined to the upper abdomen, in ileal obstruction it is generalised. Erect X-rays of the abdomen should be taken, and may be diagnostic; for example, the double-bubble of duodenal atresia, the ground-glass appearance of some cases of meconium ileus, and the calcification of an ileal atresia with prenatal perforation. In other cases fluid levels may be present but do not necessarily indicate mechanical obstruction. They will be present in functional ileus, and in a baby with ileus secondary to septicaemia.

In the neonate there are two main causes of large bowel obstruction: Hirschsprung's disease and ano-rectal anomalies. The former is the more common, and it is suggested by delay in the passage of meconium beyond 24 hours. The baby may appear otherwise well for a few days but is liable to become suddenly and acutely distended, with peripheral circulatory collapse, a feature of a 'Hirschsprung's enterocolitis'. 'Ano-rectal anomaly' is an all embracing term for a very large number of anatomical problems. There are two main types, high and low, depending on whether the bowel ends above or below the pelvic floor. All low anomalies are easily treated at birth by a perineal procedure. High anomalies require a temporary colostomy; in boys there is always a fistula to bladder or urethra; in girls there may be a fistula to the vagina. Most of these babies have no visible anus at birth:

it is extremely rare for the anal canal to be present but not communicating with the upper bowel.

Rectal agenesis

normal

'high' agenesis with or without fistula into urogenital tract

'low' agenesis—covered or anterior ectopic anus, both usually with stenosis

Anterior abdominal wall defects

Exomphalos

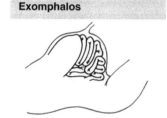

Gastroschisis

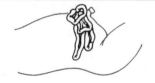

Exomphalos is a persistence of the herniation of the gut into the extra-embryonic part of the umbilical cord which is normally present between the 6th and 14th weeks of intrauterine life. Occasionally complete return of the gut into the abdominal cavity does not occur, the bowel which remains outside will be obvious at birth. In its mild form one or two loops of bowel are seen in the base of the cord, exomphalos minor; at its most severe a huge swelling occurs in the centre of the abdomen containing most of the abdominal contents (exomphalos major). The gut is covered by membrane.

In **gastroschisis** there is a protrusion of gut through a defect in the abdominal wall which is usually to the right of an otherwise normal umbilical cord. Gastroschisis also differs from exomphalos in that there is a much lower likelihood of associated chromosomal and other major malformations. The gut is however uncovered and is therefore exposed and vulnerable to damage which can complicate early management.

It is now relatively common for exomphalos and gastroschisis to be diagnosed by fetal ultrasound. It is important to differentiate the two conditions because the former merits fetal chromosomal analysis and further detailed scans to determine whether other major problems should influence the continuation of the pregnancy and postnatal management.

NEURAL TUBE ANOMALIES

Congenital abnormalities: central nervous system

Year	Numbers (England)	Rate per 10 000 births
1986	481	7.7
1991	237	3.6
1995	177	2.9
1996	154	2.5

The neural tube should be completely formed and closed throughout its entire length by the end of the 3rd week of intrauterine life. The process starts at the 14th day with thickening of the dorsal ectoderm to form the neural plate. The neural plate starts folding into a groove and by about 22–23 days complete fusion of the groove has occurred to form the neural tube. Fusion commences in the mid dorsal region and extends towards the head and tail of the embryo.

In the early 1970s neural tube defects occurred in 2–3/1000 live births and formed a large percentage of the admissions to paediatric surgical wards. The incidence has now fallen to below 1/1000, in part due to antenatal screening and termination of fetuses with severe defects and in part to a natural decline possibly due to better maternal nutrition. It is rare to encounter a child with major types of this condition in modern neonatal practice.

Anencephaly is a tragic deformity in which most of the infants are stillborn, but if liveborn survive only a few hours.

Cranium bifidum defects are relatively uncommon. The minor lesions are eminently treatable; all that is required is a good skin cover, and the prognosis is excellent, for there is no associated neurological lesion, and the incidence of hydrocephalus is low. An occipital meningocele, even when very large, is also treatable, although hydrocephalus is more likely. The overall prognosis is still good. On the other hand, a large encephalocele is not open to treatment, for surgery usually means either excision of a mass of brain tissue or a closure which results in raised intracranial pressure.

Cranial meningocele and encephalocele

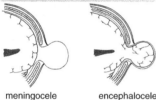

meningocele   encephalocele

Spina bifida cystica defects vary from a meningeal sac full of cerebrospinal fluid with a normal placement of the spinal cord (a meningocele), to the exposure and complete unfolding of the spinal cord on the surface of the child's back (a myelomeningocele).

Meningoceles are less common and have a good prognosis. Neurological problems with the lower limbs and hydrocephalus are rare, but partial neurological deficit affecting the bladder is not uncommon. Virtually all babies with a meningocele will be treated surgically in the first days after birth. During infancy they may develop minor foot problems and bladder dysfunction but they usually can cope well. Children with meningoceles should be followed up throughout the whole of their growing period because neurological problems may develop with growth of the spine.

Meningocele with skin cover

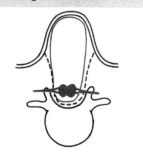

Myelomeningoceles are both more common and more serious. They are usually located in the lumbo-sacral region. The range of severity varies considerably. A child with a small lumbo-sacral myelomeningocele, which is closed on the first postnatal day, may with careful attention have good mobility, normal bladder function and intellect. On the other hand, a baby with an extensive thoraco-lumbar myelomeningocele is likely to have no functioning motor or sensory nerves distal to his nipple line. His skin will be completely anaesthetic and therefore at risk of trauma; his trunk and limbs will be paralysed and either completely flaccid or deformed as a result of reflex activity. Involuntary movement may be seen. The bladder and bowel will be paralysed and insensitive. Hydrocephalus is present in 80% of infants with myelomeningocele.

Every baby with spina bifida cystica should have full and expert assessment as soon as possible after birth to determine the extent of neurological deficit; the presence or otherwise of hydrocephalus, the

Meningocele

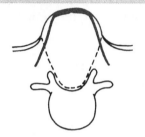

extent of bony deformity of the spine; and the coexistence of any other congenital abnormality. This permits an estimate to be made of his potential. The decision to operate can only be taken after a full and open discussion between paediatrician, surgeon and parents. Many babies with extensive defects will die within a short time whether their lesions are covered with skin or not. Early surgery is not justified. On the other hand, a baby with a lesser lesion is still at risk of infection and the complications of hydrocephalus even after surgery. It is a mistake to think that all babies will survive if operated upon and that those with uncorrected lesions will always die. One can only say that the majority of babies with minor lesions and a good prognosis will survive with treatment to adult life, and that most babies with very major lesions will die without treatment.

In the longer term the child's management should be directed by a multidisciplinary team including paediatric surgeon, orthopaedic surgeon, physiotherapist and full community child health support. The quality of life may be severely compromised.

The quality of life in children over 5 after surgery for myelomeningocele (after Lorber)

18% mild/moderate physical handicap and normal IQ
49% severe physical handicap and normal IQ
33% severe physical handicap and borderline or subnormal IQ

Spina bifida occulta and split notochord syndrome (diastomatomyelia) with meningocele

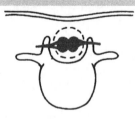

Spina bifida occulta, in contrast, is a common anomaly, said to occur in up to 20% of normal individuals, hence most people are asymptomatic. Occasionally the bony defect is associated with a hairy patch or a birth mark on the back. A few children with spina bifida occulta develop a mild spastic gait, or bladder problems with spinal growth due to tethering of the cord, a split notochord syndrome, or an associated intraspinal dermoid or lipoma.

Hydrocephalus without spina bifida. This may result from a congenital abnormality of the brain, for example aqueduct stenosis, or acquired as the result of infection or intracranial haemorrhage (especially in prematures). Early child abuse with shaking injury is another cause, which appears to be increasingly recognised. The prognosis of a child with hydrocephalus is dependent on the underlying cause and the residual integrity of the brain tissue. It is important to recognise hydrocephalus early either by careful measurement of the head circumference or by serial cranial ultrasound in infants at risk. Detailed ultrasound studies can demonstrate not only the size of the ventricles but also the flow of CSF. Ultrasound and other imaging techniques guide the neurosurgeon to the correct placement of the shunt.

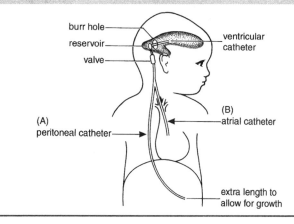

The treatment of hydrocephalus (ventriculo-peritoneal (A) and ventriculo-atrial (B) CSF shunts)

burr hole
reservoir
valve
ventricular catheter
(B) atrial catheter
(A) peritoneal catheter
extra length to allow for growth

CLEFT LIP AND PALATE

The middle third of the face develops as the result of migration and fusion of mesodermal folds covered by ectoderm. The earlier or primary palate creates the olfactory pits, and failure of fusion results in unilateral, bilateral or, rarely, median cleft lip. The secondary palate originates from folds on either side of the tongue. These rise above the tongue and fuse in the midline to form the true palate. Cleft palates occur when tissue migration is disorganised or obstructed by the tongue. It is sometimes the result of a small mandible.

Malformations of soft and hard palate

alveolus
hard palate
soft palate
uvula

normal | cleft of soft palate | + hard palate | + alveolus | + bilateral alveolus

Cleft lip/cleft palate defects in England		
Year	Numbers (England)	Rate per 10000 births
1986	794	12.7
1991	714	10.8
1995	531	8.7
1996	516	8.4

Cleft lip and palate are common—1 in 700 births. The majority are isolated abnormalities but they may be part of a chromosomal or other malformation syndrome. The family history is often positive, and most clefts are determined by polygenic inheritance which influences the threshold to ill-defined environmental factors. Occasional cases have been linked to maternal corticosteroid or anticonvulsant therapy. One-third of clefts are limited to the lip, one-quarter to the palate and the remainder involve both.

Management. The alarming facial appearance calls for prompt counselling of the parents, preferably with 'before and after' photographs to emphasise the successful outcome of corrective surgery. Feeding problems can usually be overcome by using a soft teat with an enlarged hole and by nursing the baby erect. Those with a cleft lip may cope with breast feeding. The baby should have a newborn hearing screening test. The aims of surgery are to provide a good cosmetic result and an adequate speech mechanism. The usual practice is to repair the cleft lip at 3 months of age and the palate at 6 months or later. Too early a repair may interfere with midfacial growth. In the later years additional specialist help is required to overcome Eustachian tube obstruction, speech delay and dental problems.

Pierre Robin syndrome refers to severe micrognathia with a secondary cleft palate. The affected infants are susceptible to feeding and respiratory problems, and require expert nursing until the mandible grows.

Treacher–Collins syndrome encompasses a spectrum of ear and facial malformations caused by first and second pharyngeal arch developmental failure.

Abnormal development of the face

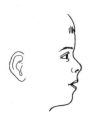 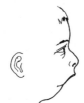 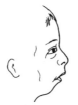 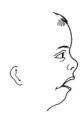 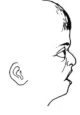

normal

Pierre-Robin
hypoplasia of
mandible
cleft palate

Treacher-Collins
hypoplasia of
mandible
deformed ears (80%)
deafness (40%)

facio-auriculo-
vertebral anomalies
unilateral (70%)
hypoplasia of
maxilla and mandible
deformed ears
deafness

Crouzon's syndrome
ocular ptosis
hypoplasia of maxilla
craniosynostosis

CLUB FOOT p. 294   DISLOCATED HIP p. 290

NEONATAL INFECTIONS

Newborn babies can die from infections before anyone is aware that they are ill. The signs of a systemic infection are generalised and often not specific to a particular system. Apparently trivial infections can rapidly lead to systemic sepsis, especially in the preterm baby.

Systemic infections

If an infant goes 'off his feeds', handles badly, has an unexpected rise or fall in body temperature, or develops unusual respiratory patterns, fits or apnoeic spells, he should be thoroughly examined at all sites for signs of possible infection. A 'septic screen' is performed in which samples of blood, urine, and CSF are taken for examination and culture, together with swabs from sites as indicated. While awaiting the results of the investigations the ill baby should be started immediately on an antibiotic combination parenterally to cover the common pathogens of the newborn period such as Group B Streptococcus, *Staphylococcus aureus*, *Escherichia coli*, and the gram-negative organisms pseudomonas, klebsiella, proteus. Widely used combinations are gentamicin and penicillin G in the first week after birth, and gentamicin and flucloxacillin thereafter; others prefer third generation cephalosporins.

When the results of the septic screen are known, the length of treatment can be decided, and the antibiotics altered to cover a particular organism more thoroughly or in accordance with the antibiotic sensitivities of the organisms grown. Serious infections include septicaemia, meningitis, pneumonia, urinary tract infections, gastroenteritis and osteomyelitis. Further investigations and follow up will be needed depending on which of these is present.

Neonatal meningitis

This has high mortality and morbidity rates. Penicillin is used to cover the possibility of Group B streptococcal meningitis, and a third generation cephalosporin such as cefotaxime or ceftazidime can be combined with gentamicin to cover the other organisms. Fits or irritability are controlled with phenobarbitone. Treatment of meningitis must continue for 3 weeks. Ultrasound scanning is used to identify any developing hydrocephalus.

Superficial infections

Conjunctivitis. Sticky eye is a common problem. Usually there is no underlying infection and, after taking swabs for culture, saline washes are all that is required. Sometimes, conjunctivitis is due to a staphylococcal infection, less commonly streptococcal or pseudomonal organisms. It may also be caused by organisms acquired from the mother's birth canal, in particular *Neisseria gonorrhoeae* and *Chlamydia trachomatis*. Both are sexually transmitted diseases. The latter is also responsible for the eye disease, trachoma. If conjunctival inflammation and pus is present, then swabs should be taken into standard and into chlamydial transport medium for Gram and Giemsa staining and appropriate cultures. Scrapings should also be taken from the inside of the lower eyelid with a swab on a stick, smeared on to glass slides, allowed to dry and examined in the laboratory for chlamydial inclusion bodies. Gonococcal eye infections can involve the cornea and damage the whole eye very rapidly, and, to prevent this, significant eye infections on the first day or two, should be presumed to be gonococcal until proven otherwise and treated vigorously with penicillin given parenterally, as well as very frequent cleaning and eye drops. Chlamydial infections are now common and must be treated with both 1% tetracycline eye drops and oral erythromycin. Ordinary bacterial infections such as caused by staphylococci are treated with chloramphenicol eye drops or ointment.

Septic spots. Small septic spots and blisters are not unusual, especially in the skin creases, and are commonly due to staphylococcal infections. The baby can be washed with a soap containing an antibacterial agent such as chlorhexidine. If there are only a few lesions, they can be cultured and cleaned with a spirit swab. More extensive lesions should be treated with systemic flucloxacillin.

Umbilical infections. The umbilical cord dries and usually drops off after a few days. The residual sticky stump usually needs no treatment but if the surrounding area becomes inflamed with an offensive discharge, swabs and a systemic antibiotic are needed.

Thrush. This is a fungal infection. Inside the mouth it is recognized by adherent white plaques on the buccal membranes and the tongue. Treatment is with nystatin oral suspension or miconazole oral gel. On the perineum the candida produces a rash with red areas around the anus and in the groins. Nystatin cream is used. The mouth should be checked for involvement.

NEONATAL CONVULSIONS

Causes of convulsions in childhood

Asphyxia
Birth injury with haemorrhage
CNS infections
CNS malformations
Hypocalcaemia
Hypoglycaemia
Hyponatraemia
Inherited metabolic disorders

Many normal newborn babies react to minor physical stimuli or loud noises with startle responses. It can be difficult to distinguish these normal 'jitters' from intermittent focal fits (twitching) and generalised tonic spasms. If the jitteriness seems excessive a blood sample is taken to exclude hypoglycaemia, and low levels of calcium, magnesium or sodium. If the baby also seems unwell an infection screen including a lumbar puncture must be carried out. If the cause is still not determined a search is made for less common inherited metabolic disorders, congenital infections and CNS malformations.

Treatment. Treatment is directed at the cause. In the presence of seizures, if the blood glucose is reduced below 2.6 mmol/l, the hypoglycaemia is corrected urgently with 10% glucose (5 ml/kg) followed by an infusion at an appropriate rate for the postnatal age. Hypocalcaemic fits are uncommon since the introduction of low phosphate milks, and normal levels vary considerably making interpretation difficult, but if fits are thought to be related to low plasma levels, 0.5 ml/kg of 10% calcium gluconate can be given intravenously, slowly and under ECG monitoring, followed up by oral supplements added to the feeds. If an infant's hypocalcaemia seems resistant to correction he may well have hypomagnesaemia as well, and this can be treated with 0.1 ml/kg of 50% magnesium sulphate intramuscularly or very slowly intravenously. Hyponatraemia responds to fluid restriction if it is dilutional, or to sodium supplements if there is a true deficiency.

If life-threatening convulsions are continuing in spite of these metabolic corrections, attempts must be made to control the fits with a loading dose of phenobarbitone 20–30 mg/kg. Rectal paraldehyde in arachis oil can be helpful if breakthrough fits still occur. Meanwhile meningitis must be excluded and investigations set in train to find any other underlying cause. The management is particularly difficult where the fits are due to severe birth trauma or hypoxia. The large doses of anticonvulsants required severely depress the baby's respiration. Surprisingly the prognosis in neonatal convulsions is favourable in the absence of meningitis and obvious cerebral damage, with 70% having normal development at long-term follow up.

BIBLIOGRAPHY

Davis J A, Richards M P M, Roberton N R C 1983 Parent–baby attachments in premature infants. Croom Helm, London
Huddart S N 1996 Acute care of the surgical neonate. Current Pediatrics 6: 257–261
Levene M I, Bennett M J, Punt J 1995 Fetal and neonatal neurology and neurosurgery, 2nd edn. Churchill Livingstone, Edinburgh
Lister J, Irving I M 1990 Neonatal surgery, 3rd edn. Butterworths, London
Macfarlane A 1977 The psychology of childbirth. Fontana, London
Remington J S, Klein J O 1997 Infectious diseases of the fetus and newborn infant, 3rd edn. W B Saunders, Philadelphia
Rennie J M 1997 Neonatal cerebral ultrasound. Cambridge Unviersity Press, Cambridge
Rennie J M, Roberton N R C 1999 Textbook of neonatology, 3rd edn. Churchill Livingstone, Edinburgh
Royal College of Paediatrics and Child Health, Royal College of Obstetricians and Gynaecologists 1997 Resuscitation of babies at birth. BMJ Publishing Group, London
Sinclair J C, Bracken M B 1993 Effective care of the newborn. Oxford, Oxford University Press
Speidel B D, Fleming P J, Henderson J et al 1998 A neonatal vade mecum, 3th edn. Edward Arnold, London

5 Nutrition

BREASTFEEDING
ARTIFICIAL FEEDING
FEEDING PROBLEMS
NUTRITIONAL DEFICIENCIES
MALNUTRITION
OBESITY

The nutrients supplied to the young in early development are uniquely and sensitively adjusted to their requirements. During intrauterine life a mixture of water, salts, proteins, carbohydrates and fats, which are drawn from the maternal blood stream and processed by the placenta, enters the fetal circulation and determines the substrates that are available for growth and energy metabolism. After birth, the breast produces a specialised total food in an acceptable and digestible form. Breast milk production is a characteristic of mammals. The mixture of nutrients in their milk varies widely from one species to another and this is to be expected, for the rates of growth of the young at birth and their motor activities are very different.

Major constituents of various mammalian milks

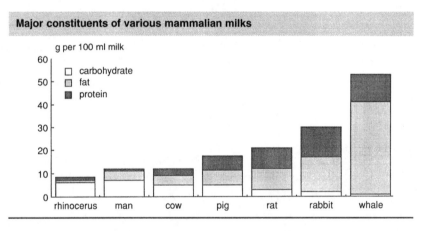

In view of this it is perhaps surprising that the young of one species can be reared effectively on the milk of another. But this is so, for some decades now it has been a common practice to rear human infants on cows' milk. So successful has it been in western societies that the advantages of human breast milk are being questioned! Breastfeeding benefits both mother and child in many ways and therefore mothers should be given every encouragement to breastfeed their infants; however for those who are unable to do so it is important to reassure them that there are other ways of rearing their infant successfully.

BREASTFEEDING

During pregnancy many endocrine agents prepare the breast for lactation. These include lactogen (human chorionic somatomammotropin), which is secreted by the placenta, and prolactin which is released by the pituitary gland and is important not only in initiating milk secretion but also in maintaining milk production after birth. Suckling is a powerful stimulus both to prolactin release from the anterior pituitary gland and to the secretion of oxytocin from the posterior pituitary gland. Oxytocin stimulates the ejection or 'let down' of milk by acting on the myoepithelial cells which surround the alveoli and ductules.

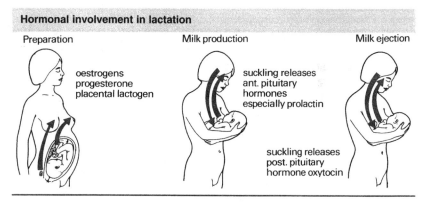

Hormonal involvement in lactation

Preparation — oestrogens / progesterone / placental lactogen

Milk production — suckling releases ant. pituitary hormones especially prolactin

Milk ejection — suckling releases post. pituitary hormone oxytocin

Technical problems

Even from this brief outline, it is obvious that breastfeeding is a complex process which might break down at a number of stages. For example, the breast and nipple may be ill formed, although appropriate care during pregnancy can do much to encourage adequate development. Milk production may not be initiated and maintained at a rate fast enough to suit a hungry baby or may flow too quickly for an ill or sleepy infant. If the full breast is not emptied then it may become engorged and inflamed, and the resulting pressure and pain will inhibit further milk production. Gentle manual expression of milk will avoid this complication. Finally, the unhappy, nervous, drowsy or sick mother may not be able to 'let down' her milk as she would wish or a lethargic, sick, newborn baby may not stimulate her to do so.

Breastfeeding does not seem to be a basic instinct; many mothers who have not seen others breastfeeding need considerable guidance initially. A simple explanation of how the breast works is often very helpful and avoids unnecessary anxiety. Should it be desirable to discontinue breastfeeding, this can be achieved most simply by firm breast support and analgesia.

Constituents of breast milk

As a food, milk has some remarkable characteristics. Most of the carbohydrate is in the form of a disaccharide, lactose, which requires a specific disaccharidase for its digestion. The fats are present mainly as triglyceride in globules surrounded by lipoproteins which are probably

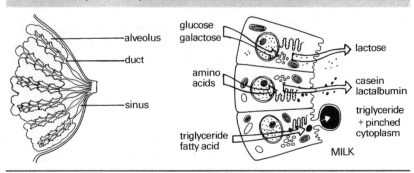

Breast anatomy and milk production

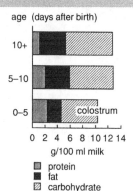

Constituents of breast milk

age (days after birth)

g/100 ml milk

- protein
- fat
- carbohydrate

probably remnants of the walls of the alveolar cells. The individual fatty acids reflect the mother's diet and her fat stores. If mothers are on low fat diets then the alveolar cells themselves make saturated fatty acid with chain lengths of 12–16 carbons. The protein content of human milk is surprisingly low but a large percentage is in the form of the more easily digestible whey, rather than the less digestible curds. Whey contains, in addition to lactalbumin, proteins which influence the infant's bowel bacterial flora, namely lactoferrin, lysozyme and IgA. Breast milk also contains vitamins, minerals, enzymes, especially lipase, and cells. The latter are predominantly macrophages and act either to keep the lacteals free from infection or to assist in the defence of the intestinal tract.

The relative amounts of the constituents vary. The first milk produced after birth, colostrum, is rich in protein and cells but the volume is small. When feeding is established, the mature milk constituents vary diurnally and from day to day. The milk at the end of a feed, hind milk, has a higher fat content than fore milk. The content of milk is also modified by the maternal diet and wellbeing, and by the mother's general level of nutrition.

Advantages of breastfeeding

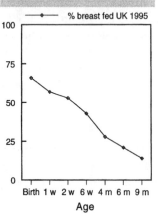

Percentage breast feeding in the UK 1995 (data from Office of National Statistics 1995

If a mother wishes and is able to breastfeed, then she should be supported in this and given every encouragement to do so. Human milk is an excellent nutrient mixture which also gives the baby some protection against infection. Its protein content is less likely to induce allergic reactions and the infant may be less at risk from unexplained sudden death. The process of breastfeeding usually gives satisfaction and pleasure to mother and child and this in itself will be of lasting benefit to both. Technically, breastfeeding is easier than bottlefeeding in as much as the mother is not required to make up the mixture according to instruction, and sterilising bottles is not a problem. In western societies breastfeeding may be economic, but elsewhere it certainly is.

Some mothers are anxious that breastfeeding or, alternatively, not breastfeeding may alter the contour of the breast, but there is little evidence one way or the other. Under non-lactating conditions the shape of the breast is largely determined by fat cells rather than the mammary gland. However, pregnancies and age are certainly two major factors leading to change. Approximately 9 out of 10 women who are feeding their babies do not ovulate; but nevertheless breastfeeding should not be regarded as a method of contraception. Cancer of the breast is less common in women who have borne children and breastfed them.

Why mothers do not breastfeed

Mothers give a variety of reasons when asked why they have chosen not to breastfeed. Some women just do not like the thought of breastfeeding and, given an alternative, they take it. Others are embarrassed or uncertain and fear that they will fail or develop sore nipples and swollen, painful breasts. Some mothers obviously believe that bottlefeeding is an easier and more certain way of ensuring their baby grows well and sleeps regularly. Others feel that bottlefeeding offers greater freedom by, for instance, making it possible for them to return to work and to take the contraceptive pill. They might, perhaps, feel differently if they were better informed and more carefully prepared during the antenatal period; for example, once lactation is established, the contraceptive pill can be taken without it influencing breastfeeding.

Contraindications

Maternal: technical. For some mothers, breastfeeding is just not possible or may be contraindicated. For example, successful breastfeeding is difficult with twins though many mothers succeed but it is virtually impossible with triplets, though to be partially fed by breast milk is beneficial.

After a premature birth, neither breasts nor baby are prepared for feeding. Nevertheless with the necessary support most mothers who wish to breastfeed their prematurely born infants are able to do so. Producing breast milk is one way that mothers can help their delicate infants over the first few weeks of life.

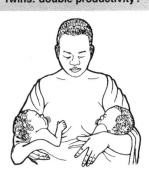

Twins: double productivity?

Maternal: health. If the mother has been chronically ill, severely undernourished, subject to severe asthmatic episodes or has limited renal function, breastfeeding *may* be an unacceptable drain on her reserves. Similarly, mothers with diabetes may find that the metabolic challenge of producing milk upsets their diabetic state. Active tuberculosis in the mother is a contraindication to breastfeeding until the infant has been immunised. HIV infection is transmitted by breastfeeding.

Drugs. Most drugs taken by the mother enter the milk. For practical purposes it can be estimated that one-tenth of the dose given to the mother enters the milk so that the possibility that a drug given to a breastfeeding mother may affect her baby must always be kept in mind. It is very rare for medication given to the mother to be a sufficient reason for stopping breastfeeding.

Infant: technical. Some babies with abnormalities of the mouth, particularly cleft palate, are unable to suckle satisfactorily and breastfeeding is virtually impossible. Tongue tie, unless it is in a very extreme form with forking of the tongue, should not interfere with the baby's ability to suckle.

Infant: health. Babies with inherited disorders of digestion or metabolism may not be able to tolerate the nutrients in human or other milks and special formulae are required. The inherited mono- and disaccharide intolerances, galactosaemia and phenylketonuria, fall into this group.

ARTIFICIAL FEEDING

Artificial feeding in babies who suck well is usually by the bottle, but a spoon, cup or plastic feeding tube may be used. The currently fashionable bottle sits on its base and has a wide neck surmounted by an artificial teat or nipple. Between feeds it must be washed with cold and then warm water and sterilised. The hole in the teat must be large enough to allow the baby to take their feeds in under 15 minutes but not so large that the feed flows so quickly as to cause the baby to splutter and choke. If a baby is unable to suck or swallow, or too weak or breathless to complete the feed, then they can be fed via a fine plastic nasogastric tube. This procedure properly performed is simple, safe and well tolerated by the infants. It has probably saved more lives than any other innovation in neonatal care. In certain situations the end of the tube may be advanced into the duodenum or jejunum.

Disadvantages of cows' milk

The feed is usually cows' milk modified in some way. Many babies have been reared successfully on ordinary pasteurised or sterilised cows' milk, reconstituted evaporated liquid, or dried powdered cows' milk, but there have been problems. Some have been due to the way cows' milk differs from human milk. Cows' milk contains more protein, in particular more curd protein or casein, and these thick curds being less easy to digest have caused bowel obstruction. Cows' milk contains more fat and phosphate. In the early weeks of life, particularly from 5 to 15 days of age, this may lead to hypocalcaemia with subsequent fitting. Cows' milk has a relatively high sodium content and this, with the tendency of mothers to make strong or concentrated feeds from powdered or condensed milks, leads to hypernatraemia, which may cause fits and brain damage, complications which are more likely during superimposed episodes of infection, particularly gastroenteritis. Some infants are allergic to cows' milk protein; they may react to feeding with perioral rashes and oedema or by vomiting or passing frequent loose stools which usually contain blood.

Makers of infant feeds now prepare a variety of modified cows' milk formulae, which have been 'humanised' in that the mixture more closely resembles that found in average mature human milk. This has posed considerable problems for manufacturers, for milk is a complex colloid mixture and, as such, it is very sensitive to any attempts to

Constituents of artificial feeds

soy feed	
whey based	
casein based	
cow's milk	

0 2 4 6 8 10 12 14
g/100 ml feed

■ protein
■ fat
▨ carbohydrate

change it. In addition, manufacturers can only modify and supplement cows' milk to resemble human milk as far as their knowledge of the constituents of human milk permits. Pyridoxine was added to formulae only after its deficiency had led to fits in artificially fed babies. The protein in cows' milk is bovine protein. New technology may allow these to be changed but it is an expensive and complicated exercise. There are claims at the moment that adding the longer chain fatty acids to artificial milk promotes neural development and, it is implied, subsequent intelligence, but the evidence is not yet convincing. However, it would seem prudent to add some unsaturated fatty acid to artificial infant feeds, because more are found in human milk than cows' milk. Manufacturers cannot of course add the 'living elements', cells and enzymes, and we do not know how important these might be.

Each manufacturer markets four standard products, a whey based formula with a whey : casein ratio of 60 : 40 like human milk, a casein based formula with a whey : casein ration of 20 : 80 like cows' milk, a soy protein based formula with no 'milk' constituents at all, and a 'follow-on' milk for weaning infants with a higher protein content. They also prepare special feeds for preterm infants, and children with rare metabolic disorders. All, as the sole nutrient, meet the infant's known requirements

Main type of non-human milk chosen by mothers who were not breast feeding (from Foster K, Lader D, Cheesbrough S 1997 Infant feeding 1995. Office of National Statistics).

Milk	6–10 weeks	4–5 months	8–9 months
Whey dominant	54	36	22
Casein dominant	44	58	35
Soy-based formula	2	2	3
Follow-on milk	0	2	24
Cows' milk	0	1	15

Nutritional requirements

If a breastfed child is content and growing, one need not trouble to consider the volume and nutrient value of each feed. There are, however, many reasons why an adequately breastfed child may not be content or may not be growing satisfactorily. The nutrient intake of artificially fed infants is as much determined by the giver as the receiver and is more easily assessed. It is this facility which tempts some mothers whose infants are not thriving on the breast to change to bottlefeeding, for then she and her health advisers can at least see the feed going in! Thus, it is essential in both breast and artificially fed infants to be able to assess their nutrient intake and their nutritional status.

Nutrient intake in breastfed babies may be assessed by weighing the baby before and after feeds, that is by carrying out a test feed. It is rarely necessary and difficult to perform. In artificially fed babies a lot may be learnt by watching while the feed is made and given. It might influence how you calculate the daily intake from the history of feed volume and frequency! Nutritional status is usually assessed from the infant's weight, a visual evaluation of the quality of the skin and by the amount and distribution of subcutaneous fat. More information can be gained by measuring length or height and skin fold thickness. Appetite and metabolic efficiency vary from infant to infant, much as they do in adults. The average intake of healthy infants can be used as a guide, but it must be remembered that the range is wide and each infant's needs must be assessed individually.

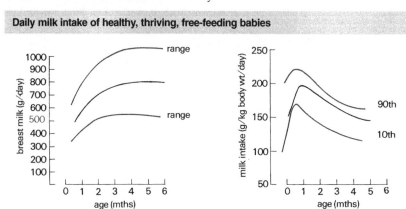

Daily milk intake of healthy, thriving, free-feeding babies

Just for interest, breast milk consumption is expressed per baby, artificial feeding is given per kg body weight

FEEDING PROBLEMS

New mothers often wish to be reassured that their babies are feeding normally. If there are problems, they may seek advice from more experienced members of the family or from shopkeepers who sell milk foods, or midwives, community nurses and health visitors, and it is to be expected that they will be given differing opinions. Occasionally, the problem is of such magnitude that medical advice is sought. The doctor must be aware of, or take advice about, the general abilities, approach and attitudes of the parents, the mother's feeding technique and the infant's nutrient intake, before considering the possibility of more serious underlying conditions.

Vomiting

Most babies swallow air with their milk. Gentle patting or massage of their backs helps them bring back the 'wind'. Most babies bring up a little milk as well; this posseting is unimportant. Occasionally, infants regurgitate large amounts of milk, either immediately after a feed or between feeds. It is rare for this to be sufficiently severe to affect the infant's nutrition but it does distress their mothers and, apart from other considerations, it makes all her clothes and furnishings smell and it fills her washing basket.

Various strategies may be tried. By not allowing the baby to cry or become too upset before a feed and using good feeding technique, excess air swallowing can be avoided. Using agents which thicken the feed like cornflour or carob seed flour also reduces the baby's ability to bring them back. Propping the baby up after a feed may also help.

Some babies enjoy bringing their feeds back, 'ruminating' like a cow. This habit may be difficult to break but it will become less of a problem as the infant's diet, abilities and interests change.

There is no clear distinction between regurgitation and vomiting. An underlying cause must be sought if a baby suddenly starts to be sick, if the vomit contains blood or bile, if the vomiting persists to the point of dehydration or malnutrition, or is associated with other signs and symptoms. Vomiting may be the first indication of a general infection; it may be the only clue to an infected throat; it is common in pyelonephritis and is usual in meningitis and gastroenteritis. Certain disorders of the oesophagus and stomach must also be considered.

Gastro-oesophageal reflux   Gastro-oesophageal reflux is very common in infancy. The lower oesophageal valvular mechanism is made up of two main components: the intra-abdominal segment of the oesophagus, and the length of the muscular component of the sphincter. Both may be relatively deficient in early life allowing for free reflux. This is regarded as innocent or physiological when it does not interfere with weight gain or health. It becomes pathological when secondary oesophagitis causes symptoms such as irritability or feeding difficulty, or results in blood loss and iron deficiency anaemia. The reflux may also lead to episodes of aspiration pneumonia, or may produce apnoea or vagus nerve mediated bradycardia. The latter can lead to apparent life-threatening events or 'near miss cot-death'. Diagnosis of significant reflux is provided by a careful history supported by barium swallow or oesophageal pH studies. Endoscopy and biopsy establish the severity of the oesophagitis.

The majority of mild to moderate cases are managed conservatively in expectation that time and the development of a more competent lower oesophageal sphincter will resolve the problem. Appropriate management includes increased time spent in a baby chair, thickening the milk feeds, addition of an alginate preparation (Gaviscon) and, if indicated by pH studies, the use of H_2-receptor antagonists or proton pump inhibitors. A small number of refractory cases and those threatening to produce an oesophageal stricture need surgical repair of the hiatus and a fundoplication. Children with severe developmental delay and mobility problems are especially liable to have reflux. Unfortunately their handicaps often delay the recognition of their reflux symptoms.

There is now less emphasis on the diagnosis of hiatus hernia of infancy. This is regarded as part of the spectrum of gastro-oesophageal reflux. Occasionally delayed gastric emptying due to mild pyloric stenosis manifests as severe reflux; the appropriate management may therefore be pyloromyotomy or pyloroplasty.

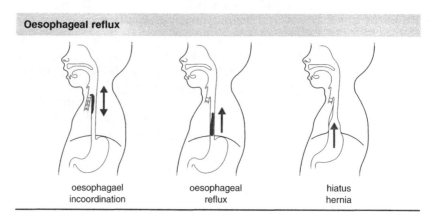

Oesophageal reflux

oesophagael
incoordination

oesophageal
reflux

hiatus
hernia

Oesophageal incoordination Oesophageal incoordination leads to dribbling, choking and aspiration of milk as well as regurgitation and vomiting. It may be due to a wide variety of conditions all of which are rare, or sometimes it may be an isolated problem. It can be recognised by cine radiography. Oesophageal incoordination can be a major problem in infants with cerebral palsy, and should be considered and excluded in all of them. Until recently this problem has not been addressed as thoroughly as it should have been and as a consequence such children have suffered unnecessarily and their growth and development has been compromised.

Pyloric stenosis Pyloric stenosis is due to hypertrophy and hyperplasia of the pyloric muscle, mainly the circular fibres. It usually develops in the first 4–6 weeks of life. The condition is inherited by the multifactorial mode and is commonest in first-born male children. Characteristically, the vomiting is projectile and may be so persistent that the baby becomes undernourished or even dehydrated. Being hungry, the baby is eager to feed again soon after he has vomited.

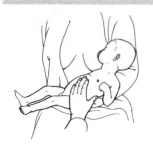

Palpation

On examination, stomach wall peristalsis may be visible and a rubbery tumour is felt by gentle deep finger palpation in the area halfway between the midpoint of the anterior margin of the right rib cage and the umbilicus. The diagnosis is primarily clinical but useful confirmation is provided by ultrasound imaging of the pylorus. Contrast X-ray studies are seldom necessary. The plasma biochemistry is also characteristic with hyponatraemia, hypokalaemia, hypochloraemia and a metabolic alkalosis. It is essential that the dehydration and biochemical disturbance are corrected before general anaesthesia and surgery. Intravenous administration of half-normal saline solution with added potassium and glucose provides for initial correction. Surgery aims to divide the pyloric muscles without penetrating the mucosa, pyloromyotomy (Ramstedt procedure).

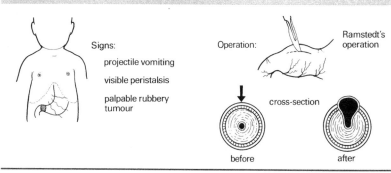

Pyloric stenosis: signs and surgery

Signs:
- projectile vomiting
- visible peristalsis
- palpable rubbery tumour

Operation: Ramstedt's operation

cross-section

before   after

Failure to thrive

Mothers are naturally anxious if their infants do not appear to be growing fast enough. In most western societies now, babies are measured at regular intervals and if they fail to grow satisfactorily compared with the average for that community, further enquiry is made. Failure to thrive can be the first indication of a serious underlying problem, such as chronic renal failure and congenital heart disease, but this is rare. More often than not it reflects difficulties in the home, limitations in the parents, unhappiness in the relationship between mother and child or uncertain feeding methods. Many women feel 'down' after pregnancy and their unhappiness and nervousness may be communicated to their babies who in turn become irritable and restless so that a vicious spiral is begun which ultimately leaves both mother and child exhausted. Bringing one or both of them into hospital to permit both to have a good night's sleep may go a long way to easing the problem. This condition is perhaps more appropriately described as 'failure to rear'.

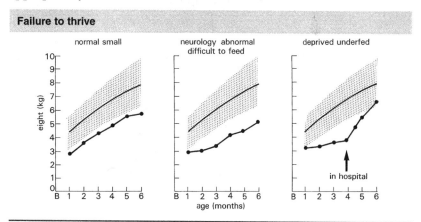

Failure to thrive

normal small | neurology abnormal difficult to feed | deprived underfed

weight (kg)

age (months)

in hospital

If a baby is undersized, and it has been established that he was of normal birth weight, that he is receiving an adequate diet in a settled home and that he has no obvious serious underlying disorder, then investigation should be made for the various causes of malabsorption. These will include food intolerance, low grade infections, cystic fibrosis (in case it has been missed by the screening procedures) and gluten enteropathy.

A crying baby and 3-month colic

Babies cry when they are hungry. They also cry for other reasons, such as cold or discomfort, and as they get older they cry when they are cross or frustrated. With experience their mothers are usually able to distinguish a cry for food and a cry in pain, but it can be difficult. Not many parents can stand their babies crying intermittently throughout the night and the temptation is to feed them, not so much for nutrition as to keep them quiet. They may react to this by vomiting.

Some babies, particularly at feeding time, but at other times as well, may have inconsolable outbursts of crying, sometimes to the point of screaming, for no obvious reason. During the attacks they may draw their knees up and go red in the face. It is difficult to believe that they are not having colic. It is possible that some infants have inflamed Peyer's patches and resulting painful bowel contractions. Drug therapy is seldom justified for the infants do not appear to come to any harm, Most parents find the crying distressful and they need reasurrance and support! This so-called '3-month colic' may last well beyond 3 months of age.

Diarrhoea, constipation and nappy rashes

There is no doubt that what infants eats influences the frequency and nature of their stool and the effect the stool has on the skin of the buttocks. It is normal for a baby to have a loose yellow bowel motion with every feed, and it is equally acceptable that they have a bowel action every other day passing a firm large brown stool. But it is not acceptable that they pass frequent stools which are green and watery, or large stools which are pale and oily, or very occasional stools which are hard enough to tear the anal mucosa causing pain and bleeding. All require investigation. They may respond to simple dietary adjustments. 'Stool gazing' is a dying art, for the information it yields is disappointingly small, but occasionally it can be instructive.

NUTRITIONAL DEFICIENCIES

When unexpected symptoms or signs appear in infants and children on odd diets or major feeding problems or severe bowel disorders, the possibility of a vitamin or mineral deficiency should be considered. Clinical syndromes due to deficiency of most vitamins and many trace elements have been reported.

Vitamin A—Xerophthalmia

Xerophthalmia due to vitamin A deficiency is a common serious nutritional disorder in the developing world and leads to blindness. In our richly endowed world many children suffer from it. Dark green leafy vegetables are the main source of vitamin A.

Vitamin C—scurvy

Scurvy is due to vitamin C deficiency. Cows' milk contains little vitamin C and most of this may disappear if the milk is stored or heated. Before artificial milks were fortified with extra vitamin C to a level similar to that in human milk, artificially fed babies were at risk of developing scurvy. In this disorder connective tissues and structural membranes break down, small vessels bleed and wounds are slow to heal. The infants present with bruises, painful periosteal bleeds or persistent superficial haemorrhages.

Vitamin D—rickets

Clinical picture

Craniotabies

Rickety rosary

Swelling of ends of long bones

Delay in walking

Curvature of ends of long bones

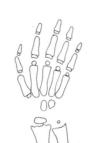

Rickets is due to vitamin D deficiency. The body obtains the vitamin by the action of ultraviolet light on the ergosterols in the deeper layers of the skin or from certain foods, including fish, eggs, butter and margarine. Lack of sunshine, a pigmented skin or a poor diet leaves a child at risk. It is important that a lactating mother has adequate vitamin D so that her milk will contain sufficient for her rapidly growing infant. Vitamin D aids the absorption of calcium from the bowel and the formation and calcification of bone. Deficiency leads to softening and deformity, particularly of the long bones. In early life rickets may be suspected if the skull bones are soft, craniotabes; in the 3–6-month-old child the enlargement of the ends of ribs produces a rachitic 'rosary'. In a child 12–18 months of age just beginning to walk, the ends of the long bones may be bowed either in or out by the strain. This is a tragedy if it occurs because the deformity is easily and cheaply avoided by vitamin D supplementation of the diet.

Radiographic appearance in rickets

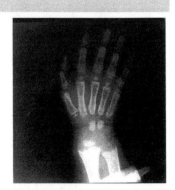

irregular metaphysis causing swelling of wrist

Secondary rickets

Vitamin D deficiency may be secondary to other disorders. It occurs in the very immature when they begin to grow and can be reversed by extra vitamin D, calcium and phosphate supplements. Rarely it develops during recovery from malabsorption (rickets occurs only in the growing child) and in children with chronic liver disease when the first hydroxylation step, vitamin D to 25(OH)D, fails. It is not uncommon in chronic renal failure when the second hydroxylation step, 25(OH)D to 1,25(OH)D, fails. This step is also limited in vitamin D dependent rickets, a rare recessively inherited disorder. In vitamin D resistant rickets (familial hypophosphataemic rickets, a sex-linked dominant condition) there is thought to be a defect in renal tubular transport of phosphate. Rickets also complicates more general disorders of tubular function, like Fanconi syndrome, renal tubular acidosis and cystinosis.

Classification of rickets and vitamin D metabolite levels

	Vitamin D	25(OH)D	1,25(OH)D
Deficient synthesis and supply —no sunlight —poor diet —immaturity	↓	↓	↓
Malabsorption	n	↓	↓
Liver disease	n	↓	↓
Chronic renal failure	n	n	↓
Vitamin D dependent rickets (recessively inherited)	n	n	↓
Vitamin D resistant rickets (sex-linked dominant)	n	n	n
Renal tubular disorders (defect of phosphate reabsorption)	n	n	n

Vitamin K—bleeding

Both the fetus and the newborn have low vitamin K status and there is little vitamin K in breast milk. Very rarely vitamin K deficiency bleeding may occur in the first 24 hours due to drugs given to the mother (early onset); more commonly it occurs in the first week of life (classical) with small bleeds from the umbilicus, mouth or bowel but occasionally a massive damaging bleed elsewhere. Rarely the bleed occurs after the first week, usually but not always by 3 months of age, and these 'late onset' bleeds are often into the brain causing death or permanent damage. There is usually a minor warning bleed and if it is recognised tragedy can be avoided. On investigation an underlying cause such as a liver disease due to α_1 antitrypsin deficiency is often found.

The routine administration of vitamin K either by injection or orally at birth prevents first week bleeding. Late onset bleeding mainly occurs in breastfed babies and a single oral dose is not as effective as a single injection in protecting against it. Giving vitamin K by injection at birth is not without risk, and it may have long-term ill effects. Therefore it is recommended that all babies are given vitamin K by mouth at birth and with regular supplements for breastfed babies until weaning. Some countries still have a policy of giving a single massive intramuscular dose to all infants at birth. What a welcome into the modern world!

Dental caries

Dental caries is due to progressive decay of teeth by organic acids produced locally by bacteria that ferment dietary carbohydrate, particularly sucrose. Fluoride reduces the incidence and severity of caries, by converting the enamel mineral, hydroxyapatite, to fluorapatite which is more acid resistant, by promoting remineralisation, and by antibacterial effects which reduce acid production. Thus, tooth decay can be considered to be a nutritional disorder, in part due to a deficiency of fluoride and in part due to excess of simple sugars. The risks of dental caries may be reduced by avoiding food between meals, particularly sticky sweets or sweet drinks in nursing bottles or pacifiers; by regularly cleaning the teeth; and by an adequate intake of fluoride either in the water, toothpaste or if necessary by tablet.

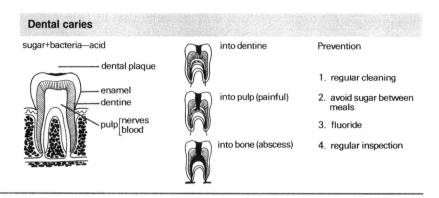

Dental caries

sugar+bacteria—acid

— dental plaque

— enamel
— dentine

pulp [nerves / blood]

into dentine

into pulp (painful)

into bone (abscess)

Prevention

1. regular cleaning

2. avoid sugar between meals

3. fluoride

4. regular inspection

MALNUTRITION

Many children in some parts of the world simply do not get enough to eat. Following a political or natural disaster, the news media have been quick to make us all more aware of the severe forms of childhood malnutrition which are prevalent during famine.

A WHO Expert Committee divided the protein-energy deficiency syndromes into marasmus, where failure to grow is associated with emaciation and a fair appetite; kwashiorkor, where malnutrition is associated with oedema and loss of appetite; and 'unspecified' where growth retardation and undernutrition are evident without frank emaciation or oedema. These terms describe the various ways by which starvation can affect the growing child. With starvation of whatever degree comes misery and an increased risk of infections. Both add to domestic problems and increase the risk of death or permanent damage.

Marasmus

Marasmus in western societies may be seen in infants born severely undernourished, or after severe chronic illnesses, particularly affecting the bowel. In poorer communities, nutritional marasmus commonly occurs due to failure of lactation in people who just cannot afford artificial milks. Thus it is more common in low-birth-weight infants, twins and in infants after infection, particularly gastroenteritis.

The infant's survival depends on the mother's ability to maintain lactation, even if the infant is unable to suckle for a few days. If food can be found, the prognosis of these infants is good. During a famine children of all ages may become marasmic and the recovery of older children may take longer. The risk of death due to superadded infection during the recovery phase is also higher.

Kwashiorkor

Kwashiorkor is a colourful word that gives the impression of a specific disease entity, however it is but one end of a spectrum. Most commonly, it occurs in children 18–24 months old at the time of weaning. The marasmic child receives a little of a balanced diet; in the child with kwashiorkor the energy intake may be just about adequate but the protein content is insufficient for growth. As a consequence there is muscle wasting but preservation of some subcutaneous fat. The infant is oedematous, listless and irritable. There may be a 'flaky paint' dermatitis of a depigmented skin and the hair is sparse and friable. The

Kwashiorkor

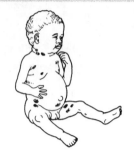

liver may be large due to fatty infiltration and the serum albumin concentration may be reduced. The complications include hypothermia, hypoglycaemia, drowsiness, severe diarrhoea, cardiac failure and all these are compounded by superimposed infections.

An inadequate supply of food is not primarily a medical problem. However the health service can help in the following ways:

1. By encouraging and supporting the lactating mother; there is no reason why breastfeeding should not be continued for 18 or 24 months.
2. By advising parents about weaning.
3. By recommending those local foods which will meet the protein needs of the growing child.
4. By the early recognition of children in difficulties so that limited food resources can be optimally deployed.
5. By the treatment of associated infections and vitamin deficiency states.

OBESITY

Obesity is a common health problem when food is in abundance and in the western world it is getting commoner. Fat parents tend to have fat children for there is a genetic component in the aetiology. Fat children tend to but do not invariably become fat adults. Fat people die on average at a younger age than thin people. In particular, fat adults are more likely to develop diabetes and hypertension; they weather chronic chest disease, heart failure and abdominal operations badly; and they have more problems with varicose veins, piles and skin crease ailments.

Obesity can be assessed reasonably well just by looking at the child and by plotting body weight on a centile chart. Contemporary reference charts for Body Mass Index (BMI = weight, kg/(height, m)^2) during childhood are now available. Skin fold thickness at standard sites can be measured if more accurate analysis is required.

Skin fold thickness

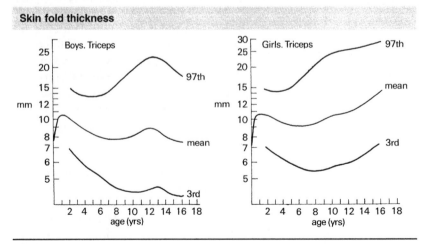

Prevention. As obesity is so difficult to treat it is best to avoid it. There is some evidence that bottlefed babies are more likely to become overweight than breastfed infants. This may be because the baby is less able to resist pressures to finish the bottle. Obesity may develop in the months after weaning when clearing the plate or emptying the cup becomes a virtue. Early weaning encourages this development. There is little virtue in commencing weaning before 4 or 5 months of age. One big meal a day appears to be more fattening than many small ones amounting to similar caloric value. Thus, the best prophylaxis for infants at risk of obesity because of fat parents is for them to be breastfed and weaned late; overfeeding should be avoided, particularly during the weaning period and the habit of taking regular exercise and eating small frequent meals should be established.

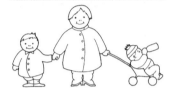

Who is for dieting?

Treatment. Obese children may be referred for medical advice for a variety of reasons. The child may be concerned because of his appearance or the clothes he is required to wear or because he is teased. Their parents may be concerned for the same reasons but also because they fear it may affect their child's health in other ways. Teachers may be concerned because of lack of physical fitness. If the child really wants to be thinner and their parents are prepared to put themselves out to help then there is some hope that a diet and exercise regimen will work. However, occasionally overeating is an outward sign of inner confusion and unhappiness. This needs to be recognised and discussed. But in the majority of cases a detailed enquiry brings little to light except bad parental dietary attitudes and practices. One mother still gave her child aged 7 years a breastfeed at night; another considered that a bumper gorge was a high treat; a third used food to settle a particularly active and demanding baby.

REFERENCE

Office of National Statistics 1995 Infant feeding.

BIBLIOGRAPHY

Mepham T B 1987 Physiology of lactation. Oxford University Press, Oxford
McLaren D S, Burman D, Belton N R, Williams A F (eds) 1991 Textbook of paediatric nutrition, 3rd edn. Churchill Livingstone, Edinburgh
Taitz L S, Wardley B 1989 Handbook of child nutrition. Oxford University Press, Oxford

6 Infection

MEASLES
RUBELLA
MUMPS
CHICKEN POX (VARICELLA)
HERPES SIMPLEX INFECTIONS
GLANDULAR FEVER
KAWASAKI DISEASE
ERYTHEMA INFECTIOSUM
ROSEOLA INFANTUM
HAND, FOOT AND MOUTH
  DISEASE
HEPATITIS A
HEPATITIS B
POLIOMYELITIS
DIPHTHERIA
PERTUSSIS
SCARLET FEVER
TUBERCULOSIS
MALARIA
HUMAN IMMUNODEFICIENCY
  VIRUS
IMMUNISATION
IMMUNE DEFICIENCY

Infections can spread readily among children. Acute respiratory infections, gastroenteritis and the main subject of this chapter, the infectious 'fevers', account for a large part of childhood illness. Scourges of the past, like diphtheria and poliomyelitis, have now virtually disappeared from many countries. But we have to stay on guard for diphtheria re-emerging in certain countries, i.e. eastern Europe. However it is hoped that soon Europe will follow the Americas and be declared polio free!

Infections are most likely to occur when children first mix with others, at a nursery, a playgroup or at primary school, and they may bring them home to their younger siblings. Usually the infectious fever is diagnosed by the mother, and the child is not very ill and can be looked after at home. If hospital admission is required it is often for social rather than medical reasons, though occasionally complications arise which are potentially damaging or life threatening.

Notifications of infectious disease in England and Wales in 1997 (Communicable Disease Report 9(1)–1998)			
Dysentery	2261	Meningococcal septicaemia	1403
Food poisoning	93353	Measles	4059
Tuberculosis	5954	Mumps	1965
Whooping cough	2974	Rubella	3397
Scarlet fever	3527	Malaria	1469
Meningitis (all)	2322		

MEASLES

Measles is a common and very infectious viral disease. The incubation period is followed by a prodromal illness with fever, coryza, conjunctivitis and cough. Generalised lymphadenopathy may be found, and tiny white spots on a bright red background, Koplik's spots, are present on the buccal mucosa of the cheeks. After 3 or 4 days a florid rash appears, and spreads downwards from the head and neck to cover the whole body. The earlier lesions are more numerous and become confluent and blotchy. The rash begins to fade by the third day and the child's general condition improves steadily.

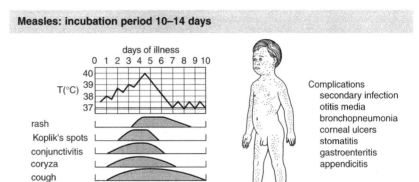

Measles: incubation period 10–14 days

Complications
secondary infection
otitis media
bronchopneumonia
corneal ulcers
stomatitis
gastroenteritis
appendicitis

Respiratory complications, particularly bronchopneumonia and otitis media, are common. Encephalitis occurs in about 1 in 5000 affected children and is manifested by headache, drowsiness and vomiting. Convulsions and coma begin 7–10 days after the onset of the illness. The course of encephalitis is unpredictable but about 15% of cases die, and 25% suffer brain damage resulting in mental retardation, fits, deafness or behaviour disorders. Measles may be associated with a disturbance of immune mechanisms, especially lymphopenia. Defective immune response may also be the basis of the rare late complication subacute sclerosing panencephalitis (SSPE), which occurs 4–10 years after an attack of measles and is characterised by slow progressive deterioration. There are very high levels of measles antibody in the blood and CSF, and measles virus antigen has been demonstrated in brain tissue.

In developing countries without the benefit of immunisation programmes, measles carries a high morbidity and mortality and also occurs at a younger age. Reported mortality rates range from 5.5% in East Africa to between 20 and 40% in a selected hospital series in West Africa. In the malnourished child, a severe form of measles may occur with a confluent rash that darkens to deep red or purple, and then desquamates. This is followed by depigmentation of the skin which lasts for several weeks and may be associated with pyodermia. A sore mouth is common during the acute illness and may lead to cancrum oris; invariably breastfeeding is disturbed. Diarrhoea is common and may persist for a long time, further aggravating any underlying malnutrition. The mortality rate from measles is directly related to socio-economic conditions, and there is a strong correlation with the distribution of kwashiorkor. In young susceptible children measles itself causes loss of weight. In a village in Nigeria almost 1 in 4 children lost more than 10% of their weight following an attack of measles, and

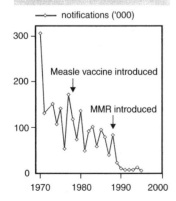

Incidence of measles in the UK

notifications ('000)

Measle vaccine introduced

MMR introduced

the average time to regain the previous weight was 7 weeks. It is therefore important to maintain the child's hydration and nutrition during the illness and afterwards. In the weeks and months following measles there is an increase in mortality from other illnesses. Another group particularly vulnerable to severe measles is the immuno-compromised child. Encephalitis and viral pneumonia can occur and there is a high mortality rate.

There is a live attenuated vaccine against measles. It was introduced in the United Kingdom in 1968. If sufficient children are immunised (perhaps 95%) epidemics of measles would cease.

RUBELLA

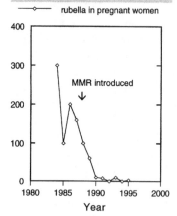

Incidence of rubella in pregnant women in England and Wales

Rubella, or German measles, is usually a mild illness, and may pass unrecognised. The incubation period is 14–21 days and there may be little or no fever or malaise before the appearance of the pink macular rash which lasts for about 3 days. Generalised lymphadenopathy, especially involving the suboccipital nodes, may be present. A rising haemagglutinin inhibition titre confirms the diagnosis. This test is seldom necessary in children but is essential when the possibility arises of rubella in early pregnancy. Complications of rubella, such as thrombocytopenia and encephalitis, do occur but they are rare. Arthritis may occur in adolescents.

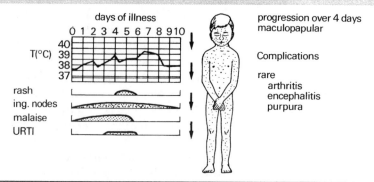

Rubella: incubation period 14–21 days

The importance of this disease lies in its devastating effect on the developing fetus if the mother contracts the infection during the first 3 months of pregnancy. A generalised viraemia may lead to fetal death and spontaneous abortion, or may affect the growth and development of the fetus resulting in a severely handicapped child with multiple congenital defects, classically including cataracts, deafness and congenital heart disease. All women should be tested for rubella immunity preferably before or in early pregnancy. There is a live attenuated vaccine against rubella and its value is in preventing rubella during pregnancy. In the United Kingdom between 1970 and 1988 the vaccination programme was aimed at girls in early adolescence. However a significant number of girls did not get the immunisation and still caught rubella in pregnancy, because there were still regular epidemics of rubella. Since 1988, the vaccine has been given early in the second year to both girls and boys to stop epidemics occurring and to protect those who cannot or have not been immunised. The vaccine is combined with measles and mumps vaccines.

MUMPS

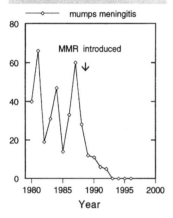

Incidence of mumps in England and Wales

Mumps is caused by a paramyxovirus. Subclinical infection is common. A long incubation period of 16–21 days is followed by fever, malaise and enlargement of one or both parotid glands, which develop over a period of 1–3 days. The child may complain of earache and difficulty in swallowing, and the glands may be painful and tender. The submandibular glands may also be affected. The swellings settle in 7–10 days and there is no specific treatment. Other causes of parotitis are rare in children and the distinction from cervical lymphadenopathy should not be difficult after careful examination.

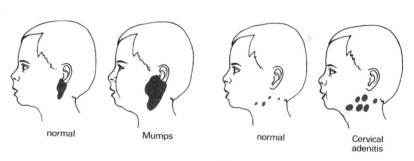

Differential diagnosis of mumps and cervical adenitis

normal   Mumps   normal   Cervical adenitis

Meningitis is a common complication, but is usually mild and characterised by headache, photophobia and neck stiffness. The CSF contains an increased number of lymphocytes and a raised concentration of protein. Recovery is almost always complete. Sensorineural deafness, usually unilateral, can occur; mumps is thought to be the commonest cause of unilateral severe deafness in children. Pancreatitis and epididymo-orchitis also occur, but epididymo-orchitis is much more common after puberty.

A live attenuated vaccine has been available for some years and was introduced in the United Kingdom in 1988 combined with measles and rubella vaccines, given at 12–18 months. There has been a noticeable fall in mumps illness since then.

CHICKEN POX (VARICELLA)

Chicken pox is a common and highly infectious disease but is usually mild in children. The same virus produces herpes zoster. The incubation period is 14–16 days. There may be no symptoms apart from the rash and a low grade fever. Chicken pox spots appear in crops, progressing rapidly from macule to papule to vesicle. The vesicle soon dries and crusts and the scabs separate without scarring. Lesions may also occur on mucous membranes, especially in the mouth where they quickly produce shallow ulcers. Now that smallpox has been eradicated from the world, problems of differential diagnosis are rare.

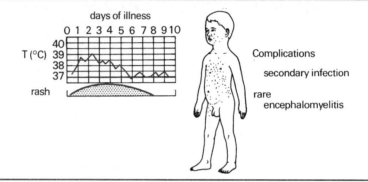

Chicken pox: incubation period 14–16 days

Complications of chicken pox are uncommon in healthy children. Encephalitis is rare but when it does occur there is often cerebellar involvement. The child presents with ataxia 3–8 days after the onset of the rash. At least 80% of affected children make a complete recovery. Pneumonia is a rare complication in children, but it may be part of the very severe form of the illness when the rash is haemorrhagic. This is more likely to occur in children with immune deficiency, in particular children treated for leukaemia. Between 1967 and 1985 there was an average of 19 deaths a year from chicken pox in the United Kingdom, often in adults and immunocompromised people.

A live attenuated vaccine is available, but is not licensed for use in the United Kingdom and at present is not routinely used. Human varicella-zoster immunoglobulin (VZIG) is licensed and recommended for those at risk of severe disease.

HERPES SIMPLEX INFECTIONS

Infection with this virus is extremely common and usually asymptomatic, less than 10% of children with primary infections becoming clinically ill. Herpes virus Type 1 is spread by infected saliva and transmission and therefore requires close personal contact.

Primary infection may affect the mouth, skin or eyes. Herpes virus Type 2 is a genital infection usually spread by sexual contact.

Newborn infants may be infected during delivery by maternal genital herpes infection (Type 2) or, less commonly, by the usual Type 1 virus in the postnatal period. Infection may result in a severe, disseminated disease characterised by lethargy, vesicular rash, hepatosplenomegaly, bleeding and neurological symptoms. Mortality is about 70% and there is a high morbidity rate among the survivors. The risk of this severe illness is about 40% if the mother has active genital herpes at the time of delivery, and an elective caesarean section should be considered.

Acute gingivostomatitis is common, particularly in preschool children from poor socio-economic circumstances. It is characterised by high fever, swelling and bleeding of gums and extensive ulceration of the buccal mucosa, tongue and palate. The cervical glands are enlarged. Eating and drinking are painful, and the child may become dehydrated. The illness lasts about 10–14 days. A vulvovaginitis may result from transfer of the infection from the mouth by the child's finger.

Keratoconjunctivitis is associated with severe oedema of the eyelids and dendritic ulcers of the cornea which may lead to scarring and loss of vision. Primary infection of the skin with vesicular lesions tends to develop in older children, often at the site of trauma. In children with eczema, an extensive vesicular rash which later scabs may occur on the eczematous skin. The child may be febrile and sometimes there is generalised infection due to blood stream spread, which is potentially fatal. Secondary infection of skin lesions is a complication. The diagnosis of local infection is not difficult, as the vesicular lesions are characteristic. Rapid confirmation can be obtained by culture of the vesicular fluid or microscopic examination of scrapings for inclusion bodies. Topical treatment with idoxyuridine is partially effective.

Cold sores. Recurrent herpes simplex infection is common and usually occurs as 'cold sores' around the mouth. The recurrence rate is very variable and though the lesions may be associated with respiratory infections, they may also be related to non-specific factors such as sunshine, menstruation and emotional stress.

Meningoencephalitis. Herpes simplex virus is a relatively common cause of meningoencephalitis. It may occur during the primary infection or due to the activation of a virus lying dormant after an earlier infection. It develops in apparently normal children and it can occur in the absence of skin lesions. The illness may be very severe and the mortality rate is high. Frontal and temporal lobe abnormalities are found, on the electroencephalogram and a brain scan may demonstrate a 'space-occupying' lesion. A rising titre of antibody in the blood or CSF confirms the diagnosis. Treatment with acyclovir, if given early, is of some benefit but the improvement in survival with active treatment has not been accompanied by a reduction in the very high rate of chronic neurological handicap.

GLANDULAR FEVER

In developed countries glandular fever, infectious mononucleosis, occurs most often in adolescents and young adults, but is not uncommon in children. Infection is usually sporadic, though epidemics can occur in schools or residential homes. The Epstein–Barr (EB) virus is the cause of the infection and is excreted in nasopharyngeal secretions. Close contact is necessary for infection to be transmitted.

The onset of glandular fever is usually insidious and occurs after an incubation period of 4–14 days. The clinical features are anorexia, malaise and fever and they are usually accompanied by a sore throat and enlarged glands in most affected children. The tonsillitis may be very severe with a thick white exudate covering the tonsils and surrounding areas. Petechiae may be seen on the palate. Cervical lymph nodes are enlarged, and the spleen is often palpable. A macular rash occurs in 10–20% of cases, especially if ampicillin has been given. Hepatitis, often with jaundice, is common, but other complications such an pneumonitis and neurological disturbances are rare.

The diagnosis is supported by the presence of atypical mononuclear cells in the blood film. These large cells have an irregular nucleus and pale-staining cytoplasm containing vacuoles, and may account for 10–25% of the total white cell count. The test for heterophil antibodies is positive in about 60% of patients in the first week of illness. These antibodies agglutinate sheep red blood cells and are not absorbed by guinea pig kidney cells. Horse red blood cells are also agglutinated and this is the basis of the monospot test. EB virus IgM is present in the early stages of the illness and is indicative of a recent infection. Liver function tests are abnormal in over half of the patients.

Glandular fever is a self-limiting disease for which there is no specific treatment. The lymphadenopathy and splenomegaly may persist for weeks or months, and there may be a long period of debility. The differential diagnosis when tonsillitis is severe includes streptococcal tonsillitis and diphtheria; when lymphadenopathy is prominent it includes leukaemia, toxoplasmosis and cytomegalovirus infection; and when jaundice or a rash are present, infectious hepatitis, measles or rubella may be suspected. The diagnosis is not difficult if the clinical features are characteristic and the appropriate laboratory tests are obtained.

KAWASAKI DISEASE (MUCOCUTANEOUS LYMPH NODE SYNDROME)

First described in Japan, this condition has now been reported from many other countries. The majority of patients are under 5 years of age and present with an acute febrile illness associated with conjunctivitis, pharyngitis and a generalised polymorphous rash. The hands and feet are typically red and oedematous, with peeling of the fingers and toes as the child recovers. Cervical lymph nodes are usually enlarged. Arthritis, urethritis and hepatitis may occur. The fever persists for 1–2 weeks and then settles.

A neutrophil leucocytosis, high erythrocyte sedimentation rate (ESR) and raised platelet counts are found but no organisms have been cultured and auto-antibodies are negative. The most important complication is cardiac involvement with clinical evidence of myocarditis or conduction defects in 20% (especially infants), and death in 1–2%. Coronary artery aneurysms may develop and are detectable by echocardiography, but fortunately slowly resolve in the majority. Post-mortem studies show a widespread vaculitis always affecting the coronary arteries. No infective agent has been isolated and there is no evidence of person-to-person transmission, even in apparent epidemics. Intravenous immunoglobulin and treatment with aspirin in full anti-Inflammatory dosage is recommended in the acute stage, and it is reasonable to continue with a small dose to reduce platelet aggregation for some weeks.

ERYTHEMA INFECTIOSUM (5th DISEASE)

This condition, caused by human parvovirus B19, is characterised by an erythematous maculopapular rash which often begins on the face giving a typical 'slapped cheek' appearance. The rash spreads to the trunk and limbs with central fading of the eruption giving a lacy or reticular appearance. It lasts about a week. There are usually no other symptoms, though arthralgia of the small joints may occur.

ROSEOLA INFANTUM (EXANTHEMA SUBITUM)

This is thought to be caused by human herpes virus 6 and 7. The patient is usually under 2 years of age. They develop a high fever, often without appearing particularly ill, though convulsions may occur. Examination reveals only a mild pharyngitis and lymphadenopathy. After 3 or 4 days the temperature drops suddenly to normal and a macular rash appears which lasts for a few hours or a day or two. The child then makes an uneventful and rapid recovery.

HAND, FOOT AND MOUTH DISEASE

This is caused by a Coxsackie virus. It is common among young children and tends to occur in epidemics. Vesicular lesions appear on the palms of the hands or fingers, the soles of the feet and in the mouth. There may be a low grade fever. Mild cases will go undetected.

HEPATITIS A (INFECTIOUS JAUNDICE)

The hepatitis A virus is an enterovirus spread by the faeco-oral route. The illness is normally mild in children. The child may be generally unwell with headache, nausea, vomiting and abdominal pain; they will often be starting to improve when the jaundice and dark urine appear; this may last for a week or two before resolving. It is rare for children to develop fulminating hepatitis. Many children do not develop the jaundice and in this situation the diagnosis is difficult. The infection often spreads round the family or to other children in a nursery or school. In these situations the level of hygiene needs to be checked.

HEPATITIS B

The hepatitis B virus is transmitted like HIV by sexual contact and intravenous drug abuse. Newborn infants may contract the infection during birth from an infected mother and therefore it is recommended that all mothers are screened during pregnancy. Vaccine given at birth cuts the risk of infection by 95%. Infection during childhood is very rare in the UK, but commoner in warmer climates. In South East Asia 80% are infected during childhood.

The incubation period is 50–160 days, the initial infection often passes unnoticed, though liver function tests may be abnormal. Fulminating hepatitis is very unusual. However in as many as 10% a carrier status develops which can lead to cirrhosis and liver cancer 30 or more years later.

There are effective vaccines available. The one currently in wide use requires three injections. WHO recommends universal vaccination either in infancy or adolescence or both. In the United Kingdom where infection during childhood is rare, the vaccine is offered to those at special risk.

POLIOMYELITIS

The introduction of successful immunisation against poliomyelitis has been one of the greatest success stories of modern medicine. A dreadful disease has been eliminated in many countries and there are hopes that it can be eradicated worldwide by the year 2000. In most people, the poliomyelitis virus produces a mild illness with fever, sore throat, headache and vomiting, lasting up to 3 days. In about one-third of affected children this is followed by improvement for 1–7 days and then a recurrence of more severe symptoms with pain and stiffness in the neck, back and legs. As in other types of viral meningitis, the CSF contains increased lymphocytes and protein. Paralysis may develop in association with muscle pain and tenderness. This is due to anterior horn cell damage, is usually asymmetrical, and varies considerably in extent, in the severe forms causing respiratory failure and bulbar paralysis. Once the fever subsides, the spread of weakness and paralysis is halted and there is then a slow improvement over a period of about 18 months. After this time any residual paralysis is likely to be permanent.

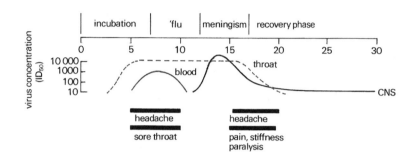

The clinical course of poliomyelitis

Two sorts of trivalent vaccines are available, oral live polio vaccine (OPV Sabin) and inactivated poliovirus vaccine (IPV Salk) which is given by injection. OPV passes through the bowel and is excreted and so it has the advantage that it can boost protection in the family. The disadvantage is that it may cause a mild episode of polio to the subject and unvaccinated contacts (less than 1 in a million).

DIPHTHERIA

Diphtheria is now very rare in countries where immunisation is practised. It is caused by one of three strains of *Corynebacterium diphtheriae*. The infection is usually in the throat and is spread by droplets from infected individuals or healthy carriers. The incubation period is 2–7 days. The child presents with a sore throat and inflamed tonsils. The pharyngeal exudate may spread with epithelial destruction and membrane formation leading to upper airway obstruction. Exotoxin released by the bacterium may cause myocarditis (second week) and neuritis with paralysis (third to seventh week).

The vaccine, a modified exotoxin, gives a very high level of protection. Treatment of the disease itself requires diphtheria antitoxin to counteract its effects and erythromycin to eradicate the organisms.

PERTUSSIS (WHOOPING COUGH)

Bordetella pertussis is the cause of a prolonged respiratory illness which is particularly dangerous in infancy. After a 7-day incubation period, there is a 'catarrhal' stage lasting 1–2 weeks, during which the child is unwell, with signs of upper respiratory tract infection. A cough develops which becomes increasingly severe and paroxysmal. Spasms of coughing may be followed by an inspiratory 'whoop', especially in older children. Vomiting may occur, and the child can become cyanosed or apnoeic during coughing spasms and be left exhausted afterwards. Between spasms there may be no obvious respiratory difficulty and the lungs are clear on examination. This phase lasts 4–6 weeks, and the cough gradually improves over another 2–3 weeks. The causative organism is cultured in early cases from a nasopharyngeal swab using Bordet–Gengou medium, but is difficult to isolate once the cough is established. A striking lymphocytosis supports the diagnosis.

The most common complication is bronchopneumonia which is especially common in infants and accounts for most of the deaths. Bronchiectasis used to be a well recognised complication but is now very uncommon. Convulsions may occur due to asphyxia from severe spasms, intracranial bleeding or encephalopathy. Subconjunctival haemorrhages and facial petechiae due to raised venous pressure during spasms may be alarming but resolve spontaneously.

The treatment of pertussis is largely symptomatic and careful nursing is required. Oxygen, suction and tube-feeding may be necessary. Erythromycin given in the catarrhal stage may abort or modify the illness but the result is often disappointing. Its use in infant contacts is justifiable. No drugs prevent the spasms once the disease is established.

A whole cell vaccine against pertussis has been available for many years. It is probably responsible for most of the local reactions and febrile responses which follow the 'triple injection' DTP (Diphtheria, Tetanus, Pertussis). Immunisation against pertussis became the subject of considerable controversy in the mid 1970s, following well publicised reports of neurological damage *associated* with reactions to the triple vaccine. The debate led to a fall in the uptake of pertussis immunisation to 31% in 1978 and as a consequence there was a bad epidemic in 1978–80. This demonstrated the effectiveness of the vaccine and the dangers of pertussis especially in infants. There were at least 30 deaths in England and Wales.

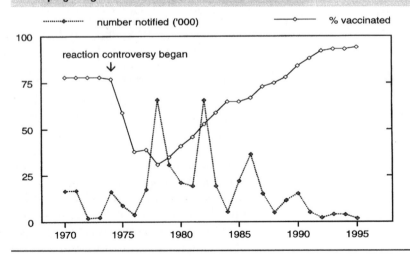

Whooping cough notifications and the effect of vaccination rates

Despite extensive study there is still no conclusive evidence that whooping cough vaccine causes an encephalopathy. Now in the United Kingdom, the vaccine is given earlier at 2, 3 and 4 months, and associated neurological illness is rarely reported. Immunisation rates have risen, and reported illness fallen. As very little maternal antibody crosses the placenta, the protection of young infants depends on the state of immunity of their older siblings, thus the need to maintain a high vaccination rate.

SCARLET FEVER

Group A haemolytic streptococci are responsible for a variety of problems in children, especially tonsillitis. Sequelae such as rheumatic fever and acute glomerulonephritis are important, but have become rare in western societies. Scarlet fever results from infection with a strain of the organism which produces an erythrogenic toxin.

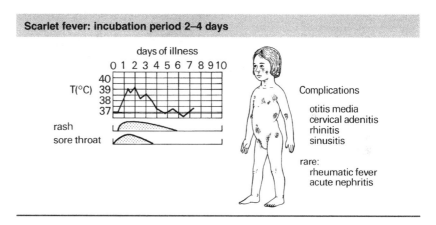

After an incubation period of 2–4 days, the child develops tonsillitis, fever, headache and malaise. The rash develops within 12 hours of the onset and rapidly becomes generalised. It consists of a fine punctate erythema which blanches on pressure. The face is spared, but the cheeks are flushed so that the child is indeed 'scarlet', apart from the area around the mouth. The tongue has a thick white coating through which the inflamed papillae project, the 'white strawberry tongue'. By day 4 or 5 the tongue peels, leaving a 'red strawberry' appearance. The skin rash fades after a few days, or sooner if penicillin is given, followed by desquamation, especially on the hands and feet. This may persist for some time and is useful in making a retrospective diagnosis. Scarlet fever may also follow infection of wounds or burns. Treatment with penicillin leads to a rapid recovery, but a 10-day course is necessary to eradicate the streptococcal infection.

TUBERCULOSIS

Tuberculosis is no longer the 'captain of the Kings of Death' in Europe, but remains a major problem in many developing countries. The incidence of TB in Europe fell steadily as a result of better social conditions and nutrition, and with the advent of effective chemotherapy. Most children with the disease are now identified because they are contacts of infected adults. In the United Kingdom children of Asian families are at special risk of infection from recent adult immigrants. Many patients with AIDs have active tuberculosis. Over the last 10 years in the United Kingdom around 5000 patients are notified each year and around 1 in 13 die. In 1991, 449 children were found to have TB and one died. As it becomes rarer the clinical possibility of TB may be overlooked.

Primary infection

Mycobacterium tuberculosis is spread by droplets, and primary infection may occur in the lung, skin or gut. One outbreak in Nottingham occurred in tooth sockets following dental extractions by a dentist with pulmonary TB. Sensitivity to tuberculin develops 4–8 weeks after infection, as shown by a positive Mantoux or Heaf test. Tuberculin tests may be negative if there is severe malnutrition or overwhelming infection.

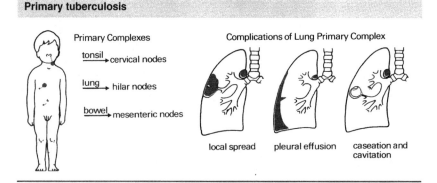

Primary tuberculosis

Primary Complexes

tonsil → cervical nodes

lung → hilar nodes

bowel → mesenteric nodes

Complications of Lung Primary Complex

local spread   pleural effusion   caseation and cavitation

Hypersensitivity reactions such as erythema nodosum (red shiny lumps on the shins) or phlyctenular conjunctivitis occur in a few instances.

Only about 1 in 20 of those infected develop disease. In these, the infection spreads locally and to the lymph nodes; together this constitutes the primary complex. Most such lesions heal slowly by fibrosis and may calcify, the process taking 12–18 months. Complications may arise from the local progression of the primary complex, especially in the lungs. An area of bronchopneumonia develops, or enlargement of the hilar nodes leads to bronchial obstruction, sometimes with rupture of the node into a bronchus. Pleural effusions occur in older children as a hypersensitivity reaction. Empyema, caseation and cavitation are seen more often in malnourished children from developing countries. Unless the lesion cavitates into a bronchus, children with primary TB do not cough up sputum and are not infectious. They may have no cough at all, but a general malaise and vague ill health. Adult pulmonary TB, characterised by cavitation, results either from new infection or a breakdown of the primary complex. Tubercle bacilli can persist in a dormant form and cause disease many years later.

Lung complications of tuberculosis

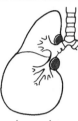 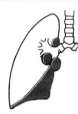 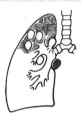

incomplete obstruction—overinflation

complete obstruction—collapse

rupture of node into bronchus—fibrosis and cavities

Gastrointestinal lesions

A primary focus in the tonsillar region may present with cervical adenitis and progress to a 'cold' abscess. This is usually due to human TB but may follow infection with a bovine strain after drinking unpasteurised milk. A similar infection in the small bowel occasionally leads to malabsorption, stricture formation and peritonitis. Cervical adenitis may also occur with infection due to atypical mycobacteria.

Miliary TB and meningitis

Blood stream spread is the most serious complication of primary TB and accounts for at least 70% of childhood deaths due to TB. The risk is greatest in young children especially in developing countries, and almost always occurs within 1 year of infection. The child presents with fever, anorexia and loss of weight. Enlargement of the liver and spleen is common and choroidal tubercles may be seen on examining the fundi. Scattered crepitations may be heard over the lungs, and the chest X-ray shows generalised mottling. There is often associated meningitis, which develops insidiously with gradual progression of lethargy, headache, convulsions and coma. Cranial nerve lesions may develop. A tuberculoma of the brain is much commoner in developing countries than in Europe and presents as a space-occupying lesion. In TB meningitis the CSF is opalescent with increased lymphocytes and protein but low sugar concentrations. A few organisms may be seen on microscopy of the deposit. A culture may take some weeks to grow so treatment should not be delayed. Unfortunately hydrocephalus and other long-term neurological damage are common in survivors.

Miliary TB

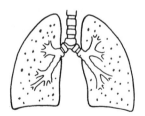

Tuberculosis of the bones and joints can develop as a result of blood stream spread within 3 years of the primary infection. Renal infection may not become apparent for 5 or more years.

Treatment. Active tuberculous infection requires prompt effective chemotherapy. The current recommendation for pulmonary infection is to give isoniazid and rifampicin for 9 months or to give these drugs for 6 months adding pyrazinamide for the first 2 months. For miliary infection or meningitis three drugs should be used for the first 2 months and then continue with isoniazid and rifampicin for 12 or 18 months. Children found to have recently converted their Heaf test from negative to positive should also be treated, mainly to prevent blood stream spread. In this situation isoniazid alone is given for 6 months or isoniazid and rifampicin for 3 months. Older children with a strongly positive tuberculin test and a clear X-ray should be kept under regular supervision and only treated if there is evidence of progression.

BCG is an intradermal injection

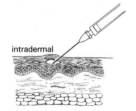

intradermal

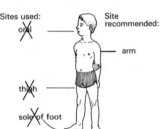

Sites used:
oral
arm
thigh
sole of foot

Site recommended:

Prevention. TB is a notifiable disease. It is essential to trace contacts of newly diagnosed patients and perform a Heaf test and chest X-ray. If the Heaf test is negative, it should be repeated after 6 weeks. If still negative BCG vaccination should be given. The aim of BCG vaccination is to produce a highly modified primary infection with attenuated organisms. It has been shown to give 80% protection against TB and to protect completely against miliary spread.

In parts of the United Kingdom BCG immunisation is offered to 11–13-year-old children who are Heaf negative; some areas have stopped doing this routinely because they consider that the risks of TB do not justify it. Newborn infants from high risk families (certain ethnic groups and those with a recent history of TB in a close relative) are offered BCG at birth. In countries with a high incidence of TB routine neonatal immunisation is advisable. Initial Heaf testing in neonates is not necessary. Following BCG the Heaf test becomes positive, though not strongly so, and it may revert to negative after some years. Natural infection gives a strongly positive reaction.

MALARIA

Malaria is endemic in many parts of the world. As a consequence of increase in international travel more children suffering from malaria are seen in non-endemic countries. 'Where have you been?' is now an important question to ask of children presenting with an unexplained high fever.

Characteristically the fever is intermittent and the spleen enlarged, but these signs are not always present. There may be associated vomiting and rigors. The treatment is normally quinine or mefloquine if the species of organism is unknown, because *Plasmodium falciparum* may be resistant to chloroquine. As sensitivity to treatment varies from place to place and from time to time, current expert opinion should be sought.

Travellers to countries where malaria is endemic should take appropriate precautions such as physical protection against bites. Chemoprophylaxis should also be taken starting a week before and continuing 4–6 weeks after return.

HUMAN IMMUNODEFICIENCY VIRUS

This virus spread worldwide in the 1980s and by the year 2000 it is estimated that 10 million children will be infected. By 1995, 300 infants in the United Kingdom were known to be HIV positive. The virus is transmitted by sexual contact or injection of infected material. The most common source in children is by vertical transmission from an infected mother at birth or less commonly via breast milk. In the past, children have been infected by contaminated blood products. Now all blood and blood products are screened for HIV and like viruses.

Infected infants may remain asymptomatic for years, they may even recover. But many develop the acquired immune deficiency syndrome (AIDS). Up to 25% die in the first year of life, in others the clinical course is more protracted. The children present with general ill health, failure to thrive and recurrent infections. Opportunistic infections are common, *Pneumocystis carinii* pneumonia (PCP), candida oesophagitis, CMV infections etc.

Children infected with HIV should be under expert management. Prophylaxis against PCP and bacterial infections, and a selective immunisation programme help. Antiretroviral agents are given to infants with symptomatic illness and to reduce transmission of infection at birth.

IMMUNISATION

Protection against some of the infectious diseases is available in the form of immunisation which is given at various stages during childhood. Immunisations for different diseases are scheduled to balance the risks of disease with the child's ability to produce a good immunological response. Immunisation should not be given if the child is acutely unwell or if a severe reaction has occurred to a previous dose of that vaccine. Live attenuated vaccines (e.g. poliomyelitis, measles, mumps, rubella, BCG) should not be given to children with immune deficiency states, including those on cytotoxic drugs and high doses of corticosteroids, because of the risk of severe generalised infection. Three weeks should elapse between live vaccines to ensure adequate immune responses to the second one.

For the recommended immunisation programme for the UK 1997 see Appendix B.

A vaccine against *Haemophilus influenzae* was introduced in the United Kingdom in 1992 and is given in three doses at the same time as the primary course of DTP. Other vaccines are available and used in particular circumstances. Influenza A, hepatitis B, anthrax and rabies, are given to certain high risk groups. Typhoid, cholera, yellow fever, meningococcus C, Japanese B encephalitis and tick borne encephalitis are recommended for travellers to countries where these illnesses are endemic. Other vaccines are being tested, for example against rotavirus gastroenteritis and meningococcal B infection, and it is likely that more will come into routine use over the next decade.

IMMUNE DEFICIENCY

In many countries children are repeatedly infected because of poor hygiene, undernutrition and lack of immunisation. In well nourished, immunised children living in clean environments, recurrent infections are more likely to be due to defects in defence: either structural abnormalities, for example vesico-ureteric reflux and recurrent urinary infection; functional abnormalities, for example abnormal ciliary activity contributing to respiratory tract infections; or specific defects of the immune system. Immunodeficiency states affecting children are most commonly congenital but acquired deficiency occurs following splenectomy and with the use of long-term corticosteroids or chemotherapy. HIV infection is discussed earlier in this chapter.

Investigation of the immune system

Innate immunity	Humoral immunity	Cell-mediated immunity	Combined immunity	Phagocytic function
Complement subtype assays	Quantitative serum immunoglobulins, including IgG subclasses	T lymphocyte numbers (CD3, CD4, CD8)	Total lymphocyte count ($<2.8 \times 10^9$/L – abnormal)	Granulocyte count in blood and bone marrow
CH50 assay – assay of classical + terminal complement pathway	Functional antibody responses to immunisations (e.g. Tetanus, HIb) common bacteria (e.g. Streptococcus) and red cell antigens	T-cell response to mitogens (e.g. phytohaemagglutinin) Skin sensitivity testing (depends upon prior exposure to antigen)	MHC Class expression Adenine deaminase (ADA) levels Purine nucleoside phosphorylase (PNP) levels	Granulocyte morphology Nitrobluetetrazolium (NBT) screening test – test of bacterial killing Chemotaxis assay
AP50 assay – assay of alternate and terminal complement pathway				Opsonisation, phagocytosis + killing assays
Natural Killer Cell numbers	Plasma B lymphocyte numbers (CD19, CD20)			Chromosomal abnormalities secondary to defects in DNA repair

Normal development of the immune system

After birth, the infant is rapidly colonised by organisms and challenged by waves of transient pathogens. Cellular immunity is active from birth, and although the neutrophil count is relatively low, infants are able to respond to bacterial infection with a leucocytosis. Humoral immunity is less well developed but the maturing system is initially supported by transplacental maternal derived IgG antibodies and potentially by breast milk factors including IgA. IgM does not cross the placenta but infants can produce it in response to infection. In an intact immune system the waning of maternally derived IgG is matched by gradual enhancement of endogenous production but there is a nadir of circulating IgG levels at age 2–3 months. The emergence of specific endogenous antibodies reflects the process of natural immunisation, and this is accelerated during the preschool years as children average 6–12 short-lived infections each year.

Abnormal development of the immune system

Immunodeficiency is suggested by a history of unusually frequent or severe infections, or by unusual patterns of infection especially if caused by organisms of low pathogenicity. A positive family history is also a powerful guide. Failure to thrive rather than overt infection may be the main manifestation. Modern immunology laboratories are equipped with the tools to test the integrity of each of the main pathways of the immune system, and the classification of disorders has become increasingly functional. Successful management depends upon swift recognition and classification of the disorder, initiation of specific treatments where indicated and meticulous attention to bacteriological and virological investigation of all infectious episodes. Where indicated, life-long immunoglobulin replacement can be very effective. Antibiotics may need to be used prophylactically for recurrent bacterial infections. Immunisations may be protective in some conditions but live vaccines should be avoided. Where there is humoral deficiency and regular immunoglobulin replacement is not being used, contact with cases of chicken pox or measles justifies preventative treatment with either zoster immune globulin (ZIG) or human immunoglobulin respectively. Pneumocystis carinii infection is a major threat and preventative cotrimoxazole is recommended.

Panhypogamma-globulinaemia

This presents as recurrent sinopulmonary infection, recurrent otitis media, bronchiectasis or giardiasis infection. It may be 'early onset' in the first two years, which is almost always the X-linked disorder described by Bruton, or 'late onset' where the presentation is more variable and the inheritance pattern less certain. Failure to thrive, gastrointestinal disorders and autoimmune disorders may complicate the clinical course. Gamma globulin replacement therapy often results in a dramatic improvement.

Selective IgA deficiency

This presents with recurrent upper and lower respiratory, and gastrointestinal tract infections. Low serum IgA levels are found in between 1 in 400 and 700 children, but the deficiency disorders only occur in around 1 in 15 000, this subgroup having associated abnormalities in IgG production. They too benefit from gamma globulin administration.

T-cell deficiencies

These conditions present with frequent and severe infections with herpes simplex, measles, varicella, cytomegalovirus, pneumocystis and fungi such as nocardia, candida and aspergillus. T-cell deficiencies may be isolated or part of extensive immunodeficiency states in which

Primary immunodeficiency disorders

Antibody defects	Combined immuno-deficiency	Immunodeficiency associated with other defects	Complement deficiency	Defects in phagocytic function
X-linked and autosomal recessive agammaglobu-linaemia	Severe combined immunodeficiency (SCID — reduced T- and B-cell numbers)	3rd & 4th arch anomalad — Di George syndrome	Family deficiencies of C1r, C2, C3, C4, C5, C6, C7 and C8	Neonatal neutrophilis
				Chronic granulomatous disease
	Reticular dysgenesis	Wiskott–Aldrich syndrome	Complement pathway dysfunction	
Common variable immune deficiency	Adenosine deaminase (ADA) deficiency	Ataxia telangiectasia	(e.g. neonates, SLE, diabetes	Chediak–Higashi syndrome
			mellitus, C5	Specific granule deficiencies
Ig deficiency with increased IgM (Hyper IgM syndrome)	Purine nucleoside phosphorylase (PNP) deficiency	Transcobalamin II deficiency	dysfunction, chronic haemodialysis glomerulonephritis)	Leucocyte adhesion deficiency
		Partial albinism		
IgA deficiency	MHC Class I and II deficiency	Hereditary defective response to EBV		
IgG subclass deficiency				
kappa chain deficiency				

humoral immunity is also impaired. Di George syndrome is an example of T-cell deficiency associated with congenital absence of the thymus. T-cell function is defective in Wiskott–Aldrich syndrome, ataxia telangiectasia and chronic mucocutaneous candidiasis. Bone marrow transplantation may be used to replace T-cell deficiencies, although it is of high risk especially in patients with a strong previous history of recurrent infections.

Severe combined immune deficiency

This presents with failure to thrive in the first year of life, recurrent sinopulmonary infection, persistent candidiasis, pneumocystis infections, persistent diarrhoea, severe recurrent systemic infections and disseminated viral infections. It is a rare condition and is inherited as autosomal recessive or X-linked. First cases in families are difficult to diagnose and almost always have established infection. A low lymphocyte count ($<2.8 \times 10^9/l$) is an important clue worthy of further investigation. Subsequent pregnancies may be offered antenatal diagnosis and immediate postnatal investigation. Deficiency of adenine deaminase (ADA) or purine nucleoside phosphorylase (PNP) are found in certain subtypes. For children with severe combined immune deficiency (SCID) successful treatment depends upon the presence of an HLA matched bone marrow donor.

Complement (C 5, 6, 7 and 8) deficiencies

In general deficiencies do not normally present with recurrent infections but are found as a result of investigation of the immune system for other disorders, for example vasculitis. Recurrent neisseria infections can be a presenting feature because of the specific need for components of complement to clear this group of organisms.

Chronic granulomatous disease

This presents as recurrent staphylococcal infections with abscesses in and around liver, lungs and bones, or infection with uncommon organisms, or chronic lymphadenopathy and hepatosplenomegaly. Chronic granulomatous disease (CGD) is an X-linked disease in which phagocytes can ingest pathogens but are unable to mount the oxidative burst of intracellular metabolism necessary to kill them. It used to be fatal but continuous administration of antibacterial agents like trimethoprim together with vigorous antibiotic therapy for each new infection has improved the outlook in children diagnosed early and monitored closely.

BIBLIOGRAPHY

American Academy of Pediatrics 1996 Report of the Committee on Infectious Diseases ('The Red Book'), 26th edn. American Academy of Pediatrics
Department of Health 1996 Immunisation against infectious disease. HMSO, London
Graham Davies E, Elliman D A C, Hart C A, Nicoll A, Rudd P T 1996 Manual of childhood infections. W B Saunders, Philadelphia

Hazards

INJURIES
BURNS
DROWNING/NEAR DROWNING
CHOKING AND SUFFOCATION
POISONING
ENVIRONMENTAL HAZARDS

Children are more susceptible to the hazards of everyday life than adults because of their different physical abilities and psychological responses. They are still learning but are adventurous, do not always appreciate dangers, and want to impress their friends. They require protection and guidance until they acquire the maturity to deal with these dangers appropriately. This protection can be achieved by cooperation between different groups in society, including parents, teachers, health workers and town planners.

Injury and poisoning are the commonest causes of death in children over 1 year of age in the United Kingdom. Recently the number of deaths from these causes has declined, but there are still approximately 600 'accidental' deaths annually in this country. Road traffic accidents are the commonest cause, followed by burns, drowning, choking, poisons and playground accidents.

For every child who is killed in an accident, approximately 20 are seriously hurt, and 120 suffer minor injuries. One child in four attends a local accident and emergency department annually, and nearly 10% of these will require admission. The cost of accidents is therefore high financially, as well as physically and psychologically.

The risks of environmental hazards are influenced by three factors: the causative agent or situation, for example a road or a swimming pool; the circumstances of the child such as the degree of parental supervision or family support; and, most important of all, the child themselves—sex, intelligence, social circumstances, personality, physical and mental development. Boys have more accidents than girls at every age, as do children from socially deprived areas. The Government 'Health of the Nation' targets include at least a 30% reduction in deaths from accidents among children under 15 years of age by 2005, that is from 6.7 to 4.5/100 000. Understanding the cause of accidents may lead to strategies for prevention. Toddlers are most at risk in the home and they do not understand reason. They must be actively protected by their carers and those responsible for home design (e.g. by constant adult supervision, fire guards, smoke alarms, cooker-guards, safety gates, window locks and child-resistant containers).

The young school child can be taught about the dangers of traffic and encouraged to use cycle helmets and appropriate car seats and

Accidental deaths 1995: 0–14 years	
Total number	590
Road accidents	
pedestrians	130
passengers	80
cyclists	60
Burns	64
Drowning	34
Choking and suffocation	22
Falls	19
Poisoning	6

restraints, but equally those who design schools, playgrounds and roads must take account of the child's inexperience. Accidents in parks and playgrounds, 89 000 in 1995, are a significant problem and require attention to the design and maintenance of playgrounds and equipment in order to prevent unnecessary injury. A third of these accidents occur in July and August when children spend more time outside their homes. Bouncy castles are a relatively new hazard and caused 6500 injuries requiring hospital treatment in 1995.

Older children have wider boundaries, enjoy risk taking and may resent adult interference. They can be taught to swim and guided towards supervised but challenging sports or pastimes.

Death by accident: (On the State of Public Health 1997. The Annual Report of Chief Medical Officers. HMSO, London)

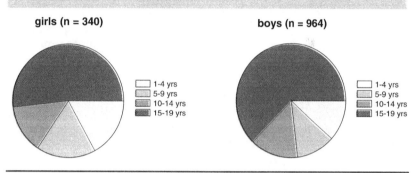

girls (n = 340)   boys (n = 964)

- 1-4 yrs
- 5-9 yrs
- 10-14 yrs
- 15-19 yrs

INJURIES

Road traffic accidents

Over 50% of all accidental deaths in children are a result of road traffic accidents, most of which occur on the way to, or from, school. Children are unable to judge the speed or dangers of traffic or to foresee dangerous situations. Education, the use of cycle helmets and laws to ensure the use of correctly fitted car seats and restraints are all useful but town planning to facilitate the separation of vulnerable children from cars would appear to be the best way forward.

Speed and fatality	
at 20 m.p.h	5% die
at 30 m.p.h.	45% die
at 50 m.p.h.	85% die

Road accident fatalities

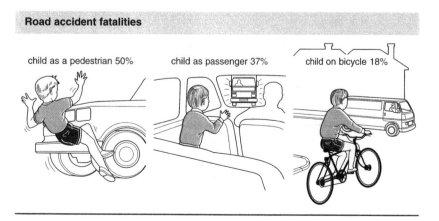

child as a pedestrian 50%   child as passenger 37%   child on bicycle 18%

Falls

Children frequently suffer head injury as a result of falling out of windows, trees, beds or cots, down stairs or from climbing frames. While such injuries are not usually fatal, 19 fatalities in 1995, they are a common cause of presentation for medical attention.

Head injury

Injury to the brain is the major cause of death in childhood accidents, and many of those who do survive are left with permanent damage.

Management. Most head injuries are minor requiring only reassurance and simple analgesia. Many children can be allowed home with instructions for their carers on warning signs and symptoms indicating deterioration. Hospital admission is indicated if the injury was associated with loss of consciousness, if there is a penetrating injury or clinical or radiological evidence of a skull fracture. The latter is not in itself an indication of the severity of injury—many serious brain injuries occur in the absence of a fracture. Pallor and vomiting are very common after minor head injury in young children and result from vagal stimulation. Persistent vomiting is an indication for admission, as is a convulsion or any abnormal neurological sign.

The aim of treatment is to stabilise the child and prevent secondary brain injury due to hypoxia, poor perfusion, hypothermia or raised intracranial pressure.

Paediatric Glasgow Coma Scale

Glasgow Coma Scale (4–15 years)		Children's Coma Scale (< 4 years)		
Response	Score	Response		Score
Eyes		Eyes		
Open spontaneously	4	Open spontaneously		4
Verbal command	3	React to speech		3
React to pain	2	React to pain		2
No response	1	No response		1
Best motor response		Best motor response		
Verbal command:		Spontaneous or obeys verbal		
Obeys	6	command		6
Painful stimulus:		*Painful stimulus:*		
Localises pain	5	Localises pain		5
Flexion with pain	4	Withdraws in response to pain		4
		Abnormal flexion to pain		
Flexion abnormal	3	(decorticate posture)		3
		Abnormal extension to pain		
Extension	2	(decerebrate posture)		2
No response	1	No response		1
Best verbal response		Best verbal response		
Orientated and		Smiles, orientated to sounds,		
converses	5	follows objects, interacts		5
Disoriented and		*Crying*	*Interacts*	5
converses	4	Consolable	Inappropriate	4
		Inconsistently		
Inappropriate words	3	consolable	Moaning	3
Incomprehensible				
sounds	2	Inconsolable	Irritable	2
No response	1	No response		1

The pupillary size and reaction, the central and peripheral nervous system and the Glasgow Coma Scale need to be examined regularly to identify any signs of deterioration. A fall of 2 or more points in the Glasgow Coma Scale is significant and requires neurosurgical assessment. Infants whose cranial sutures are still open require especially careful assessment as they may develop large focal intracerebral lesions or severe oedema of the brain before neurological deterioration becomes evident.

A Glasgow Coma Score of less than 8 requires urgent protection of the airways by endotracheal intubation. A cranial CT or MRI scan will show whether an increase in intracranial pressure (ICP) is due to oedema, contusion or haemorrhage (and will identify the origin of the latter). If there is localised bleeding surgery is necessary to decompress the brain, remove the clot and treat the source of bleeding. If not, raised ICP is monitored, directly and treated by cooling, hyperventilation and drugs such as mannitol, to reduce brain swelling.

BURNS

Fire is the second most common cause of accidental death in the United Kingdom, 40 deaths in 1995, with most being due to the effects of smoke inhalation. The majority of incidents occur at home, particularly in areas of social deprivation and overcrowding. The inquisitive toddler is fascinated by matches and flames, may go too close to open fires, grasp a saucepan of boiling water by the handle or the flex of an electric kettle and pull it over themselves. Burns outside the home involving bonfires and fireworks tend to happen to older children, who are therefore more likely to have additional injuries.

Causes of home accidents: fires, hot liquids and cleaning fluids

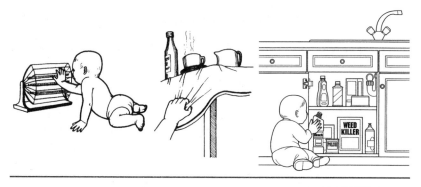

First aid treatment for minor burns is to hold them under cold water for 5–10 minutes to reduce the temperature of the deeper structures, then cover with a clean tea towel or cling film until they can be assessed. No creams or ointments should be applied at this stage.

The immediate medical management is to ensure an adequate

airway, relieve pain, and then assess the extent of the burns. This can be done with a Lund and Browder chart or by using the child's palm and adducted fingers which approximate to 1% of their body surface area.

Percentage body surface area of a child

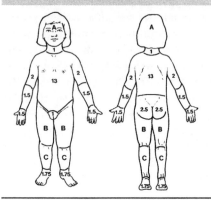

Area indicated	Surface area at				
	0	1 year	5 years	10 years	15 years
A	9.5	8.5	6.5	5.5	4.5
B	2.75	3.25	4.0	4.5	4.5
C	2.5	2.5	2.75	3.0	3.25

The depth of the burn is often difficult to assess initially. Superficial burns are painful and cause erythema with no skin destruction. Partial thickness burns are painful when exposed and there is damage to the top layers of skin with blistering leaving the dermis intact. Full thickness burns are painless and the dermis is destroyed, leaving the skin white or charred.

Large quantities of fluid, blood and protein are lost from the burned areas and must be replaced. If more than 10% of the child's surface area is burned, intravenous fluids (plasma and saline) are necessary. The child's urine output and haematocrit should be closely monitored. If more than 50% of the child's surface area is affected, the chances of survival are poor.

Antibiotics as prophylaxis against toxic shock syndrome are recommended even for relatively minor burns, and tetanus toxoid should be given when existing cover is not adequate. The burn should be covered with an appropriate non-adhesive dressing and arrangements made for review. Full thickness burns or those to special areas usually require assessment at a specialist unit. Skin grafting may be necessary at a later date and remember that children who have been burned are often psychologically scarred too. Prevention and education are the best ways to reduce the 60 000 paediatric attendances for burns at accident and emergency departments annually. Campaigns for firework and Bonfire Night safety, the fitting of smoke detectors and the use of flame resistant materials are important, but supervision of toddlers and anticipation of problems are essential.

DROWNING/NEAR DROWNING

Drowning is the third commonest cause of accidental death in childhood. Three-quarters of drowning incidents occur in inland waters, swimming pools and, in the very young, in domestic baths. The remaining quarter occur in the sea. Boys are three times more commonly involved than girls in all types of accidents in water. Swimming and life-saving lessons at school, wearing life-jackets on boats, and supervised pools and beaches are important preventive measures. Children die during drowning either as a result of laryngeal spasm, when the cause of death is cerebral anoxia (dry drowning), or else water may enter the lungs, rapidly leading to respiratory failure with cardiac arrest (wet drowning). In either situation, the child may respond well to prompt resuscitation with mouth to mouth ventilation and cardiac massage. Unfortunately, if the water is muddy or polluted, the child may be revived only to die later with progressive pneumonia and pulmonary oedema, secondary drowning. The type of water, sea or fresh, does not affect the prognosis. All surviving victims should be observed in hospital for at least 24 hours. Hypothermia has a protective effect and resuscitation should be continued until the core temperature is above 32°C.

CHOKING AND SUFFOCATION

Children may choke on small toys, beads, or food such as peanuts, or suffocate on a carelessly discarded plastic bag. A child who is choking is distressed, makes violent respiratory efforts and becomes progressively cyanosed, but makes little noise as the obstruction lies at the level of the larynx, wedged between the vocal cords. Death results if the child is unable to remove the obstruction by their own efforts. The traditional first aid measure of violent slaps on the back is often unsuccessful, but abdominal compression (the Heimlich manoeuvre) can be life-saving. The rescuer places a clenched fist in the epigastrium and covers it with the other hand—a short sharp squeeze directed inwards and upwards compresses the residual air in the lungs and may dislodge the obstruction. This can be performed with the victim standing, sitting or lying but is not recommended for young children or infants as it may cause intra-abdominal injury. In this group back blows and chest thrusts using the finger position as for cardiac massage should be used.

Treatment of choking

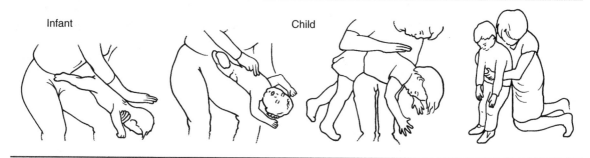

Infant   Child

POISONING

Few children die as a result of poisoning, but many thousands attend hospital each year for treatment. Occasionally a child may intentionally ingest a poison, but in most cases the self-poisoning is accidental. Children may also be poisoned deliberately by their parents, or inadvertently by their doctors. Most children who ingest a poison are fearless, inquisitive toddlers, peak age 2–3 years, who are attracted by the appearance of tablets, medicines, household or garden substances, berries, seeds or fungi. They will eat almost anything, regardless of taste. It has been shown that a child is particularly likely to ingest a poison when the family is under some sort of stress, presumably because of decreased supervision.

Common accidental poisons	
Cleaning agents	20%
Caustic agents	11%
Paracetamol	10.5%
Plants	6.5%
Cough medicines	2.5%
Vitamins	1.5%
Antidepressants	1.5%
Alcohol	1%
Iron	1%
Contraceptive pill	1%
Unknown	12%

Some poisonous berries

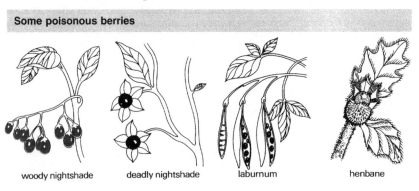

woody nightshade   deadly nightshade   laburnum   henbane

The management of a poisoned child is to treat the acute symptoms, maintain adequate ventilation and circulation, limit the absorption of the poison, and observe for the anticipated symptoms and signs. The way to limit absorption is to give activated charcoal which offers an alternative binding site for toxins. It is relatively unpalatable when given orally so the child may require a nasogastric tube. Occasionally gastric lavage is indicated, for example when a large quantity of iron or aspirin has been ingested. This is only recommended when the child presents promptly, and after the airway has been protected by intubation. It is never appropriate after ingestion of corrosive substances or volatile agents, for example paraffin or turpentine, which may be inhaled and cause lung damage.

If the side effects of a poison are not known, information can be obtained at any time of day or night from one of the regional poison centres. Many ingested substances, for example vitamins, oral contraceptives, most antibiotics and simple antacids, are non-toxic and can be managed by reassurance. Most plants and berries are not harmful, causing only a mild gastrointestinal upset; an exception being deadly nightshade which classically gives dilated pupils, dry skin and mouth, fever, tachycardia, abdominal distension, excitement and confusion due to its anticholinergic effects. Children likely to have ingested a toxic agent, or those with symptoms, should be admitted to hospital for observation and treated with an antidote if available. All those who have taken a poison intentionally should be assessed by a

Age of children admitted with poisoning	
Age (yr)	No. Children
< 1	24
1	190
2	168
3	88
4 & 5	61
6 & 7	24
8 & 9	10
10 & 11	17
12 & 13	61
>14	78

child psychiatrist before discharge and health visitors should be informed of all accidental ingestions.

Paracetamol

This is the commonest poison ingested by children, because it is readily accessible. It is available as a paediatric elixir, which is rarely ingested in a dangerous amount, or as various adult preparations. Nausea and vomiting are the only acute symptoms but hepatic failure is a risk if appropriate treatment is not given. A blood paracetamol level should be checked at least 4 hours after ingestion and compared with the nomogram to assess the need for treatment. The antidote acetylcysteine may be effective up to 24 hours after ingestion. If liver failure develops the child should be transferred to a specialist centre.

Aspirin

Aspirin is a respiratory stimulant and a cell poison. When taken in large quantities it produces nausea, vomiting, tinnitus and dehydration. Hyperventilation with deep sighing respiration is a consequence of both metabolic acidosis and respiratory stimulation. Hypoglycaemia, hyperglycaemia and an increased prothrombin time may occur in cases of severe poisoning. Since aspirin was withdrawn from paediatric treatment, because of its association with Reye syndrome, overdose is rare except in the group of children who take it deliberately. When blood levels of salicylate are high, excretion should be enhanced by inducing a diuresis and reducing tubular reabsorption of the drug by making the urine alkaline. As with most poisons, there is no specific antidote.

Iron tablets

Iron tablets are frequently swallowed by toddlers because they are likely to be available, for example prescribed during pregnancy, and because they look like sweets. A small child can be fatally poisoned by as little as 2 g of iron. There are four phases recognised after iron poisoning. Firstly, within an hour of the ingestion the child develops severe gastrointestinal symptoms, diarrhoea, vomiting, haematemesis and melaena. These symptoms may gradually subside so that the child seems well. However, some hours later, the serious third phase may develop with iron encephalopathy manifested by coma and fits, liver damage and circulatory collapse. Finally, a child who survives this may develop scarring of the stomach and pylorus as a consequence of local irritation. Iron ingestion is an indication for gastric lavage if the presentation is within the first few hours. The iron chelating agent desferrioxamine is useful. It can be left in the stomach to prevent further absorption of iron and it can be administered parenterally to enhance iron excretion and lessen the severity of the poisoning.

Tricyclic agents

Tricyclic agents such as amitriptyline and imipramine are among the most dangerous drugs consumed by young children and are responsible for most of the deaths. They may be available because one of the parents is taking them for depression, or because a child in the family is being treated for bed-wetting. The effects of poisoning include respiratory and cardiovascular depression, as well as cerebral stimulation leading to irritability, excitation, hallucinations and fits, with exaggerated tendon reflexes. Tricyclic antidepressants also have a marked atropine-like action, giving fixed dilated pupils, a dry red skin, sinus tachycardia, urinary retention and paralytic ileus. Their most serious effect is on heart rhythm, resulting in atrial and ventricular tachycardias, fibrillation or heart block. There is no specific antidote, only symptomatic treatment. Diazepam is used to treat convulsions and antiarrhythmic drugs are occasionally necessary.

Alcohol

Alcohol is a dangerous poison in young children who drink it accidentally, or older school children who drink it experimentally. The acute encephalopathy is often enhanced by severe hypoglycaemia which is particularly common in children and occasionally causes death. Blood glucose must be carefully monitored and intravenous dextrose given if it falls to low levels. Alcohol is also a factor underlying risk-taking behaviour.

Child-resistant containers

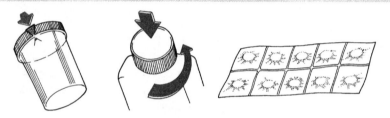

Important developments have led to a decrease in the incidence of severe accidental poisoning in children. Child-resistant containers have been developed which can only be opened by lining up an arrow on the lid with an arrow on the bottle or by pushing the lid down and twisting it open at the same time. In the United Kingdom it is compulsory for all aspirin and paracetamol tablets to be prescribed in this way, and pharmacists are encouraged to dispense other dangerous tablets in this form too. Recent legislation has limited over-the-counter sales of these drugs to a maximum of 16 tablets. 'Blister packs' are also helpful as it takes the child some time to eat sufficient tablets to cause symptoms, and they frequently lose interest, or are discovered in the act.

ENVIRONMENTAL HAZARDS

The risk of a noxious agent producing permanent damage is highest in the earliest phase of development, embryogenesis. A number of such agents have been identified as being associated with a high incidence of congenital abnormalities. Harmful environmental factors after birth are less easy to identify because many children are exposed to potential hazards, and the ill effects may be quite subtle, making an association difficult to prove.

Smoking

The harmful effects of smoking on those who actually smoke are well known. Chronic bronchitis, lung cancer and coronary heart disease are three common conditions whose incidence is greatly increased in smokers. Many school children now smoke regularly and are, therefore, at risk. It is obviously important to try to dissuade children from taking up smoking by appropriate health education in schools and by reducing the 'glamour' often associated with particular brands aimed at children. It is also known that the children of smoking parents have a higher incidence of bronchitis, pneumonia and serous otitis media; this applies particularly to babies and young children. Exposure to smoke in the home and maternal smoking antenatally significantly increase a baby's risk of Sudden Infant Death syndrome.

Carbon monoxide

Sources of carbon monoxide include car exhausts, poorly ventilated heating systems and smoke from all types of fires. Haemoglobin has a much higher affinity for carbon monoxide than for oxygen, leading to a lack of oxygen for the tissues. The toxic effects are headache, nausea, vomiting, confusion, coma and death. The severely poisoned victim classically has a 'cherry red' appearance of the skin and lips. The management is to remove the victim from the gas and give 100% oxygen.

Lead

Lead is an environmental element which is undoubtedly harmful. If it is ingested or inhaled in large quantities it can produce a serious illness, which may be lethal or result in brain damage. It is probable too that chronic exposure to environmental lead has a harmful effect on mental development. There are several sources of lead. It used to be present in paint, so that children who chewed painted surfaces were liable to be poisoned. Water in lead pipes may contain sufficient lead to cause poisoning. Lead fumes produced by burning car batteries may produce toxic symptoms. Asian families use lead salts ('surma') in cosmetics applied regularly to the conjunctivae of the child. More recently, there has been concern about atmospheric lead. Lead is present in exhaust fumes from vehicles and blood lead levels are higher in urban children and in those living close to major roads. It has been suggested that this chronic exposure to moderate amounts of atmospheric lead may produce permanent intellectual impairment. The change to unleaded fuel has been in response to public concern.

A child who has ingested lead may show symptoms of encephalopathy, with irritability, drowsiness, convulsions and eventually coma. Papilloedema may be present. Colicky abdominal pain is common and an abdominal X-ray may actually show radio-opaque lead fragments in the gastrointestinal tract. The diagnosis is made on the clinical picture, a history of exposure to a source of the lead and investigations. Blood lead levels can be measured and are a guide to the severity of poisoning. Lead affects many enzyme systems, but particularly those involved in haem synthesis There may be hypochromic anaemia and basophil stippling of neutrophils. In chronic poisoning, lead interferes with the growing ends of bones producing dense metaphyseal plates on X-ray, 'lead lines'.

The treatment of a poisoned child is directed at removing lead from the body. This is achieved by using lead-chelating agents which form non-toxic lead compounds. In severe cases with encephalopathy, calcium edetate (EDTA) and dimercaprol are given parenterally. In less severe cases oral D-penicillamine is used. If there are signs of raised intracranial pressure, cerebral oedema can be lessened by intravenous mannitol or dexamethasone. The source of the lead must obviously be identified and removed. Severe lead poisoning carries a high mortality, and survivors are often neurologically handicapped.

REFERENCE

On the state of public health 1997 The Annual Report of Chief Medical Officer, HMSO, London

BIBLIOGRAPHY

Advanced paediatric life support. The practical approach 1993 BMJ Publishing Group, London

Blumer J L, Reed M D 1986 Pediatric toxicology. Pediatric Clinics of North America vol 33: (2). W B Saunders, Philadelphia (chapters on gastric lavage and all the common poisons)

Department of Health 1992 The health of the nation: a strategy for health in England. HMSO London

Health Committee's Second Report 1997 The specific health needs of children and young people. February 1997

Meadow R 1989 ABC of child abuse: poisoning. British Medical Journal 298: 1445–1446

Office for National Statistics, Mortality Statistics Childhood, Infant and Perinatal 1995 Series DH3 no 28.

Office for National Statistics, Mortality Statistics 1993, 1994 Series DH2 no 21

Piomelli S, Rosen J F Chisholm J J 1984 Management of childhood lead poisoning Journal of Pediatrics 105: 523–532

Roberts I, Power C 1996 Does the decline in child injury mortality vary by social class? British Medical Journal 313: 784–786

Sharples P M et al 1990 Causes of fatal childhood accidents involving head injury in Northern region, 1979–86. British Medical Journal 301: 1193–1197

Sharples P M et al 1990 Avoidable factors contributing to death of children with head injury. British Medical Journal 300: 87–91

Airways and lungs

UPPER RESPIRATORY TRACT
   INFECTIONS
STRIDOR
INHALED FOREIGN BODY
ACUTE LOWER RESPIRATORY
   TRACT INFECTION
CYSTIC FIBROSIS
ASTHMA

Normal range for respiratory rate in children	
Age (yr)	Respiratory rate (breaths/min)
< 1	25–35
1–5	20–30
5–12	20–25
>12	15–25

Respiratory problems in children are common. Upper respiratory tract infections account for almost half of children's visits to their general practitioners. Up to 15% of school children in the United Kingdom have symptoms of asthma. However respiratory illness is commonly misdiagnosed and it is important to take a careful history and to look for signs of acute or chronic respiratory disease.

When you take a history establish precisely which respiratory symptoms have been observed. Make sure that children and their parents know what you mean when you use words such as 'wheeze'. (One child was asked whether he had wheeze at night and replied that he didn't if he went to the toilet before he went to bed!) Describe exactly what you mean by a symptom, for example wheeze is 'a whistling noise in the chest when your child breathes out'. Clarify vague terms such as 'chesty'. Do not forget to ask about parental smoking and illness in parents and siblings.

Any child with an acute illness may be febrile, miserable and may vomit and so it is important to observe sick children closely for signs of respiratory distress. Take the time to measure the respiratory rate and look for signs of respiratory distress before you touch the child. These signs will identify the presence and severity of an acute respiratory illness and you must then determine the precise diagnosis and appropriate management. Look also for signs of a chronic problem, for example hyperinflation of the chest, finger clubbing and 'Harrison's sulci' (a permanent indrawing of the lower ribs anteriorly). Only when you have gained as much information as possible by observing the child should you risk upsetting them with palpation, percussion and auscultation. Simple bedside investigations such as measurement of peak flow are invaluable in the school age child and some children will already be recording this in a diary at home. Chest X-ray is an over-used investigation but in some cases is justified, for example with a first attack of asthma.

UPPER RESPIRATORY TRACT INFECTION

Upper respiratory infections are common and on average preschool children will have between five and eight episodes per year. However most of these infections are viral and antibiotics are not usually indicated. It is often difficult to distinguish viral and bacterial infections clinically.

Otitis media

This an acute infection of the middle ear. Most children will be febrile though younger children may not localise the pain. Full examination of the ears and throat should be routine in any febrile child. Inspection with an auroscope may reveal the bulging tympanic membrane which is suggestive of bacterial infection. In viral infection, the common appearance is of a leash of dilated blood vessels around the circumference of the ear drum and the handle of the malleus. Viral otitis media is usually bilateral and accompanied by viral pharyngitis. In bacterial infection the tense tympanic membrane may perforate, discharging pus and a perforation may be seen with the auroscope. In rare occasions infection may spread to structures adjacent to the middle ear, causing meningitis or mastoiditis. However, the most frequent complication of otitis media is a persistent middle ear effusion ('glue ear'). This may lead to conductive deafness which can have a detrimental effect on language development. Drainage and insertion of grommets may be necessary. Antibiotics must be used sparingly. If no antibiotics are prescribed, over half of children with acute otitis media will be pain free in 24 hours.

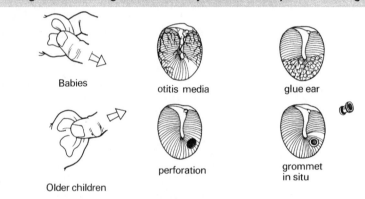

Pulling the ear to straighten the auditory canal and four possible findings

Babies

Older children

otitis media

perforation

glue ear

grommet in situ

Tonsillitis

The child may have a poor fluid intake due to discomfort on swallowing. He will have enlarged, inflamed tonsils and the tonsillar lymph nodes may also be enlarged. The presence of a white exudate on the tonsils does not distinguish bacterial from viral infection. Viral tonsillitis, often due to adenovirus, is more common in preschool children, whereas a higher proportion of school age children will have streptococcal infection. Epstein–Barr virus ('glandular fever') causes a florid tonsillitis, and petechial haemorrhages may be present on the palate. All children should have a throat swab taken for culture. Some laboratories can perform rapid antigen detection for group A beta-haemolytic streptococci. Where the illness has been more than a few days or there is marked lymph node enlargement, blood should be sent for a glandular fever screening test (e.g. the 'monospot test'). Infection with group A beta-haemolytic streptococci may be complicated by glomerulonephritis or rheumatic fever. The latter is rarely seen in the United Kingdom but remains a substantial problem in developing countries. Rarely tonsillitis may be complicated by peritonsillar abscess (quinsy). All children should have symptomatic treatment with paracetamol and should be encouraged to drink fluids. Antibiotic treatment should be reserved for those children in whom results of a throat swab are available.

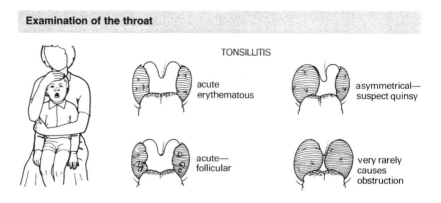

Examination of the throat

TONSILLITIS

acute erythematous

asymmetrical—suspect quinsy

acute—follicular

very rarely causes obstruction

STRIDOR

Stridor is a harsh noise during breathing which originates in the upper airway. It may be inspiratory or expiratory. Acute stridor is dealt with in the section on croup below. Some babies have stridor from birth, or shortly after and this will be considered here.

Congenital stridor

Congenital stridor arising from a problem with the larynx is inspiratory and most commonly due to laryngomalacia or a 'floppy larynx'. When the child has stridor plus signs of respiratory distress then a laryngoscopy or flexible bronchoscopy is indicated. Where there is a history of cough and vomiting a barium swallow should be performed to exclude a vascular ring, an abnormal blood vessel compressing the trachea and oesophagus.

Barium swallow (lateral view) showing indentation of the oesophagus from behind caused by a vascular ring

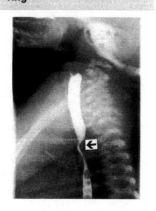

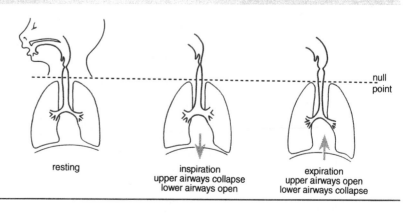

Airways collapse

resting

inspiration
upper airways collapse
lower airways open

expiration
upper airways open
lower airways collapse

null point

Expiratory stridor may mimic wheeze but it is a harsher sound and the symptoms will not respond to bronchodilators. The symptom is often due to floppy airway ('tracheomalacia' or 'bronchomalacia') which collapses as the child breaths out. Tracheomalacia is seen in children who have had a repair of tracheo-oesophageal fistula. Stridor should be distinguished from stertor which is obstructed nasal breathing seen in babies with upper respiratory infections or rarely with abnormal nasal airways.

Findings on bronchoscopy/laryngoscopy

 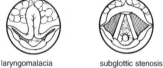

| laryngomalacia | subglottic stenosis | congenital web | juvenile papillomatosis | rt. recurrent nerve palsy | bilateral recurrent nerve palsy |

INHALED FOREIGN BODY

Chest radiograph showing left-sided hyperinflation with mediastinal shift to the right, due to a foreign body (peanut) in the left main bronchus

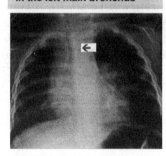

From the age of 6 months children will place small objects in their mouths. The older child may chew a pen top or try to catch a peanut in their mouth. Any of these may be inhaled. There is usually a history of choking followed by dyspnoea and examination may reveal unilateral wheeze or occasionally stridor. Children may present months or years afterwards with haemoptysis. Chest X ray may reveal unilateral hyperinflation and it is usually not necessary to perform inspiratory and expiratory films. The foreign body should be removed by an experienced bronchoscopist, using a rigid bronchoscope.

ACUTE LOWER RESPIRATORY INFECTION

Causes of acute lower respiratory infection in 40 Nottingham children

Respiratory syncytial virus	9
S. pneumoniae	4
Mycoplasma pneumoniae	4
Influenza virus	2
Adenovirus	2
No organism found	19

Worldwide, 4 million children die from acute lower respiratory infections every year. It is the commonest cause of death in children under 5 and most deaths are in children under 1 year old. In developing countries, the majority of children with lower respiratory infection have bacterial pneumonia. In the United Kingdom, viral bronchiolitis is more common. Mortality in the United Kingdom is low and largely confined to children with pre-existing cardiac or respiratory disease.

Bacterial pneumonia

In the developing world, the most common causative organisms are *Streptococcus pneumoniae* and *Haemophilus influenzae*. These organisms are also important in the United Kingdom but atypical organisms such as *Mycoplasma pneumoniae* are responsible for a substantial number of cases. Children usually present with a short history of cough, fever and dyspnoea—though mycoplasma has a more insidious onset. Parents of children under 1 year may say that their baby is not finishing milk feeds or is breastfeeding poorly. Children may have signs of respiratory distress but localising signs such as bronchial breathing or crackles will be difficult to detect in young children. Oxygen saturation should be recorded in all children, when they are initially assessed, and facial oxygen given where the saturation is less than 93% in air. A chest X-ray will establish whether the child has a lobar pattern (suggesting *S. pneumoniae* or *H. influenzae* infection) or a more diffuse pattern (suggestive of mycoplasma). It is important to identify the organism responsible, where possible, and a nasopharyngeal aspirate should be collected for bacterial culture and viral immunofluorescence, together with samples for blood culture and serology. In most cases antibiotics can be given orally unless the child is unable to drink. In uncomplicated cases, antibiotics are given for about a week. A follow-up X-ray should be taken after at least a month where lobar collapse is present.

Chest radiographs of children with pneumonia

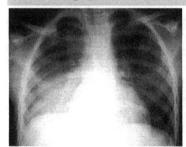 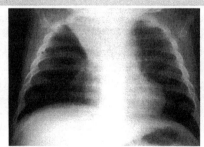 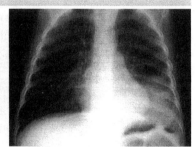

Right lower and middle lobe consolidation

Right upper lobe collapse

Left lower lobe consolidation

Small pleural effusions are a common complication of pneumonia. Occasionally such an effusion may become secondarily infected and pus accumulates in the pleural cavity. This is termed an empyema. Fibrous septae may form in an attempt to wall off the pus and the empyema is said to be loculated. This can be seen on ultrasound of the chest. Empyema should be suspected when an effusion is seen on the X-ray and the temperature has not settled after several days of antibiotics. The diagnosis should be confirmed by means of pleural tap. The aim of treatment is to drain pus (before this becomes impossible due to loculation) and a chest drain should be inserted.

Chest radiographs showing a right-sided effusion subsequently found to be an empyema.

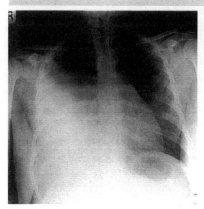 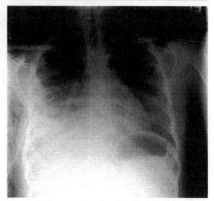

After drainage showing lower lobe collapse

Measles

Measles is now uncommon in the United Kingdom as a result of immunisation but is an important cause of death in the developing world. Measles infection may be followed by croup, otitis media or bronchopneumonia. In 1 in 4 children who die from pneumonia, their infection has arisen as a complication of measles. It is vital to improve immunisation—WHO aims for 90% coverage by the year 2000. However, giving high doses of vitamin A to children with measles reduces deaths from both pneumonia and diarrhoea.

Croup

Croup or laryngotracheobronchitis is caused by a viral infection, usually with parainfluenza virus, and commonly occurs in spring or autumn. Children present with a sudden onset of barking cough and stridor. Some children with asthma and atopic disease suffer frequent attacks of spasmodic croup which may have an allergic basis. It is important to differentiate children with croup from other causes of stridor of sudden onset like epiglottitis. Epiglottitis is fortunately now rare due to HiB immunisation. Children with epiglottitis have a sudden onset of high fever without preceding coryza. They are often unable to drink or swallow secretions and may drool. When the diagnosis is suspected the throat should not be examined. These children require urgent intubation by an experienced anesthetist and prompt antibiotic treatment.

Children with croup who have a cough but no respiratory distress or stridor at rest, require no treatment. Those with more severe croup should be given steroids. Oral dexamethasone and nebulised budesonide are equally effective though dexamethasone is easier to administer and much cheaper. Some children with severe croup will require intubation until the inflammation of the upper airway has resolved. This may take up to a week.

Bronchiolitis

Bronchiolitis is an acute viral infection of the airways below 1 mm in diameter. It chiefly affects children under 1 year. The commonest virus implicated is respiratory syncytial virus (RSV) but parainfluenza, influenza and adenoviruses can also be responsible. The illness occurs in winter epidemics and is mostly mild and self limiting. However 2% of children under 1 year will require hospital admission. Serological surveys show that almost all children will have had an infection with RSV by 2 years. There is currently no effective immunisation against RSV infection and the first vaccine used in trials led to more severe disease, rather than protection. The virus is highly infectious and cross-infection in hospital is common. Children must be nursed in cubicles or 'bronchiolitis bays'.

Chest radiographs of a child with acute bronchiolitis showing hyperinflation and patchy areas of collapse

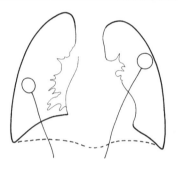 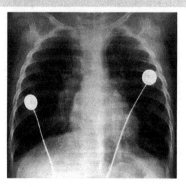

The parent may say that their infant has been feeding poorly and has developed a cough. Copious nasal secretions are common and wheezing is usually obvious. Infants under 6 weeks old may have life-threatening apnoeas which are central in nature (rather than obstructive). When he is examined, the child will be tachypnoeic and have signs of respiratory distress. In addition the chest will be hyperinflated and the liver may be palpable. Fine crackles are usually heard when listening at the lung bases. A chest X-ray will confirm hyperinflation and may show patchy areas of consolidation which usually resolve without antibiotic treatment.

Treatment is symptomatic and bronchodilators are ineffective. Oxygen saturation should be measured and oxygen administered if the saturation is less than 93%. A head box or nasal cannulae can be used. If the child is not feeding then nasogastric or intravenous fluids may be needed. The illness will usually run its course over about a week, though in the first few days the child may deteriorate. Some children deteriorate despite adequate supportive treatment and require mechanical ventilation. Those at greatest risk are children with chronic respiratory disease (e.g. bronchopulmonary dysplasia) and congenital heart disease. The antiviral agent ribavirin has been given in nebulised form to these high risk infants and produces some clinical improvement. However it has not been shown to reduce the number of high risk children needing mechanical ventilation and it should not be used in otherwise healthy infants. Over half of infants with bronchiolitis will go on to have further episodes of cough and wheeze. Even 10 years after the initial infection, one-third of children will suffer from episodes of wheezing requiring bronchodilators.

Pertussis

Although immunisation coverage is now high, children still develop whooping cough and may require admission to hospital. Those at greatest risk are infants under 2 months old who will not yet have had their first immunisation, although full immunity does not develop until the third dose of triple vaccine has been administered at 5 months. The incubation period is 1–2 weeks, with a prodromal coryzal phase lasting up to 10 days. This leads to a 6–8 week period when the child has spasmodic cough and may vomit or feed poorly. In young infants apnoea may be the main symptom and mechanical ventilation may be required. Diagnosis depends on isolation of *Bordetella pertussis* on a pernasal swab, taken from the nasopharynx. Antibiotic treatment with erythromycin is effective only if given during the coryzal stage of the illness. Otherwise treatment is supportive. Oxygen is administered where necessary and the infant may need to be fed nasogastrically.

CYSTIC FIBROSIS

Cystic fibrosis (CF) is responsible for the majority of deaths from lung disease in childhood, in developed countries. It is a genetic disorder, inherited in an autosomal recessive fashion. The incidence is around 1/2500 live births, with a carrier prevalence in the population of around 1/25. CF is a multisystem disorder affecting lung, gastrointestinal tract, sweat glands, hepatobiliary system, pancreas and reproductive system. Most deaths from CF are however from respiratory failure. Survival has improved greatly over the last 30 years and many patients now survive well into adult life.

Genetics. The CF gene is located on chromosome 7. One mutation, DF508, accounts for 68% of all abnormal CF genes but over 350 other mutations have been identified—some so rare that they occur in only one family. The gene product is a protein which spans the apical membrane of epithelial cells—the CF transmembrane conductance regulator. This regulates the cyclic AMP dependent movement of chloride ions across epithelial surfaces. Where an individual has two abnormal genes, the protein is defective and chloride transport is disrupted.

Pathogenesis. In the mucus producing glands in the airways of CF patients, there is a failure of chloride transport from the cell into the lumen. Water is drawn into the cell by osmosis to follow the chloride ions, and the mucus within the lumen becomes dehydrated. This disrupts the action of the mucociliary escalator and leads to bacterial colonisation of the airway, with chronic inflammation. A similar mechanism underlies the production of viscid secretions in the biliary tract, pancreas and reproductive system. In the lung, the abnormal chloride content of lung lining fluid may lead to inactivation of small bactericidal molecules ('defensins'). Failure of these mechanisms leads to recruitment of neutrophils which destroy bacteria but which cause considerable 'innocent bystander' damage through the release of proteolytic enzymes. Much CF sputum is composed of viscid DNA from lysed neutrophils.

Diagnosis. In some areas of the United Kingdom, neonatal screening programmes for CF operate. These rely on a dried blood spot sample, collected on the 'Guthrie card' at 5 days of age, on all newborn infants. The CF screening test is performed at the same time as tests for phenylketonuria and congenital hypothyroidism. The fetal pancreas is damaged in utero leading to leakage of trypsin into the blood stream and a raised immunoreactive trypsin test. When this test is positive, further confirmation is sought by looking for the ΔF508 gene. When a diagnosis is made by screening, a sweat test should still be performed when the baby is about 6 weeks old. The sweat test detects the high levels of chloride and sodium in sweat found in CF patients and it should be performed by an experienced technician. Pilocarpine is allowed to diffuse into the skin of the child's forearm using an electric current (pilocarpine iontophoresis) and stimulates sweating via cholinergic receptors in sweat glands. The sweat is then collected on filter paper and the weight of sweat, as well as the chloride and sodium concentrations, are then calculated. At least 100 mg of sweat is needed. Results highly suggestive of CF are: concentrations of chloride and sodium of greater than 60 mmol/l and a chloride concentration greater than the sodium.

Clinical presentation. Screening for CF is not yet universal and, even with screening, cases will be missed. It is therefore important to recognise the clinical features of CF and make an early diagnosis. The commonest mode of presentation in the newborn period is meconium ileus (10–15% of CF diagnoses). This occurs when there is difficulty in passing thick, sticky meconium, leading to small bowel obstruction. The baby may present with abdominal distension and bilious vomiting. In some cases this is complicated by perforation, which may occur antenatally when peritoneal calcification is seen on abdominal X-ray.

The majority of patients with CF will have pancreatic malabsorption and this may present in infancy with failure to thrive. Stools may be pale and greasy and around 10% of children will have rectal prolapse. Late diagnosis may occur where malabsorption is missed and in the 15% of children with CF who have normal pancreatic function. Children may then present with respiratory symptoms such as troublesome wheeze in infants and productive cough in older children. In these children, diagnosis may only be made after substantial lung damage has occurred. It is therefore important to perform a sweat test in any child with chronic respiratory symptoms which are unexplained.

Presenting features of CF in 144 Nottingham patients		
Presenting feature	*<1 yr*	*>1 yr*
Neonatal screening	45	0
Meconium ileus	34	0
Respiratory symptoms	11	16
Diarrhoea and failure to thrive	22	4
Affected sibling	4	5
Rectal prolapse	2	1

CF: complications

Respiratory
Nasal polyps
Persistent wheeze
Bronchiectasis
Haemoptysis
Pneumothorax
Allergic bronchopulmary aspergillosis
Cor pulmonale

Non-respiratory
Weight loss and failure to thrive
Cirrhosis and portal hypertension
Diabetes mellitus
Distal intestinal obstruction syndrome
Fibrosing colonopathy
Rectal prolapse
Heat exhaustion
Subfertility in women
Infertility in men

Management. With early diagnosis and meticulous daily treatment, children with CF should grow and develop normally, attend school, and participate in sport or social activities. Most children will require pancreatic enzyme supplements. These come in the form of capsules ('creon' or 'pancrease') containing tiny granules of enzyme, coated to prevent activation until they reach the small intestine. Babies may need half a capsule per milk feed while older children often require up to a dozen capsules per meal. Even with good pancreatic enzyme supplementation, malabsorption may occur. In older children, partially digested material, with a high fat content may accumulate in the ascending colon causing intestinal obstruction ('distal intestinal obstruction syndrome'). Vitamin supplementation with fat-soluble vitamins (usually vitamins A and E) is routinely given. Good calorie intake is vital and so fat intake is not restricted despite the problems of fat malabsorption. Dietary supplements are often required, and in some cases nasogastric or gastrostomy feeds are necessary for normal growth.

Signs of inflammation and infection are evident in the lungs of babies with CF in the first year of life. Routine, daily chest physiotherapy is therefore started at the time of diagnosis. In infants and young children, this is by percussion and postural drainage, whereas teenagers and young adults should use a technique which gives them greater independence such as a positive end-expiratory pressure ('PEP') mask. The enzyme DNase, given by nebuliser, breaks down neutrophil derived DNA in the sputum and helps make secretions less viscid.

Physiotherapy for CF children

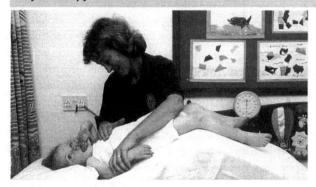

Percussion and postural drainage

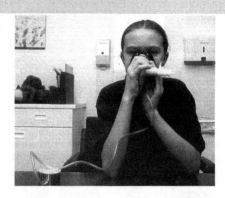

'PEP' mask physiotherapy in a teenager

Young children with CF suffer recurrent infection with *Staphylococcus aureus* and *Haemophilus influenzae* and prophylactic antibiotics against *S. aureus* are often used. Older children may acquire chronic infection with *Pseudomonas aeruginosa* which will lead to increased symptoms and will affect prognosis. If infection is detected at an early stage, chronic infection may sometimes be prevented with oral antibiotics such as ciprofloxacin and nebulised antibiotics such as colistin. Once chronic infection with *P. aeruginosa* has become established, patients may still benefit considerably from appropriate antibiotics although the infection is not eradicated. Chronic infection may also be caused by *Burkholderia cepacia*, a plant pathogen, which is transmissible between patients and resistant to most antibiotics.

As patients with CF live longer, complications other than lung disease are becoming an increasing problem. Thick secretions may lead to obstruction of the bile ducts with 'sludge' and ultimately biliary cirrhosis, portal hypertension and oesophageal varices, which may bleed. The water-soluble bile acid ursodeoxycholic acid is a promising preventative agent in CF liver disease. In older children, failure to gain weight may be the first manifestation of diabetes. Regular insulin therapy is usually required. In adult life the reproductive implications of CF become an important issue for patients and male infertility should be discussed with teenage boys. Pregnancy is no longer discouraged in women with CF but timing is important to allow intensified treatment of pulmonary infection.

The only definitive treatment of end-stage respiratory failure is lung or heart–lung transplantation. However at present the demand for donors outstrips supply and over half of patients needing transplant die on the waiting list. Gene therapy and strategies aimed at improving chloride transport offer promise but have not yet been developed into practical treatments which benefit patients. The dying patient with CF needs expert nursing and control of pain and dyspnoea. Some families will prefer to do this at home, in which case good community nursing support and involvement of the general practitioner is essential.

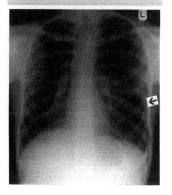

Chest radiograph of a patient with moderately severe CF lung disease showing hyperinflation and a left-sided pneumothorax

Bronchiectasis

Although CF is the commonest cause of bronchiectasis in children, the condition does occur in other groups. The bronchi in the affected area of lung are dilated and filled with purulent secretions. The child will have a productive cough. Causes include a previous lower respiratory infection, for example pertussis; recurrent aspiration due to swallowing difficulties; and lung disorders such as ciliary dyskinesia. Treatment is similar to CF with regular physiotherapy and antibiotics.

ASTHMA

Epidemiology. Asthma is reversible airways obstruction which causes intermittent wheeze. The condition is common—15% of school age children will have had at least one episode of wheeze in the last year. The prevalence of asthma in children is increasing and this may be because doctors are more willing to use the term asthma in a wheezy child. However the number of children with objective evidence of asthma, such as bronchospasm in response to histamine, has also increased, suggesting that diagnostic labelling is not the only reason for the rise. Although rates of hospital admission for asthma have been rising in the United Kingdom, this trend has now levelled off. Asthma is a heterogeneous condition. Babies who wheeze in the first 3 years of life but then improve often do not have atopic features, though they may have mothers who smoke. However children who continue to wheeze are more likely to have raised IgE levels and to have mothers who also have asthma.

Pathogenesis. The symptoms of asthma are due to spasm of smooth muscle in the bronchial wall and mucosal inflammation, with oedema and increased amounts of secretions. In the pathogenesis of asthma there are two important questions:

1. What factors lead to a child developing asthma?
2. What factors trigger an asthma attack in an asthmatic child?

Children with asthma have an increased activity of a group of T helper cells which produce cytokines such as interleukin 4, the so called 'Th2 phenotype'. Interleukin 4 encourages IgE production, which in turn allows degranulation of mast cells and release of histamine and other inflammatory mediators, which induce bronchospasm. Any factor which encourages the Th2 phenotype may lead to a child developing asthma and exposure to infections early in life may be important. As asthma symptoms become chronic, the airway structure changes so that there is more smooth muscle and there may be a poor response to bronchodilators.

In approximately 80% of primary school children a respiratory viral infection (commonly with rhinovirus) acts as the trigger to their asthma attack. Important allergen triggers include the faeces of the ubiquitous house dust mite *Dermatophagoides pteronyssimus*, pollens, fungal spores and occasionally pets. Inhaled irritants such as cigarette smoke can act as triggers and parents (and teenage patients) should be advised not to smoke. The diurnal trough in cortisol secretion in the early morning explains night-time attacks and premenstrual asthma in teenage girls may also have an endocrine basis. Problems in school or at home may explain poorly controlled asthma and this should be sought in the history.

Differential diagnosis of persistent cough and wheeze in infants

Cough
Chronic collapse
Pertussis

Cough & wheeze
Asthma
Cystic fibrosis
Gastro-oesophageal reflux
Foreign body in the airway

Wheeze
Postbronchiolitis wheeze
Bronchomalacia

Assessment. Diagnosis relies on a good history. If the child does not wheeze or the wheezing is not intermittent, consider other diagnoses. A history of night-time cough or exercise-related symptoms supports the diagnosis of asthma. Ask about atopic symptoms (such as eczema, hay fever and urticaria), whether there is a family history of asthma and about smoking. It is important to establish how disabling the symptoms are. Does the child wake at night? How many acute exacerbations has he had? How much school has he missed? Supportive evidence for the above history should then be sought by giving the parents a symptom diary and, in the school age child, asking them to record peak flow measurements at home. If the child has already been started on medication check the precise number of puffs and strength of each inhaler—this is a common source of confusion.

Management

Chronic asthma. The British Thoracic Society guidelines have been devised to encourage a stepwise approach to asthma management. The guidelines for school age children are summarised in the illustration below. Although the details differ slightly, the same steps apply broadly to the under fives.

Step 1:   Occasional use of relief bronchodilators

E.g. salbutamol, terbutaline (which act on β_2-adrenergic receptors) or ipratropium bromide (which is an anticholinergic agent). Ipratropium is commonly used in infants.

If the 'as required' medication is needed more than once per day move to step 2.

Step 2:   Regular inhaled anti-inflammatory agents.

These divide into two categories: sodium cromoglycate and the inhaled steroids, e.g. beclomethasone, budesonide and fluticasone. Sodium cromoglycate has almost no side effects but must be given 3–4 times per day. Few side effects are seen with low doses of inhaled steroids but oral candidiasis can result from drug deposition in the mouth.

Step 3:   High dose inhaled steroids or low dose inhaled steroids plus a long acting inhaled beta agonist

For most inhaled steroids 'high dose' is >400 µg/ day, though for the more potent steroids (e.g. fluticasone) the threshold is lower. Salmeterol is a long acting beta agonist which may be particularly helpful with night-time and exercise-induced symptoms.

Step 4:   High dose inhaled steroids and regular bronchodilators

A sequential trial of other medication should be tried at this point, e.g. inhaled salmeterol (if not used already on step 3), sustained release oral theophylline, regular inhaled ipratropium bromide, sustained release salbutamol tablets, sodium cromoglycate.

Stepwise approach to asthma management in school age children (adapted from the British Thoracic Society guidelines for asthma management)

Step 1 Occasional use of relief bronchodilators

Step 2 Regular inhaled anti-inflammatory agents

Step 3 High dose steroids or low dose inhaled steroids plus a long acting beta agonist

Step 4 High dose inhaled steroids and regular bronchodilators

Step 5 Addition of regular steroid tablets

Stepping down (getting better!) Review treatment every 3-6 months if control is achieved reduce treatment.

Step 5:   Addition or regular oral steroids

In combination with as required bronchodilators and high dose inhaled steroids. Whenever possible, oral steroid treatment should be for short periods only and alternate daily rather than continuous. (Adapted from the 1997 British Guidelines on Asthma Management. Thorax 1997; 52(suppl 1): S1–S21)

Step down when stability is achieved

In children under 5 years, step 5 is omitted. In step 3 salmeterol or slow release theophylline should be tried in addition to high dose inhaled steroids. Children should never take their drugs directly from a metered dose aerosol. A large volume spacer (e.g. 'volumatic' or 'nebuhaler') gives the most effective drug delivery to the lungs. Children under 2 will require a mask attached to the spacer device. Dry powder devices (e.g. 'accuhaler' and 'turbohaler') are convenient for use at school or nursery. Older children may prefer the breath-actuated devices. Inhaler technique should always be checked before moving to the next step of treatment. There is no point in trying more potent treatment if current medication is not being given effectively. Nebulisers are seldom required for prophylactic medication or for bronchodilators unless the child is very dyspnoeic.

Children should avoid known allergens. In most cases this can be assumed from the history, but skin testing may be helpful. School age children on step 3 and above of the guidelines may benefit from a self-management plan. These are usually based on peak flow measurements allowing the parent or the older child to increase their medication and treat exacerbations early.

Children using inhaler devices

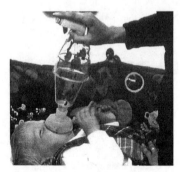 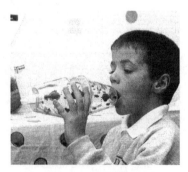 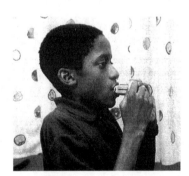

Large volume spacer with face mask in a child under 3 (note that the spacer has been tipped so that the valve is open)

Large volume spacer without the face mask in an older child

Dry powder device in a teenager

Acute asthma. Even with the best possible asthma management, exacerbations will still occur. Children often begin to improve once they are in a calm, controlled environment. Assess the child carefully and look for the following clinical signs: tachypnoea, signs of respiratory distress, cyanosis, inability to complete sentences (in a school age child), signs of dehydration. Measure oxygen saturation— if in doubt start face mask oxygen immediately.

If the child is not too dyspnoeic, and uses a large volume spacer at home, then give up to 10 puffs of salbutamol slowly via this route. Otherwise use a nebulised bronchodilator but remember nebulisers can cause transient hypoxaemia and may worsen tachycardia. If the child needs oxygen, then a bronchodilator should be nebulised via wall oxygen. Oxygen should never be stopped to allow salbutamol to be nebulised via a compressor. The frequency with which nebulisers are given varies from every 4 hours in moderate attacks to continuous nebulised treatment in severe attacks. All but the mildest cases will need treatment with oral prednisolone—usually for 3 days. Before discharge from hospital, children should be changed back to medication via aerosol and spacer and should have been stable for 24 hours. In the school age child, peak flow should be above 75% of predicted without marked fluctuations.

BIBLIOGRAPHY

British Thoracic Society, National Asthma Campaign, Royal College of Physicians of London et al 1997 The British guidelines on asthma management. 1995 review and position statement. Thorax **52**: S1–S21
Dinwiddie R 1997 Diagnosis and management of paediatric respiratory disease, 2nd edn. Churchill Livingstone, Edinburgh
Martinez F D, Wright A L, Taussig L M, Holdberg C J, Halonen M, Morgan W J 1995 Asthma and wheezing in the first 6 years of life. New England Journal of Medicine **332**: 133–138
Shale D J (ed) (1996) Cystic fibrosis. BMJ Publishing Group, London
World Health Organisation 1990 Acute respiratory infections in children: case management in small hospitals in developing countries WHO Geneva:

9 Heart

ACYANOTIC LESIONS WITH A LEFT
  TO RIGHT SHUNT
OBSTRUCTIVE LESIONS
AORTIC STENOSIS
CYANOTIC HEART DISEASE
ARRHYTHMIAS
SUBACUTE BACTERIAL
  ENDOCARDITIS
RHEUMATIC FEVER
HYPERTENSION
HYPERLIPOPROTEINAEMIA

The incidence of congenital heart disease is falling

Year	Numbers (England)	Rate per 10 000 births
1986	676	10.8
1991	432	6.5
1995	404	6.6
1996	395	6.4

Aetiology

The nine commonest congenital heart defects

Acyanotic
Ventricular septal defect
Atrial septal defect
Patent ductus arteriosus
Pulmonary stenosis
Aortic stenosis
Coarctation of the aorta
Hypoplastic left heart

Cyanotic
Transposition of the great vessels
Tetralogy of Fallot

Antenatal detection

Now that rheumatic fever is rare, congenital abnormalities have become the main cause of heart disease in children. Acquired heart disease still occurs but it is not common; congenital heart defects, however, occur in approximately 7–8 infants per 1000 live births and heart disease thus forms the commonest single group of serious congenital abnormalities. Less than a quarter of affected children will die in the first year of life, the majority within the first month. These children have severe cardiac abnormalities which, in many cases, are complex and inoperable. However, the number of children with severe lesions who are now surviving beyond the first year is increasing, a tribute to the skill and ingenuity of cardiac surgeons. Between 10 and 15% of children with congenital heart disease have more than one cardiac abnormality. Also 10–15% have an associated non-cardiac abnormality; the skeletal, gastrointestinal and genito-urinary systems are the most commonly involved. There are nine common congenital heart lesions which together make up 90% of all cases. The remaining 10% consist of numerous rarer, more complex anomalies.

As with most congenital defects, the precise aetiology is unknown but both genetic and environmental factors have been identified. Family studies suggest that the mode of inheritance is polygenic, although occasionally single gene mutations occur. If a mother has a child with a congenital heart defect, the chances of a second child being affected are about three times higher than if her child had no heart defect. Children with chromosomal abnormalities have a greatly increased incidence of congenital heart disease; nearly half of all children with Down syndrome have a cardiac lesion. Maternal rubella in the first trimester of pregnancy, maternal diabetes and drugs in pregnancy (like thalidomide, alcohol, phenytoin) are environmental factors associated with an increased incidence of congenital heart disease.

Severe congenital heart disease can be detected at 16–18 weeks' gestation by fetal echocardiography. Increasingly, this is being used as a screening test for severe heart abnormalities but it is particularly useful in the case of families where a previous baby has had a heart abnormality.

Presentation

Congenital heart disease usually presents in one of the three following ways.

Heart murmur. This is the commonest mode of presentation. Most murmurs are detected in the first year of life, either on routine examination in the newborn period or in the child health clinics. A minority are not discovered until the child starts school or on coincidental examination.

Heart failure. A number of lesions will cause heart failure, commonly in the first year of life. The symptoms and signs are similar to those found in an adult. The baby becomes breathless, particularly after the exertion of feeding or crying. He may have difficulty completing feeds and as a consequence fails to thrive. Sweating is often a prominent symptom. On examination, the baby has a rapid respiratory rate and a rapid pulse rate. Heart enlargement is usually present and can be detected clinically; a thrill or murmur may be present and there is often a gallop rhythm due to a third heart sound. Invariably the liver is enlarged due to venous congestion. Oedema of the dependent parts of the body is rarely seen. Fine moist sounds of pulmonary oedema are less easily heard in babies than in adults. If frank pulmonary oedema is present, the baby may be centrally cyanosed and the cyanosis will disappear when oxygen is given.

Heart failure in infancy

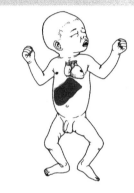

Symptoms
breathlessness on exertion
(especially feeding and crying)
sweating
failure to thrive
Signs
rapid breathing
rapid heart rate
enlarged heart
murmur
enlarged liver

Cyanosis ('blue baby'). If the heart defect results in unsaturated venous blood bypassing the lungs, central cyanosis will be present and is not corrected while breathing 100% oxygen. This lack of response to oxygen helps to distinguish cyanosis due to heart disease from cyanosis due to severe lung disease, especially in the newborn period when this distinction can be difficult. Longstanding central cyanosis results in clubbing of the fingers and toes and secondary polycythaemia. A child with cyanotic congenital heart disease often has a reduced exercise tolerance and fails to grow normally.

Investigations

Investigations must be carried out urgently in symptomatic infants. A chest X-ray and electrocardiogram are useful investigations in the assessment of a child with suspected heart disease. Echocardiography using ultrasound is a non-invasive investigation which gives detailed information about the anatomy of the heart and great vessels. The additional use of Doppler ultrasound provides haemodynamic information. Almost all lesions which cause heart failure or cyanosis in infancy, and many of those which produce a murmur, can be confidently diagnosed by echocardiography. Cardiac catheterisation is an invasive investigation, only performed in specialist units; it enables the pressures and saturations within the cardiac chambers to be measured and, with angiocardiography following injection of radio-opaque dye, permits precise anatomical and physiological diagnosis. As a diagnostic tool it has largely been replaced by echocardiography but it is particularly useful for the therapy of certain lesions which previously could only be treated surgically.

The innocent murmur

Many babies and children have heart murmurs without any structural abnormality of the heart. Indeed, in one reported series, a cardiologist detected a heart murmur in the majority of healthy school children on routine examination! Such murmurs are termed innocent, or functional. They are diagnosed as being innocent on the basis of their characteristics and are associated with a normal chest X-ray, cardiac ultrasound and ECG. If a murmur is obviously innocent, no follow up is necessary. If there is uncertainty an expert opinion should be sought as soon as possible, before the seeds of cardiac neurosis are sown. There are three types of innocent murmur:

Innocent murmurs
- venous hum
- pulmonary flow murmur
- vibratory murmur

Venous hum. This is a blowing, continuous murmur heard at the base of the heart, often just below the clavicles. It varies both with respiration and the position of the head, and disappears when the child lies down. It is due to blood flow through the systemic great veins and is sometimes confused with a patent ductus arteriosus.

Pulmonary flow murmur. This is a soft, systolic ejection murmur heard in the pulmonary area (the second left intercostal space). It is due to rapid flow of blood across a normal pulmonary valve and is especially prominent when the cardiac output is high, for example after exercise, in febrile children or in cases of anaemia.

Vibratory murmur. This is a short, buzzing murmur heard in systole at the left sternal edge or at the apex of the heart. It is variable and changes with position.

If a murmur is pansystolic, diastolic, loud or long, associated with a thrill or with cardiac symptoms, it is not innocent.

Congenital heart disease can conveniently be classified into two groups:

1. Acyanotic due to either a left to right shunt or obstructive lesion.
2. Cyanotic with either increased or diminished pulmonary flow.

ACYANOTIC LESIONS WITH A LEFT TO RIGHT SHUNT

A common type of congenital heart defect is a hole between the two sides of the heart, at the level of either the atria, the ventricles or the great arteries. In fetal life, pulmonary blood flow is small and the pressures in the right ventricle and pulmonary artery are high. With the onset of regular respirations, the pulmonary vascular resistance falls, with a consequent fall in the pressures on the right side of the heart. Since the pressure on the left side of the heart now exceeds that on the right side, blood will start to flow from the left side to the right side through the hole. The fall in pulmonary vascular resistance occurs rapidly in the first few days after birth and then more slowly over the next few weeks, so that by the age of about 3 months the left to right flow of blood reaches a maximum. There is therefore an additional circulation of blood from the left side of the heart to the right side, thence to the lungs and back to the left side of the heart again. This is termed a shunt. If the hole is small, the shunt may be trivial, but if it is large, it may represent the majority of the cardiac output, so that the blood flow through the pulmonary artery may be several times greater than the flow through the aorta. A large shunt imposes an added burden on the heart, with consequent hypertrophy, dilatation and sometimes failure. Because of the high pulmonary vascular resistance immediately after birth, frequently a murmur is not heard and in babies with a simple left to right shunt, heart failure is uncommon in the first few weeks of life.

A left to right shunt, if appreciable, will give rise to a number of consistent findings, regardless of the site of the hole. Clinical examination may show an enlarged heart with hypertrophy of one or both ventricles. Signs of ventricular hypertrophy will be present on the electrocardiogram. A chest radiograph will reveal an enlarged heart with a prominent pulmonary artery and an increase in vascular markings (pulmonary plethora) due to the high pulmonary blood flow.

ATRIAL SEPTAL DEFECT (OSTIUM SECUNDUM)

In the majority of atrial septal defects, the hole is in the atrial septum in the region of the fossa ovalis, the site of the foramen ovale: this is the ostium secundum defect. Because the right ventricle is less muscular and easier to fill with blood than the left ventricle, blood will flow from the left atrium to the right atrium through the defect, thence to the right ventricle and the lungs. The right side of the heart therefore takes the whole of the added burden of the shunt.

Natural history. Symptoms are rare in infancy and uncommon in childhood, even if the shunt is large. However in the third or fourth decade, heart failure, pulmonary hypertension or atrial arrhythmias may occur.

Clinical features. Because symptoms are unusual in childhood, most children with atrial septal defects present with a heart murmur. The murmur is often quite soft and frequently not detected until the child is at school. If symptoms do occur, they are of breathlessness or tiredness on exertion, or recurrent chest infections.

Atrial septal defects

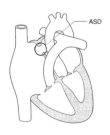

Examination. The child is well, pink and has normal pulses. The right ventricle may be easily felt. There is a systolic murmur at the second left interspace. This is due not to flow of blood across the defect, but to a high flow of blood across a normal pulmonary valve. If the shunt is large, a mid-diastolic tricuspid flow murmur may be heard too. The aortic and pulmonary components of the second sound are widely separated because the excessive filling of the right ventricle delays closure of the pulmonary valve. Furthermore, the time interval between these two sounds does not vary with respiration ('fixed splitting') because the two atria function as a single unit and respiration affects them both equally.

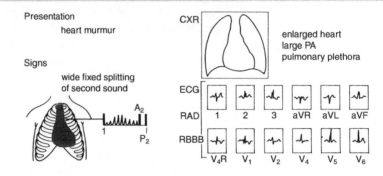

Presentation, examination and investigation of atrial septal defect

Presentation
    heart murmur

Signs
    wide fixed splitting
    of second sound

CXR — enlarged heart, large PA, pulmonary plethora

ECG — RAD, RBBB

Investigations. The chest X-ray shows cardiomegaly with prominent atrium and pulmonary artery, and pulmonary plethora. The electrocardiogram shows right axis deviation, right ventricular hypertrophy and in most cases right bundle branch block. The diagnosis is confirmed by echocardiography.

Treatment. If the defect is moderate or large, closure is advisable, using cardiopulmonary bypass. Repair is by simple suture or by insertion of a patch of pericardium. Occlusion of the defect with a device passed by cardiac catheter is now being practised.

ATRIAL SEPTAL DEFECT (OSTIUM PRIMUM)

Although less common than secundum defects, ostium primum defects are more serious. The hole is situated low down in the atrial septum and represents a failure of development of the septum primum in fetal life. The defect is just above the atrioventricular valves, and usually extends to the insertion of the anterior leaflet of the mitral valve, so that the latter is cleft and frequently incompetent. An ostium primum atrial septal defect represents the mild end of the spectrum of developmental abnormalities involving the central portion of the heart, atrioventricular septal defects. In the most severe form, the defect extends from the atrial septum, through the origin of both atrioventricular valves into the ventricular septum. This is described as an atrioventricular canal defect and gives rise to a large left to right shunt and both mitral and tricuspid incompetence. The atrioventricular septal defects are particularly common in children with Down syndrome.

Clinical features. Heart failure commonly develops in infancy and childhood and there is a high mortality without surgery. The development of severe pulmonary hypertension is common, especially in Down syndrome. There are commonly signs of heart failure with marked cardiac enlargement. The child is often breathless at rest, with deformities of the lower ribs (Harrison's sulci). He is pink, with normal pulses. Clinically, the heart is large with increased activity of both ventricles. In addition to the auscultatory signs of an atrial septal defect there may be an apical pansystolic murmur signifying mitral regurgitation.

Investigations. The chest X-ray shows marked cardiomegaly, prominent pulmonary arteries and pulmonary plethora. The electrocardiogram is frequently diagnostic, showing left axis deviation and right bundle branch block. Catheterisation is required to assess the size of the shunt and the degree of mitral incompetence.

Treatment. Early surgery is usually advised for children with ostium primum defects. The defect is closed and the cleft mitral valve repaired. It is a more difficult and risky operation than that for a secundum defect.

VENTRICULAR SEPTAL DEFECT

This is the commonest of all congenital heart lesions. Usually a single defect is found in the membranous portion of the ventricular septum, adjacent to the tricuspid valve, or below the aortic valve. Less commonly, single or multiple defects are found in the muscular part of the septum. In 25–30% of affected children other heart defects are also present.

Natural history. There are four possibilities:

1. The hole may close spontaneously. This occurs in perhaps as many as 50% of cases, usually in early childhood but sometimes in later childhood, adolescence or adult life.
2. The hole may remain the same size. Since the heart is growing throughout childhood, the defect becomes relatively smaller.
3. Stenosis of the outflow tract of the right ventricle (the infundibulum) may occur. This raises the pressure in the right ventricle and steadily reduces the size of the left to right shunt. Eventually the shunt may reverse and the child will become cyanosed. The child in effect develops Fallot's tetralogy.
4. Progressive pulmonary hypertension may develop. If the left to right shunt is large, the torrential pulmonary blood flow may irreversibly damage the smaller pulmonary vessels, giving rise to pulmonary hypertension. This makes the defect inoperable and considerably reduces the child's life span. It is rarely seen with isolated ventricular septal defects.

Clinical presentation depends on the size of the defect and whether pulmonary hypertension is present.

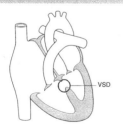

Ventricular septal defect

VSD

Small ventricular septal defect

Since the shunt through the defect is small, the child is symptom free and the heart murmur is often picked up on routine examination. The child is well, pink and has normal pulses, and the heart is not enlarged. Frequently there is a thrill at the lower left sternal border. On auscultation a harsh, pansystolic murmur is heard at the same site due to flow of blood through the defect. The heart sounds are normal.

Investigations. The chest X-ray and electrocardiogram are usually normal. The defect can be identified with Doppler echocardiography.

Treatment. There is a risk of bacterial endocarditis and antibiotic prophylaxis is therefore necessary at the time of dental extractions, etc.

Moderate ventricular septal defect

Symptoms usually occur in infancy, with breathlessness on feeding and crying, failure to thrive and recurrent chest infections. As the child gets older, the symptoms tend to improve and may disappear altogether, because of actual or relative closure of the defect.

Examination. The baby is breathless at rest but is pink, with normal pulses. The heart is enlarged clinically with prominent activity of both ventricles. There is a systolic thrill at the lower left sternal border. On auscultation there is a loud, harsh pansystolic murmur, maximal at this site but heard all over the chest. There is frequently an apical mid-diastolic murmur, caused by an increased flow of blood across a normal mitral valve. The second heart sound is noticeably split and the pulmonary component may be louder than normal.

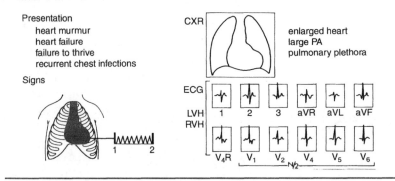

Clinical features of ventricular septal defect

Investigations. The chest X-ray shows cardiomegaly, prominent pulmonary arteries and pulmonary plethora. The electrocardiogram shows biventricular hypertrophy, since both ventricles are involved in the shunt. The defect can be seen on echocardiography.

Treatment. If symptoms are prominent, diuretics should be given. Surgery should be avoided because of the tendency to spontaneous improvement. Exceptions are continuing symptoms and the development of pulmonary hypertension.

FREE RETURN POSTAGE FOR STUDENTS & FY DOCTORS!

Use this label for the **FREE** return of books to the BMA Library

BMA Library

Freepost RTKJ-RKSZ-JGHG
British Medical Association
PO Box 291
LONDON
WC1H 9TG

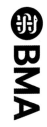

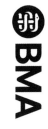

BMA

BMA Library

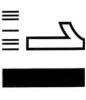

Freepost RTKJ-RKSZ-JGHG
British Medical Association
PO Box 291
LONDON
WC1H 9TG

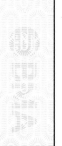

Large ventricular septal defect

When the pulmonary vascular resistance falls to its lowest level at about 3 months of age, the shunt through a large defect is great and results in heart failure. Symptoms of breathlessness on feeding usually start earlier than this and sweating is very common. Affected babies may be severely ill with congestive cardiac failure, and they have an increased tendency to chest infections which often precipitate episodes of failure.

Examination. The baby is usually underweight, breathless and ill. If there is frank pulmonary oedema, cyanosis will be present. The heart is large clinically with increased ventricular activity and a systolic thrill. Signs of heart failure will be present. On auscultation, there is a harsh systolic murmur which is caused by increased flow across the pulmonary valve. A pulmonary systolic ejection and a mitral mid-diastolic flow murmur are usually heard and the pulmonary second sound is loud.

Investigation. The chest X-ray shows very marked cardiomegaly, large pulmonary arteries and pulmonary plethora. The electrocardiogram shows biventricular hypertrophy. Echocardiography will display the defect but catheterisation is sometimes carried out to measure the size of the shunt and the pulmonary artery pressure.

Treatment. The initial treatment is medical. The infant in heart failure is nursed in a semi-sitting position. Diuretics (usually frusemide or a thiazide) are given, together with potassium supplements or a potassium sparing diuretic such as spironolactone. The success of treatment can be gauged by regular weighing and by recording the size of the liver.

As the heart failure responds to treatment there will be a rapid weight loss and a progressive decrease in liver size. If the baby does not respond to treatment, surgical closure is necessary as a single stage operation, using cardiopulmonary bypass. An alternative method of surgical treatment is to place a constricting band around the base of the pulmonary artery, thus reducing the size of the shunt.

A second operation is required to remove the band and close the defect.

PATENT DUCTUS ARTERIOSUS

Patent ductus arteriosus

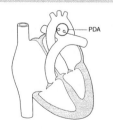

This is a common congenital heart lesion, either singly or in combination with other heart defects. It is more common in girls, in children whose mothers had rubella in early pregnancy and in babies who are born prematurely. In fetal life the ductus arteriosus, which is a large vessel with a muscular wall, diverts blood from the right ventricle and pulmonary artery into the descending aorta. Within 24 hours of birth, it closes in response to oxygenated blood. Spontaneous closure of a ductus arteriosus which remains patent after the first few days of life is unlikely, except in the premature baby in whom closure of the ductus may still occur at any time up to the expected date of delivery. As the pulmonary vascular resistance falls after birth, a left to right shunt of blood from the aorta to the pulmonary artery occurs through the ductus (the opposite direction to the flow in fetal life).

Small ductus

The child is symptom free and a heart murmur is detected routinely or coincidentally. He is pink with normal pulses. On auscultation there is a loud, continuous murmur heard best below the left clavicle. The murmur extends through systole into diastole because the pressure in the pulmonary artery is lower than that in the aorta throughout the whole cardiac cycle. It has a rough 'machinery' quality.

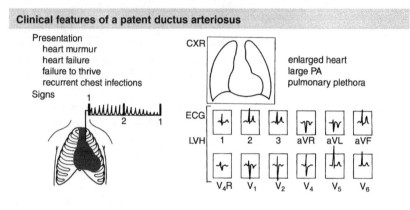

Clinical features of a patent ductus arteriosus

Investigations. Chest X-ray and electrocardiogram are normal. Echocardiography with Doppler demonstrates the duct.

Treatment. Closure is recommended because of the cumulative risk of bacterial endocarditis. The duct can be surgically ligated. Alternatively, it can be occluded by means of an umbrella device which is placed in the duct by cardiac catheter.

Large ductus

The severity of symptoms is related to the size of the shunt. The child may be underweight with a reduced exercise tolerance and increased tendency to chest infections. At the other end of the spectrum, severe heart failure may develop in infancy. On examination the child is often small and thin. An increased respiratory rate is common. There is no cyanosis, but the pulses are easily felt, being full and collapsing in nature. The diastolic blood pressure is low and pulse pressure is wide. The heart is enlarged clinically with a prominent left ventricle and there is a systolic thrill in the pulmonary area. On auscultation, there is a harsh systolic murmur which may extend through the second sound into early diastole. The length of the murmur depends on the pulmonary artery pressure. This is high in large shunts so that blood only flows from left to right during systole. The pulmonary second sound is loud. A mitral (mid-diastolic) flow murmur may be heard.

Investigations. The chest X-ray shows the typical features of a left-to-right shunt. The electrocardiogram shows left ventricular hypertrophy. The diagnosis is confirmed by echocardiography.

Natural history. If the duct is small, the only risk to the patient is from bacterial endocarditis, or more accurately, endoarteritis. This is appreciable. If the duct is larger, heart failure may occur in infancy, or may occur for the first time in adult life. Pulmonary hypertension and shunt reversal can occur.

Treatment. If heart failure is present, medical treatment is necessary. Ligation or catheter occlusion should be carried out as soon as the child's condition allows.

PULMONARY HYPERTENSION

A large left to right shunt with a high pulmonary blood flow may produce an elevation of pulmonary artery pressure simply because of the increased flow (hyperdynamic pulmonary hypertension). Following surgical closure of the defect, the pulmonary artery pressure returns to normal. Persisting high pulmonary blood flow may result in permanent damage to the smaller pulmonary vessels with consequent narrowing and irreversible pulmonary hypertension. If the defect is closed under these circumstances, the pulmonary artery pressure remains elevated. When the pulmonary artery pressure reaches systemic levels the left to right shunt ceases and may actually reverse.

Clinical features. The child becomes mildly cyanosed, with clubbed fingers and toes, but otherwise may appear remarkably well. However, exercise tolerance is usually reduced. On examination, the right ventricular impulse is prominent, and the pulmonary second sound is palpable. On auscultation there is usually a systolic ejection murmur in the pulmonary area (caused by blood flow through the huge pulmonary artery, not through the shunt), and sometimes an early diastolic murmur signifying pulmonary incompetence. The pulmonary component of the second sound is very loud.

Investigations. A chest X-ray shows an enlarged heart with a prominent right atrium. The pulmonary artery is greatly increased in size but its smaller branches are not seen. The electrocardiogram shows right axis deviation, right atrial hypertrophy and right ventricular hypertrophy. Cardiac catheterisation is needed to demonstrate the site of the shunt and to measure the pulmonary artery pressure.

The development of severe, irreversible pulmonary hypertension as a result of a large left to right shunt is called the Eisenmenger syndrome. Although it was originally described in association with a ventricular septal defect (Eisenmenger complex), it may occur with a left to right shunt at any site. It is particularly likely to occur in cases of large ventricular septal defects, atrioventricular canal defects and transposition of the great arteries where there is a large shunt. No surgical correction is possible and the life expectancy of affected children is considerably reduced. Heart–lung transplantation may be an option although success with this procedure is currently disappointing.

OBSTRUCTIVE LESIONS

The commonest examples are aortic stenosis, coarctation of the aorta and pulmonary stenosis. The chamber of the heart proximal to the obstruction hypertrophies in an attempt to overcome it. If the obstruction is severe, heart failure may result.

AORTIC STENOSIS

This is a common congenital heart lesion which may occur in isolation or in combination with other heart defects. In the majority of cases the aortic valve itself is narrowed by congenital deformity. The deformed valve may be bicuspid instead of tricuspid and the cusps are frequently fused at the edges. The degree of stenosis may worsen as the child gets older, with thickening and calcification of the cusps. A bicuspid aortic valve may open normally in childhood, but become thickened and narrowed in adult life. If the aortic valve is particularly narrowed and rigid, a degree of aortic incompetence is common too.

Occasionally, aortic obstruction may be above or below the aortic valve. In supravalvular stenosis, the ascending aorta above the valve is narrowed. This is often associated with an unusual facial appearance, mental handicap and hypercalcaemia in infancy (Williams syndrome). In subvalvular aortic stenosis, there may be a fibrous or muscular diaphragm below the valve obstructing the flow of blood from the left ventricle to aorta, or there may be excessive hypertrophy of the left ventricle and interventricular septum which obstructs the outflow tract of the left ventricle during systole (hypertrophic obstructive cardiomyopathy, HOCM).

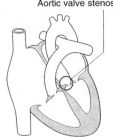

Aortic stenosis

Aortic valve stenosis

Clinical features. Severe aortic stenosis may cause heart failure in infancy. In less severe cases a heart murmur is detected routinely.

A minority of older children with severe aortic stenosis may feel faint or dizzy on exertion, and lose consciousness. This is an indication for urgent treatment. Bacterial endocarditis is a complication of aortic stenosis of any degree.

Examination. The child appears well and is pink. The pulses are often small in volume and slow rising. The systolic blood pressure may be low. On palpation, the left ventricle is prominent and a thrill may be palpable at the lower left sternal border, in the suprasternal notch and in the neck over the carotid arteries. On auscultation there is a systolic ejection murmur heard at the apex and lower left sternal edge, which is conducted upwards into the neck. There is usually an ejection click immediately before the murmur. The aortic second sound is soft and delayed. If the stenosis is severe the aortic second sound may actually occur later than the pulmonary component so that there is reversed (paradoxical) splitting of the second sound with respiration.

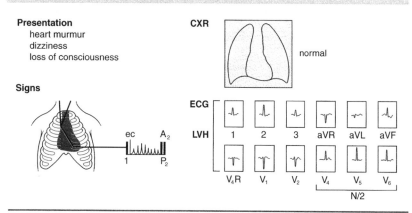

Clinical features of aortic valve stenosis. ec = ejection click

Presentation
    heart murmur
    dizziness
    loss of consciousness

Signs

Investigations. A chest X-ray may show a prominent left ventricle with post-stenotic dilatation of the ascending aorta. An electrocardiogram shows varying degrees of left ventricular hypertrophy relating to the severity of the stenosis. The aortic valve gradient can be measured by Doppler ultrasound.

Treatment. If echocardiography shows a gradient across the aortic valve greater than 40 mmHg, cardiac catheterisation is necessary to confirm the findings. The stenosis can be relieved by balloon valvuloplasty—with a catheter tip passing through the aortic valve from the femoral artery, a balloon is inflated to widen the stenosed valve. If this is unsuccessful or the aortic stenosis is severe, an open aortic valvotomy is necessary. Residual stenosis and incompetence are common, but aortic valve replacement is avoided where possible until children have stopped growing. Aortic stenosis is the one congenital heart lesion in which strenuous activity should be avoided because of the risk of sudden death. Prevention of bacterial endocarditis is important.

COARCTATION OF THE AORTA

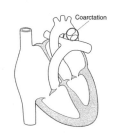

Coarctation of the aorta

This is a localised narrowing of the descending aorta, close to the site of the ductus arteriosus and usually distal to the left subclavian artery. Arterial blood bypasses the obstruction reaching the lower part of the body through collateral vessels which become greatly enlarged. The left ventricle hypertrophies to overcome the obstruction and heart failure may result. The systolic blood pressure in the upper part of the body is usually elevated.

Clinical presentation. If the narrowing is severe, heart failure may occur in the first few weeks of life. In most cases, however, the diagnosis is made on routine or coincidental examination, either because a murmur is heard, or the femoral pulses cannot be felt or because of the discovery of hypertension. Occasionally, a child or adult may present with a complication such as a subarachnoid haemorrhage from rupture of an intracranial aneurysm or bacterial endarteritis.

Examination. The child is well and pink. The brachial and radial pulses are normal but the femoral pulses are either absent or weak and delayed. There is usually systemic hypertension and the left ventricle may be prominent. On auscultation, a systolic ejection murmur is usually heard over the left side of the chest, especially at the back. Collateral arteries are often palpable over the scapulae.

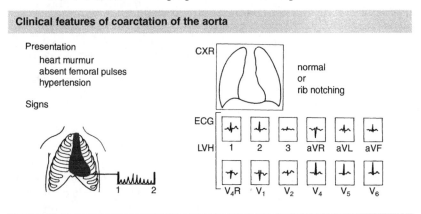

Clinical features of coarctation of the aorta

Presentation
heart murmur
absent femoral pulses
hypertension

Signs

CXR
normal
or
rib notching

ECG
LVH   1   2   3   aVR   aVL   aVF
V₄R   V₁   V₂   V₄   V₅   V₆

Investigations. A chest X-ray may show a prominent left ventricle. In older children rib notching may be seen where the enlarged intercostal arteries have eroded the underside of the ribs. An electrocardiogram may show left ventricular hypertrophy.

Treatment. Surgery is recommended in all but the mildest cases and should be carried out soon after the diagnosis is made. The narrowed segment of aorta is resected and the two ends sewn together. In infants, the proximal portion of the left subclavian artery can be used to widen the aorta (subclavian flap aortoplasty). Early surgery is more effective in correcting the hypertension but as the child grows there is a risk that relative narrowing at the site of the coarctation will occur again. This is treated by balloon dilatation.

HYPOPLASTIC LEFT HEART

In this condition, the left ventricle is underdeveloped, frequently with hypoplasia or atresia of the mitral valve, aortic valve and arch of the aorta. The ductus arteriosus is patent and blood therefore bypasses the left-sided obstruction. Affected babies present in the first few days after birth with severe heart failure when the ductus closes. They are pale and shocked, with very weak pulses. Diagnosis is made by echocardiography. Unfortunately this is a relatively common condition. No curative surgery is possible although heroic palliative surgery may offer the possibility of survival and the option of later heart transplantation. Symptomatic relief is important to relieve the distress of acute heart failure. Death occurs within days or weeks. Increasingly the condition is being recognised in pregnancy by routine fetal echocardiography.

PULMONARY STENOSIS

Pulmonary stenosis

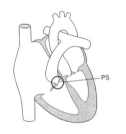

In this condition the pulmonary valve is congenitally deformed, thickened and narrowed. The right ventricle hypertrophies in an attempt to overcome the obstruction. The muscular outflow tract of the right ventricle, the infundibulum, also hypertrophies and this may increase the degree of obstruction.

Clinical presentation. If the stenosis is severe, the infant presents with right-sided heart failure. There may be cyanosis from a right to left shunt of blood through the foramen ovale. In mild and moderate cases a heart murmur is heard on routine examination. Symptoms are rare in childhood. However, in cases of moderate stenosis, dysfunction of the right ventricle and arrhythmias are liable to occur in adult life.

Examination. In mild to moderate cases the child is well, pink and has normal pulses. The right ventricle is heaving and a systolic thrill is palpable in the pulmonary area. On auscultation, there is usually an ejection click followed by a systolic ejection murmur caused by blood flowing across the narrowed valve. The murmur is heard in the upper part of the left chest anteriorly and is conducted to the back. The pulmonary component of the second sound becomes softer and more delayed as the stenosis increases.

Clinical features of pulmonary valve stenosis

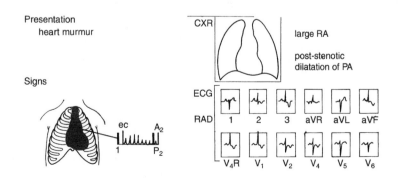

Investigations. A chest X-ray shows post-stenotic dilatation of the pulmonary artery. An enlarged right atrium and right ventricle are seen in severe cases. An electrocardiogram shows varying degrees of right axis deviation, right atrial hypertrophy and right ventricular hypertrophy, according to the severity of the stenosis. The pulmonary valve gradient is measured by Doppler ultrasound.

Treatment. If the Doppler gradient across the valve exceeds 40–50 mmHg cardiac catheterisation with balloon valvuloplasty is carried out. This is highly successful—the narrowing is reduced by 75% or more and does not usually recur.

CYANOTIC HEART DISEASE

A minority of babies or children with congenital heart disease are centrally cyanosed because unsaturated blood is bypassing the lungs. An affected child may be quite well at rest, even though he may be very blue. However, when the body's demand for oxygen increases during exercise, he becomes very easily tired and breathless. Even though the arterial oxygen saturation may be very low, the child's intelligence is usually normal. Secondary polycythaemia follows chronic hypoxia. This is to the child's advantage at first because it increases the amount of oxygen that can be transported in the blood. However, when the packed cell volume exceeds a certain limit, the viscosity of the blood increases with a resultant tendency to thrombosis, particularly in cerebral vessels. Bacteria in the systemic veins bypass the pulmonary capillaries and enter the arterial system. Cerebral abscesses are therefore a well described complication. Cyanotic heart disease can be subdivided into two types. In the first type the lungs are underperfused as blood shunts from right to left bypassing the lungs. Tetralogy of Fallot is the commonest example. In the second type, the lungs are normally filled or even over-perfused with blood, but cyanosis results because there is inadequate mixing of the systemic and pulmonary circulations. Transposition of the great arteries is the commonest example.

TETRALOGY OF FALLOT

The two essential features of this condition are a large ventricular septal defect, usually sited high up in the membranous part of the septum beneath the aortic valve, and stenosis of the pulmonary valve or infundibulum. There is therefore resistance to the flow of blood through the pulmonary valve with a consequent shunt of blood from the right to left ventricle and thence to the aorta. In fact, as the septal defect is just below the aortic valve, the aorta appears to override the

Fallot tetralogy

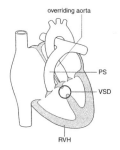

right ventricle and the shunt is directly from the right ventricle to the aorta. Pulmonary or infundibular stenosis leads to right ventricular hypertrophy. The overriding of the aorta and right ventricular hypertrophy, in combination with the ventricular septal defect and pulmonary stenosis, make up the tetralogy originally described by Fallot. The main pulmonary artery is small and in the most severe cases may not be patent (pulmonary atresia with a ventricular septal defect).

Clinical features. Affected children are usually pink in the newborn period, though a heart murmur due to blood flow through a narrow infundibulum or pulmonary valve may be detected. Cyanosis develops and increases over the next few weeks or months. Sometimes the baby may be quite pink when at rest, only becoming cyanosed with the exertion of crying or feeding. Sometimes cyanotic 'attacks' or 'spells' occur. An affected baby is relatively well most of the time but is prone to attacks during which he becomes extremely cyanosed and pale often with loss of consciousness. Such spells result from increased infundibular narrowing and reduced systemic vascular resistance, increasing the right to left shunt and preventing blood from reaching the lungs. As the child becomes older, cyanosis at rest becomes more obvious, exercise tolerance is reduced and the typical squatting may occur. The latter is a manoeuvre to gain symptomatic relief after exercise in which the child squats down on his haunches with his knees up to his chest. This traps unsaturated venous blood in the legs preventing it from returning to the heart and also raises systemic pressure by obstructing the femoral arteries, with a consequent reduction in size of the right to left shunt.

Heart failure is extremely rare in tetralogy of Fallot but the thromboembolic complications of polycythaemia, bacterial endocarditis and cerebral abscess may occur.

Examination. The affected child may be cyanosed at rest with clubbing of the fingers and toes. The heart is not enlarged clinically but the right ventricle is easily felt and there may be a systolic thrill in the pulmonary area. On auscultation, there is a systolic ejection murmur in the pulmonary

Clinical features of tetralogy of Fallot

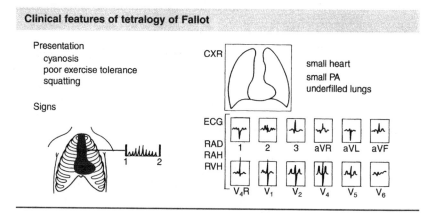

area and a single second heart sound. No murmur arises from blood flow through the septal defect because the pressures in the two ventricles are similar.

Investigations. The chest X-ray shows a normal size heart with the apex above the left diaphragm but the left heart border is concave because the main pulmonary artery is small and the heart is said to look like a boot. The lung fields are oligaemic. The electrocardiogram shows right axis deviation, right atrial hypertrophy and right ventricular hypertrophy. The diagnosis is made by echocardiography.

Treatment. This is surgical in all cases. Symptomatic infants require a palliative shunt to improve their symptoms until they are old enough for a total correction. A shunt operation is the creation of a communication between the pulmonary and systemic circulation (an artificial ductus arteriosus). The most commonly performed type is the modified Blalock procedure where a tube of Goretex is used to connect the subclavian and the pulmonary arteries on either the left or right side. After the age of 6 months, a total correction is carried out using cardiopulmonary bypass—the hole is closed and the pulmonary valve and infundibulum are widened. Results of surgery are excellent.

TRANSPOSITION OF THE GREAT ARTERIES

In this heart lesion, the aorta and pulmonary artery are 'transposed' so that the aorta arises from the right ventricle and the pulmonary artery from the left ventricle. This means that there are two isolated circulations, pulmonary and systemic, working in parallel. Obviously this is not compatible with life—there must be some mixing between the two circulations. In fetal life, the baby is in no difficulty because the pulmonary blood flow is very small. After birth however, as the ductus arteriosus and foramen ovale begin to close, progressive cyanosis develops. The severity of the symptoms depends on the degree of mixing of the two circulations through these fetal channels. In some cases, a large ventricular septal defect or a large patent ductus arteriosus may be present, in which case there is a high pulmonary blood flow and only slight cyanosis. In the simple form however, progressive cyanosis develops in the first hours or days after birth. Without treatment, few children survive the first year of life.

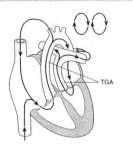

Transposition

Clinical features. Progressive cyanosis develops within the first few hours or days of life. The affected baby becomes increasingly blue. Breathlessness and heart failure may follow.

Examination. Cyanosis is the major physical sign and persists even if the baby is given 100% oxygen. There are usually no heart murmurs but the second sound is loud because the transposed aorta lies anteriorly, close to the chest wall.

Clinical features of transposition of the great arteries

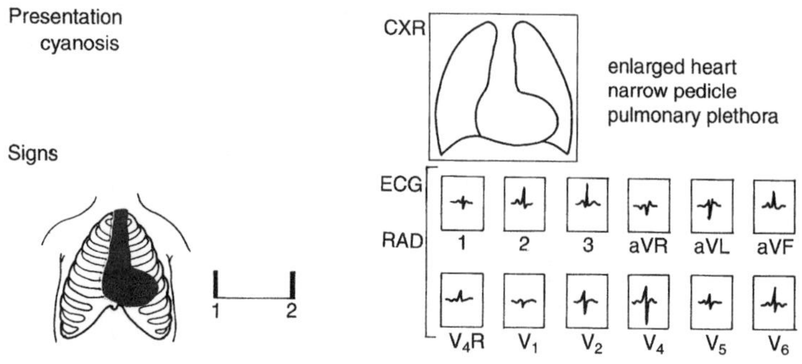

Presentation
cyanosis

Signs

CXR — enlarged heart
narrow pedicle
pulmonary plethora

ECG
RAD   1   2   3   aVR   aVL   aVF
V₄R   V₁   V₂   V₄   V₅   V₆

Investigations. The chest X-ray is often typical. The heart is slightly enlarged and is said to look like an egg lying on its side. The vascular pedicle of the heart is narrow because the aorta and pulmonary artery lie one in front of the other. The lung fields are normally filled or plethoric. Diagnosis is made by echocardiography.

Treatment. A communication between the systemic and pulmonary circuits is urgently needed. It is created by means of a balloon atrial septostomy (Rashkind procedure). A special double lumen catheter is passed via the umbilical vein, inferior vena cava, right atrium and foramen ovale into the left atrium. A balloon near the catheter tip is inflated with contrast medium and catheter and balloon are then pulled sharply back through the atrial septum, tearing it and creating a large septal defect. This allows mixing of blood and improves the cyanosis.

The definitive corrective operation is an anatomical repair, in which the pulmonary artery and aorta are switched to their rightful ventricles. It is usually carried out in the first week or two of life.

CARDIAC ARRHYTHMIAS

Children often have cardiac arrhythmias which are of no clinical significance; sinus arrhythmia is the most common example. A number, however, have symptoms which are a direct result of an abnormality of heart rhythm.

Paroxysmal supra-ventricular tachycardia

This is a regular, rapid rhythm at the rate of 180–300 beats per minute. It is caused by impulses from the atrioventricular (AV) node re-entering the atria either within the AV node itself or via an accessory pathway and thus exciting the AV node prematurely. Since the heart rate is so rapid, diastolic filling of the ventricles is impaired and cardiac failure arises. The younger the patient, the faster the heart rate in supraventricular tachycardia (SVT), the less well it is tolerated and the earlier heart failure develops. The tachycardia is paroxysmal and frequently recurs. A minority of children with this disorder have an underlying cardiac defect, either congenital or acquired.

Clinical features. Paroxysmal tachycardia may be noted in utero or occur at any time in infancy, childhood or adult life. As the heart rate suddenly becomes rapid, the baby may go pale, start to breathe quickly and vomit. After a few hours, symptoms of heart failure occur and death may occasionally result. Older children tolerate SVT more readily and can usually recognise its onset by describing palpitations. Paroxysms may occur spontaneously or be precipitated by illness. Return to sinus rhythm produces a diuresis.

Examination. The child looks pale but may be otherwise well. A baby is more likely to show signs of heart failure. The pulse is very rapid, regular and weak. It does not gradually slow when carotid sinus or eyeball pressure is applied.

The ECG in supraventricular tachycardia

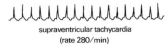

supraventricular tachycardia
(rate 280/min)

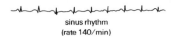

sinus rhythm
(rate 140/min)

Investigations. The electrocardiogram shows a heart rate greater than 210 beats per minute in a baby or greater than 180 in a child. The P waves may be present, abnormal, or absent, and the QRS complexes are normal. Between paroxysms, the electrocardiogram shows normal sinus rhythm. A number of children show the Wolff–Parkinson–White syndrome, an electrocardiographic abnormality comprising a short P–R interval and slurring of the beginning of the QRS complex.

Treatment. In some cases an attack can be terminated by vagal stimulation. In an infant this is best achieved by eliciting the diving reflex—the infant's face is immersed for a few seconds in ice-cold water. In a child, straining (the Valsalva manoeuvre), carotid sinus massage or eyeball pressure can be tried. If this fails, then anti-arrhythmic drugs are used; adenosine is the drug of choice. This drug has a very short half life and has to be given as a rapid intravenous bolus. Digitalisation is often effective but slow. In an emergency DC shock may be necessary. Recurrent attacks can be prevented or suppressed by regular digoxin, beta-adrenoreceptor blockers or other anti-arrhythmic agents.

Complete heart block

Complete heart block with atrioventricular dissociation may occur in otherwise normal children or in children with underlying congenital or acquired heart disease. It is often congenital and may be suspected before birth. There is an association with maternal systemic lupus erythematosus because auto-antibodies of the IgG type cross the placenta and damage the conduction system of the fetal heart. The ventricular rate of contraction is in the region of 50 per minute and may increase with exercise. Many affected children lead normal, healthy lives and remain symptom free. A minority have classical Stokes–Adams attacks in which they fall to the ground and lose consciousness. They need an artificial pacemaker.

SUBACUTE BACTERIAL ENDOCARDITIS

This is a well recognised complication of congenital as well as rheumatic heart disease. The risk is highest with those lesions which result in a turbulent jet of blood, such as a ventricular septal defect, coarctation, patent ductus and aortic stenosis. The endocardium becomes infected in the presence of a bacteraemia which may occur during dental treatment or cardiac surgery. As in adults, *Streptococcus viridans* is the commonest infecting organism.

Clinical features. Fever, malaise and anorexia are usually the presenting symptoms. Peripheral signs include clubbing of the nails and splinter hemorrhages. The spleen may be palpable and the physical signs of the heart defect can change rapidly as the endocarditis damages the heart valves.

Investigations. The diagnosis is made on one or more positive blood cultures. Microscopic haematuria is common, and the white count and ESR are usually raised.

Treatment. Bacteriocidal antibiotics are given parentally in large dose for a period of 6 weeks. The combination of benzylpenicillin and gentamicin is particularly useful for *St. viridans* but frequent monitoring of serum levels for killing activity against the organism is necessary.

Prevention. Any child known to have a congenital heart lesion, no matter how trivial, needs antibiotic prophylaxis with dental treatment and should carry a card to show to his dentist. The card states that the child has congenital heart disease and that in the event of dental treatment (extraction, fillings or scaling) antibiotics should be given. The usual practice is to give oral amoxycillin as a single large dose 1 hour before the treatment. Similar prophylaxis is also necessary before surgery involving the middle ear, tonsils or adenoids.

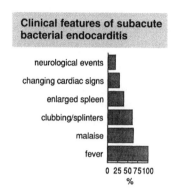

Clinical features of subacute bacterial endocarditis

neurological events
changing cardiac signs
enlarged spleen
clubbing/splinters
malaise
fever

0 25 50 75 100
%

RHEUMATIC FEVER

There has been a dramatic decline in this disease which used to cause much illness in children and permanent valvular damage in adults in the western world. It remains common, however, in the Middle East and Africa. The decline of the disease is probably the result of diminished virulence of the group A beta-haemolytic streptococcus, the introduction of antibiotics and improved social conditions. Rheumatic fever may represent an abnormal immunological response to the beta-haemolytic streptococcus, an organism commonly responsible for sore throats and tonsillitis. It is thought that the body confuses its own antigens with those of the organism, thereby causing an autoimmune reaction.

Clinical features. Between 1 and 3 weeks after a throat infection, the child (usually of school age) develops a fever, malaise and an acute migratory polyarthritis involving the medium-sized joints (knees, ankles, wrists and elbows). Carditis is common, involving all the layers of the heart. Pericarditis produces a friction rub or a pericardial effusion. Myocarditis produces a tachycardia, cardiac enlargement and arrhythmias. Endocarditis causes systolic and diastolic murmurs. Skin rashes, especially erythema marginatum, and subcutaneous nodules over the occiput or extensor surfaces of the elbows, wrists and fingers are less common. Chorea is a neurological manifestation of rheumatic fever which is rarely associated with carditis.

Investigations. There is usually evidence of a recent streptococcal infection (raised ASO titre and/or positive throat swab) with a raised white count and ESR. The P–R interval is commonly increased in the presence of carditis, often above 0.2 seconds.

Treatment. Penicillin is given to eradicate the streptococcus and high doses of aspirin lower the fever and relieve the arthritis. Steroids shorten the illness but do not reduce the incidence of permanent cardiac damage from the carditis—they are used in particularly severe cases of rheumatic fever. Rheumatic fever tends to recur and carditis is common in subsequent attacks if it occurred in the initial illness. Such recurrent episodes of carditis produce severe rheumatic valvular disease and should be prevented by penicillin prophylaxis for life. On the other hand, children who have no carditis with their initial rheumatic fever have a reduced risk of further relapses and a very low chance of carditis in future episodes.

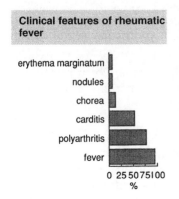

Clinical features of rheumatic fever

HYPERTENSION

Unfortunately blood pressure measurement is often overlooked when assessing a child's problems. This attitude arises from the difficulties of making accurate measurements in a restless young child with equipment which is designed for adults and also because the yield of abnormal readings is very low. With attention to correct technique using suitable cuff sizes and making repeated attempts in a relaxed atmosphere, reliable measurements can be made using a mercury sphygmomanometer. In infants the Doppler method may be used to determine systolic pressure. Automated measurement by oscillometry is increasingly popular in all age groups. Blood pressure increases with age, height and weight, although it should be remembered that the fat arm may give an artificially high reading. Too narrow a cuff in a normal arm also causes this error. There is no precise definition of

Normal blood pressure in childhood		
Age (years)	Mean mmHg Systolic	Diastolic
0-2	95	55
3-6	100	65
7-10	105	70
11-15	115	70

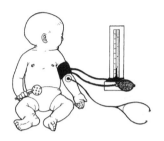

hypertension in childhood and although the figure of 130/85 mmHg is often used, this overlooks those children who fall in the top 5% of the blood pressure distribution for age. A proportion of these high rankers, particularly those with a family history of hypertension, become the adult population at risk from symptomatic hypertension, ischaemic heart disease and cerebrovascular disease. No child should be regarded as having an abnormal blood pressure until this has been confirmed on several occasions.

Surveys in several countries have demonstrated that the majority of children with mild asymptomatic hypertension fall into the primary or essential category. In contrast almost all those with severe symptomatic hypertension have some underlying cause, most commonly renal parenchymal disease. Greater attention to blood pressure measurement will bring these underlying problems to attention more promptly and may avoid life-threatening complications. Hypertension may manifest itself as persistent headache, dizziness, disturbed vision, unexplained irritability, convulsions, and other neurological signs like facial palsy. Naturally, blood pressure should always be measured in the presence of cardiac and renal disorders. Paroxysmal episodes of palpitation and sweating raise the possibility of a phaeochromocytoma.

HYPERLIPOPROTEINAEMIA

The morbidity and mortality arising from atherosclerosis has reached such epidemic proportions in industrial societies that paediatricians can no longer evade their responsibilities in this direction. Fatty streaks are already present in the aortas of children aged 10–11 years and the coronary arteries start to show involvement in the early twenties. Both genetic and environmental factors contribute towards atheroma. Currently there is great interest in preventive measures. Some measures, such as antismoking campaigns, the prevention of obesity and the encouragement of regular exercise are well validated although not always easy to implement; others such as the widescale modification of diet in infants and young children must be approached with caution. Hyperlipidaemia, and in particular hypercholesterolaemia, has been linked to the development of atheroma. The majority of serum cholesterol is transported as beta-lipoprotein, a low density lipoprotein (LDL).

Hyperbetalipoproteinaemia (familial hypercholesterolaemia) This is an autosomal dominant condition in which homozygote individuals have a severe disease. They develop tuberous and tendon xanthomata in early childhood and die of ischaemic heart disease in the second or third decade. The heterozygote condition is relatively common, affecting approximately 1 in 280 in England and Wales. Fifty-one per cent of heterozygote males and 12% of heterozygote females have a heart attack by the age of 50 years. There is therefore a case for detecting this disorder in early life so that dietary and drug treatment can be introduced before ischaemic disease is established. Cholesterol screening is justified in at-risk families but as yet has no place in routine child health surveillance programmes. Children with elevated LDL-cholesterol levels need to be referred to specialist clinics for more detailed lipid and lipoprotein analysis. Diet remains the main component of lipid-lowering strategies. Anion-exchange resins such as cholestyramine are effective in lowering LDL-cholesterol but compliance is a problem. A new class of drugs which block cholesterol synthesis may be useful but are still undergoing trials in children.

Diet and hypercholesterolaemia. The majority of hypercholesterolaemia in affluent society is not due to a single, genetically inherited disorder but reflects the impact of a high animal fat diet on a polygenically susceptible population. Within families there is a significant correlation between the serum cholesterol concentrations of children and those of their parents. The family history should include details of the occurrence and age of onset of ischaemic heart disease so that advice can be offered in an attempt to safeguard at-risk children. It is obviously sensible to reduce the fat intake, particularly from dairy products, but there is no evidence for the radical exclusion of cholesterol. Children tend to acquire the tastes of their parents and habituation to high fat or salt diets, smoking, and lack of exercise may well contribute to the future toll of atherosclerosis.

BIBLIOGRAPHY

Anderson R H, Macartney F J, Shinebourne E A, Tynan M (eds) 1987 Paediatric cardiology, vols 1 and 2. Churchill Livingstone, Edinburgh
Jordan S C, Scott O 1989 Heart disease in paediatrics, 3rd edn. Butterworths, London

10 Gut

ACUTE ABDOMINAL PAIN
RECURRENT ABDOMINAL PAIN
GASTROENTERITIS
MALABSORPTION
CHRONIC DIARRHOEA
INTESTINAL PARASITES
CONSTIPATION
LIVER DISEASE

Disorders of the gut are common in children and are usually readily recognised because of abdominal pain, vomiting, diarrhoea or constipation. Most are short lived and do not interfere with the overall health of well nourished children. However chronic gut disease may have profound effects on health because of poor food intake and malabsorption and should always be considered in infants and children with unexplained misery and growth failure.

Normal function of the gastrointestinal tract depends on a carefully regulated balance between motility, sphincter tone, exocrine secretion and integrity of the absorptive surfaces. These functions begin to evolve early in fetal life: digestive enzymes and primitive swallowing movements are first detectable in the 12-week fetus and regular flow of amniotic fluid into the gut occurs from 20 weeks; by term this amounts to half the total amniotic fuid volume, around 500 ml. Gut function must undergo abrupt adjustment and maturation with birth and the onset of intermittent oral feeding. There is a marked increase in small intestinal mucosal surface area and this is at least partially mediated by gut hormones and growth factors which are released in response to milk feeds. Digestive enzymes show a varied pattern of maturation, with lactase activity being fully developed at term, whereas trypsin takes 12 months to reach maximal levels. Although the gut is probably sterile at birth, it is rapidly colonised by bacterial entry through the mouth and anus. A normal microflora contributes to the available supply of vitamin K, folic acid and biotin. Immunological protection is provided to the newborn by secretory IgA antibodies in the maternal milk which supplement the transplacental passage of IgG antibodies.

Key features of abdominal pain

Time and mode of onset
Site, radiation and shifting
Character
Severity
Duration
Frequency and periodicity
Aggravating and attenuating factors
Precipitating events
Child/parent perception of the cause

ACUTE ABDOMINAL PAIN

In children the 'acute abdomen' is a common and testing problem. Surgical conditions which require prompt diagnosis and treatment have to be distinguished from a large number of medical disorders. Careful history taking, general examination and urinalysis are essential. A key diagnostic step is to encourage the child and parents to describe the pain in their own way and then to define nine key features.

The localisation of pain is more difficult to assess in children. The viscera are derived from midline embryonic structures and intestinal pain is localised vaguely in the midline. Thus when the appendix is inflamed the pain is initially periumbilical, but when the parietal peritoneum becomes involved the pain migrates to the right iliac fossa.

Acute appendicitis

Appendicitis is the commonest acute surgical emergency of childhood, 3 or 4 children in every 1000 have their appendix removed each year and many more are admitted for observation for abdominal pain. It can occur at any age but is usually seen in children over 5 years of age.

The characteristic triad of clinical features seen in adults, abdominal pain, low grade fever and tenderness with guarding in the right iliac fossa, is seen in the older child but in infants recognised pain may not be a feature; they are more likely to present with a history of a recent respiratory infection followed by anorexia, vomiting, irritability and a high fever. This often leads to diagnostic confusion and delay so that the incidence of perforation with resulting peritonitis or abscess formation is higher in the younger child. The course of the disease in the young child is extremely rapid, a 2 year old can progress from apparent normality to perforation in 6 hours! There is no place therefore for prolonged observation in the young patient.

Causes of acute abdominal pain

Surgical	Medical (relatively common)	Medical (rare but important)
Acute appendicitis	Mesenteric adenitis	Lead poisoning
Intussusception	Constipation	Diabetes
Intestinal obstruction	Gastroenteritis	Sickle cell crisis
Torsion of ovary or testis	Lower lobe pneumonia	Acute porphyria
Hydronephrosis	Acute pyelonephritis	Pancreatitis
Renal calculus	Henoch–Schönlein purpura	Primary peritonitis
	Hepatitis	Meningitis

Non-specific abdominal pain (mesenteric adenitis)

Vague central or generalised abdominal pain commonly accompanies viral upper respiratory tract infections. The mechanism is uncertain but may reflect non-specific inflammation in the mesenteric lymph nodes causing tenderness and increased motility of adjacent intestine.

It is usually possible to distinguish non-specific abdominal pain from acute appendicitis, but if there is any doubt 4–6 hours after the child is first seen, and in all cases where there is persisting local tenderness, the child must be surgically explored.

Primary peritonitis

Primary peritonitis, usually due to pneumococcus, is considerably rarer than peritonitis secondary to appendicitis. Patients with nephrotic syndrome, liver disease and immune deficiency states are more susceptible.

Features which distinguish appendicitis and non-specific abdominal pain

Acute appendicitis	temperature	Non-specific abdominal pain

37-38°C		above 38°C
—	pharyngitis, cervical adenitis	+
—	headache	+
—	vomiting	—
++	abdominal pain	+
++	guarding	+
—	shifting tenderness	+
+	rebound tenderness	—

upper respiratory tract infection and appendicitis can occur simultaneously

Malrotation

Malrotation refers to anomalous movement of the midgut loop around the superior mesenteric artery in the embryo. In normal embryological development the midgut loop herniates into the umbilical cord from the sixth to the fourteenth intrauterine weeks. The apex of the midgut loop communicates with the yolk sac by the vitelline duct and in about 2% of people there is a remnant of this duct called the Meckel diverticulum. While still in the extra-embryonic coelom a counterclockwise rotation of 270 degrees around the superior mesenteric artery occurs. At about 14 weeks the gut starts to return to the abdominal cavity, the proximal jejunum leading and lying in the left upper abdomen. The caecum is the last portion of the gut to re-enter the abdomen, lying in the subhepatic position before descending to the right iliac fossa.

Arrested caecal descent is the most common abnormality diagnosed. It can cause bile-stained vomiting in the neonate due to duodenal obstruction by Ladd bands, and partial recurrent volvulus in the older child due to the narrow mesenteric attachment between the caecum and the duodenojejunal flexure. Often it is asymptomatic but it causes severe technical difficulty if the patient develops acute appendicitis.

Maldescent and malrotation

arrested caecal descent   incomplete rotation   reverse rotation

Incomplete rotation. The second anomaly causing clinical problems is correctly called incomplete rotation of the gut. Here rotation in the extra-embryonic coelom only amounts to 90 degrees counterclockwise, and the colon and caecum return first to the abdomen and occupy the left side. The small bowel fills the right side. The whole small bowel is suspended by an extremely narrow mesenteric attachment between duodenojejunal flexure and caecum. A volvulus in early infancy is a high risk and can result in total small bowel infarction.

True malrotation can occur when embryonic rotation is 90 degrees clockwise instead of 270 degree counterclockwise but this is rare. The duodenum will be anterior to the transverse colon. Clinical problems are unusual.

Meckel diverticulum

This diverticulum is a remnant of the vitello-intestinal duct. It arises from the antimesenteric border of the terminal ileum and usually gives no trouble, but rarely it may become inflamed and then the symptoms and signs mimic acute appendicitis. More commonly the diverticulum causes an intussusception or a volvulus. It may also contain ectopic gastric mucosa in which peptic ulceration can produce haemorrhage or perforation. A technetium scan may help to identify ectopic mucosa.

Intussusception

Intussusception is an invagination of bowel into an adjacent lower segment. The usual origin is the terminal ileum or ileocaecal valve, resulting in an ileocolic intussusception. Although uncommon, 2 in 1000 live births, it is the most frequent cause of intestinal obstruction in the first 2 years of life. Typically, parents describe their infant as crying inconsolably for a period, going pale then returning to normal before repeating the sequence. The infant may vomit with the paroxysmal pain which causes the periodic crying. On examination a sausage-shaped mass is often palpable in the right upper abdomen, and bloodstained mucus (the redcurrant jelly stool) may be found on rectal examination. If there is delay in diagnosis the child will develop fever, a distended abdomen and will pass bloodstained mucus rectally. The diagnosis is usually based on clinical suspicion supported by a plain abdominal X-ray showing a mass and an absent gas pattern over the caecum and ascending colon. Abdominal ultrasound is increasingly

Intussusception: plain abdominal radiograph and barium enema reduction

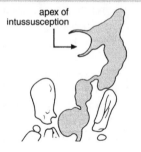

apex of intussusception

Bowel obstruction due to hernia

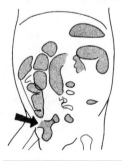

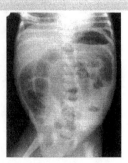

Distended small bowel

note air in Rt. inguinal sac

used to confirm the diagnosis and guide treatment. If the history is for less than 24 hours and there are no signs of peritonitis, it is appropriate to attempt reduction of the intussusception by hydrostatic pressure using either air or barium. Hydrostatic reduction has a success rate of approximately 75%, the remaining children require immediate surgery. In older children an underlying cause such as a Meckel diverticulum is more likely and may justify a surgical approach. Rarely a recurrent non-obstructive intussusception may be the cause of chronic diarrhoea.

RECURRENT ABDOMINAL PAIN

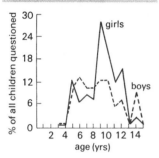

Age of 200 children with recurrent abdominal pain (Apley 1975)

Episodic pain, lasting 3 months or more and disrupting the child and family's lives, is a common problem affecting at least 10% of school children at some time. Although no organic cause is found in over 90%, it is essential to identify those with an organic condition promptly. This enables specific management of the problem and confident counselling of children with functional disorders. The majority of children are adequately evaluated on the basis of a careful history and examination. Allow the child to describe the pain but check the details with the parents. Key issues are the pain's periodicity and coexistent symptoms. Intervening good health and normal growth reinforce the innocence of the problem. Successful reassurance requires the doctor to take the child and family's concern seriously, and there needs to be an opportunity to explore unspoken anxieties about serious disease. Only a minority justify investigation beyond a blood count and a urinalysis.

In planning management the child's pain has to be accepted as real in the same way that an adult with headaches merits sympathy and support. The family will be helped by an explanation of possible mechanisms, for example that the pains represent amplified awareness of normal gut movement.

Cyclical vomiting and childhood migraine. Children who go on to have classical migraine commonly present with recurrent episodes of prolonged midline abdominal pain associated with nausea or vasomotor symptoms. A positive family history of migraine is an important clue.

Renal tract infection must be excluded by urine culture and microscopy. Loin pain in the absence of urinary abnormality may still be an indication for urinary tract ultrasound examination in the case of hydronephrosis due to pelviureteric junction obstruction.

Peptic ulcers are now being diagnosed more often in children, partly as a consequence of the wider application of endoscopy. Waking because of epigastric pain and a family history of peptic ulceration are useful clues. *Helicobacter pylori*, a curved gram-negative micro-aerophilic bacterium which can multiply under the mucus lining the stomach, is a cause of gastritis and duodenal ulceration in children as well as adults. The natural history is for acquisition of the infection within the family, development of gastritis and later in life a duodenal peptic ulcer. The organism can be eradicated by a week's triple therapy of omeprazole, metronidazole and clarithromycin. Bacterial suppression results in resolution of gastritis but may not cure abdominal pain, suggesting that there is an overlap between *H. pylori* infection and non-organic recurrent abdominal pain. The diagnosis of suspected peptic ulceration is by endoscopy and antral biopsies for *H. pylori* can also be taken. The organism produces a urease which splits urea forming carbon dioxide, the basis of direct tests on antral biopsies and carbon labelled urea breath tests.

Features pointing to an organic cause for recurrent abdominal pain

Organic causes		Non-organic causes
−	family history (abdominal pain, headache)	+
−	tense personality	+
+	headache	++
+	vomiting	+
++	abnormal signs	−
++	abnormal growth	−
++	abnormal investigation (TBC, ESR, Urinalysis)	−

Chronic recurrent pancreatitis. Although rare, it may be suggested by a family history and by episodic central abdominal pain radiating through to the back with vomiting. Clinical suspicion is confirmed by finding elevated blood amylase levels during an episode.

GASTROENTERITIS

Diarrhoeal illness, frequently superimposed on malnutrition, extracts a terrifying toll from the world's children: at a conservative estimate 10–15 million deaths annually. WHO has committed itself to 'Health for All by the Year 2000', major targets being the universal availability of safe water supplies, simple but life saving oral rehydration treatment and promotion of breast feeding. One successful programme is the 'Child-to-Child' approach which exploits the potential of children to spread health ideas and practices through their communities. In the developed world gastroenteritis is common and usually mild but should not be underestimated with the risk of morbidity or death in vulnerable infants.

Management of the child presenting with an acute episode of diarrhoea and/or vomiting requires assessment and treatment of dehydration, confirmation of the diagnosis preferably with identification of the infective agent, and observation in case of complications. There may also be public health implications. In the initial diagnosis it is important to remember that vomiting and diarrhoea may be the presentation of a range of systemic illnesses, and also of surgical conditions such as appendicitis, Hirschsprung disease and intussusception.

For the majority of infective gastroenteritis, treatment is aimed at correction of dehydration. Antimicrobial treatment has a very limited role unless systemic bacterial spread is likely. Antidiarrhoeal agents such as loperamide are contraindicated in acute diarrhoea.

Bacterial gastroenteritis

Differential diagnosis of diarrhoea and/or vomiting

Gastroenteritis
Other infections
 Urinary tract infection
 Upper or lower respiratory tract infection
 Necrotising enterocolitis
 Septicaemia
 Meningitis
Surgical disorders
 Appendicitis
 Pyloric stenosis
 Intussusception
 Hirschprung disease
Malabsorption
 Coeliac disease
 Cows' milk protein intolerance
 Immune deficiency
 Inborn absorptive enzyme deficiency
Drugs and toxins

Bacteria can be pathogenic by interfering with mucosal integrity by direct invasion, by toxin release, or by adherence to and disruption of the enterocyte brush border. Groups of E. coli operate by all three mechanisms, the genetic determinants of virulence being carried in chromosomes or in plasmids. Gene probes have been developed to facilitate the laboratory identification of pathogenic E. coli.

Campylobacter jejuni, often derived from uncooked meat, is now a common cause of diarrhoeal illness in developed countries. Fever and blood in the stool are common in invasive bacterial gastroenteritis and in particular in shigella infection. Shigella can release a neurotoxin causing pyrexial convulsions and marked meningism which may precede overt enteric symptoms. Some invasive strains of E. coli such the 0157 strain release a verotoxin which can trigger endothial damage and the haemolytic uraemic syndrome.

Food poisoning may arise due to the ingestion of the exotoxin produced by coagulase-positive staphylococcus.

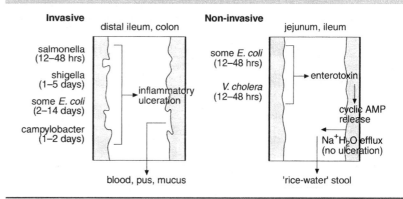

Mechanisms of invasive or non-invasive bacterial gastroenteritis

Viral gastroenteritis

In developed countries viral infection is responsible for 50–60% of acute gastroenteritis in children under the age of 5 years. Rotavirus, a double stranded RNA virus, is the main agent responsible for winter epidemics of gastroenteritis. There are several different strains of rotavirus and of other agents, for example astroviruses and caliciviruses, and this diversity is an obstacle to the development of both host immunity and effective vaccines. Vomiting may be the only obvious presenting feature as diarrhoea may not occur for several hours and even then a watery stool is liable to be confused with urine in the wet napkins. Colicky abdominal pain with ill defined tenderness and exaggerated bowel sounds is common.

Dehydration

The water loss associated with gastroenteritis places a relatively greater stress on the young infant with a higher percentage of body water (80% at term and 60% at 12 months), a higher metabolic rate and a larger surface area to volume ratio. The assessment of dehydration relies upon a series of clinical signs which reflect changes in body water and circulatory status. These changes are more easily recognised in thin than in overweight infants. A recent reliable weight is a better guide to body fluid loss. The clinical estimate indicates the percentage of the expected body weight which needs to be replaced, so that 10% dehydration in a 5 kg infant indicates a replacement volume of 500 ml.

Clinical assessment of dehydration

Sign	5% dehydration	10% dehydration
Skin	Loss of turgor	Mottled, poor capillary return
Fontanelle	Depressed	Deeply depressed
Eyes	Sunken	Deeply sunken
Peripheral pulses	Normal	Tachycardia, poor volume
Mental state	Lethargic	Prostration, coma

The dehydration may be hypotonic (serum sodium below 130 mmol/l), isotonic or hypertonic (also termed hypernatraemic when the serum sodium is above 150 mmol/l). The plasma electrolytes should be measured if the infant has features suggesting hypertonic dehydration or has signs of more than 5% dehydration.

Features which differentiate isotonic and hypertonic dehydration

lethargic ; hypotonic ; depressed fontanelle : sunken eyes ; loss of skin turgor

irritable ; hypertonic ; normal or full fontanelle ; normal eyes ; doughy skin

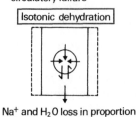

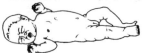

dehydration recognised before circulatory failure

circulatory failure due to masking of dehydration

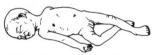

Isotonic dehydration

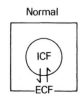

Normal

Hypertonic dehydration

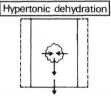

Na^+ and H_2O loss in proportion

H_2O loss greater than Na^+

Mild dehydration (under 5%) can be corrected at home by an oral rehydration solution of salt and glucose over 12–24 hours followed by reintroduction of a normal diet. The discovery that a combination of glucose with sodium chloride in solution results in even damaged mucosa absorbing water more effectively is justifiably claimed to be the greatest life saving medical advance of this century. It utilises the mechanism of the coupled sodium-glucose transporter to remove sodium and glucose from the gut lumen and then water follows by osmosis. A range of formulations available exploit the principle that oral rehydration therapy is considerably more efficient when glucose or sucrose is added to an electrolyte solution. In impoverished cultures effective rehydration solutions can be created using cheap local ingredients, for example salt and boiled rice water. It is essential to advise families how to make up these solutions appropriately and that unnecessarily prolonged use places the child at risk of malnutrition.

Oral rehydration therapy

Formulation	UK (mmol/l)	WHO mmol/l
Na	30–50	90
K	20	20
Cl	30–50	80
Citrate	10	10
Glucose	200	100
	for use in UK to replace mild faecal electrolyte loss, reduced risk of hypernatraemia	for use in developing world to replace substantial faecal electrolyte loss, to be used in addition to water and milk

Moderate to severe dehydration (over 5%) requires urgent intravenous fluid, especially when there are signs of peripheral circulatory failure. When initial resuscitation is complete rehydration can be continued with oral rehydration solution (ORS). Appropriate management demands an understanding of normal maintenance requirements as well as an assessment of the fluid deficit and continuing losses. Metabolic acidosis may accompany severe dehydration and is corrected by providing about half the calculated deficit as sodium bicarbonate solution: deficit (mmol) = weight (kg) $\times 0.3 \times (24 -$ observed plasma bicarbonate mmol/l).

Maintenance requirements

Age (months)	H_2O (ml/kg)	Na (mmol/kg)	K (mmol/kg)
0–6	150	2.5	2.5
6–12	120	2.5	2.5
12–24	100	2.5	2.5
Over 24	80	2.0	2.0

Complications

Diarrhoea commonly continues for a few days after the acute illness. It is a potential problem if it causes recurrence of dehydration, goes on beyond 14 days or interferes with weight gain. Continuing or repeated infection requires re-examination of stool particularly for giardiasis. Transient lactase deficiency leads to unabsorbed lactose causing osmotic diarrhoea. If lactose, a reducing substance, is persistently found in the stool then a lactose-free milk is prescribed for about 4 weeks. Secondary cows' milk protein intolerance is possible if the above have been excluded and is confirmed by finding of a patchy partial villous atrophy on small bowel biopsy which responds to a cows' milk free diet. Acute gastroenteritis may provoke convulsions because of fever, hypo- or hypernatraemia, hypoglycaemia and hypocalcaemia. An encephalopathy may signify haemolytic-uraemic syndrome. Cerebral damage may also follow hypotension or vascular thrombosis.

Principles of intravenous therapy

Total fluid requirements

maintenance	0.2 saline in 4.3% glucose plus KCl
+	
deficit	Normal saline plus KCl
+	
ongoing loss	Normal saline plus KCl

Scheme

0–0.5 hours	Treat shock immediately	Plasma or Normal saline 20 ml/kg
0.5–4 hours	Initial replacement	0.5 Normal or Normal saline 10 ml/kg/h (awaiting serum electrolyte results)
4–24 hours	Continuing replacement	
	(a) Serum Na under 150 mmol/l	0.2 Normal saline in 4.3% glucose plus KCl 30–40 mmol/l plan correction in 24 hours
	(b) Serum Na above 150 mmol/l	0.2 Normal saline in 4.3% glucose plus KCl 30–40 mmol/l restrict fluid to 150 ml/kg in first 24 hours and plan total correction over 48 hours

---

Solutions	Na	K	(mmol/l) Ca	Cl	Lactate
Normal saline (0.9%)	150	—	—	150	—
0.5 N saline in 5% dextrose	77	—	—	77	—
0.18% N saline in 4.0% dextrose	30	—	—	30	—
Ringer's lactate solution (Hartmann's solution)	130	5	4	112	27

MALABSORPTION

Enzymatic degradation of the major nutrients occurs within the gut lumen, at the microvilli and in the cytoplasm of the columnar epithelial cells. Disorders in the lumen may be due to failure of exocrine secretion, for example pancreatic insufficiency in cystic fibrosis, or disrupted bile salt circulation as in cholestatic liver disease. The mucosa may suffer non-specific epithelial damage in a variety of conditions, including coeliac disease and post-gastroenteritis. Other more specific inherited disorders interfere with individual pathways in the epithelium, for example primary congenital alactasia and familial chloride diarrhoea. Malabsorption may also occur due to obstruction of lymphatics in the intestinal wall as in congenital lymphangectasia.

Investigation of malabsorption is relatively complex and must not be initiated until it has been established that the child is failing to gain weight on a normal diet, does not have other systemic diseases and is being cared for in an adequate environment. Stool microscopy may reveal abundant fat globules. Quantitative measures of faecal fat are now largely redundant. Relevant investigations include a sweat test to exclude cystic fibrosis, and abdominal imaging to rule out malrotation and other structural abnormalities. Intestinal endoscopy and biopsy are useful procedures in suitably selected patients.

Coeliac disease

Clinical features of gluten enteropathy

failure to thrive
vomiting
diarrhoea
irritability
anorexia
anaemia
hypotonia
abdominal distension
wasted buttocks
rickets
delayed bone age
short stature
delayed puberty

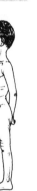

Coeliac disease is the permanent inability to tolerate dietary wheat or rye gluten. Exposure to gluten results in morphological and functional abnormality of the proximal small intestine which can be reversed by exclusion of gluten. The incidence is about 1 in 2000 in the UK and as high as 1 in 300 in west Ireland. Susceptibility to coeliac disease is inherited but disease manifestation probably depends on early dietary and environmental factors. Breastfeeding and delayed gluten exposure appear to delay presentation to later life. There is a suggestion that gastroenteritis particularly with adenovirus infection may trigger the disease. The majority of children with coeliac disease present before the age of 2 years. The weight record may show progressive growth failure dating from the introduction of gluten-containing solids. In a few, overt malabsorption may not occur for many years, and the diagnosis only comes to light after recognition of late growth failure and delayed puberty. Positive IgA gliadin and endomysial antibodies provide a useful screening test for coeliac disease. A diagnostic duodenal or jejunal biopsy is essential before restricting a child to a gluten free diet. Children with coeliac disease usually show a prompt response when

Normal and abnormal jejunal mucosa

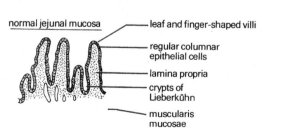

normal jejunal mucosa
— leaf and finger-shaped villi
— regular columnar epithelial cells
— lamina propria
— crypts of Lieberkühn
— muscularis mucosae

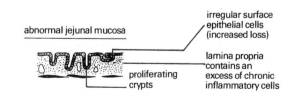

abnormal jejunal mucosa
— irregular surface epithelial cells (increased loss)
— lamina propria contains an excess of chronic inflammatory cells
— proliferating crypts

placed on a gluten free diet; parents certainly appreciate the improved mood. Children over 2 years with positive antigliadin and anti-endomysial antibodies and with a good response to a gluten free diet will not require further challenge and should continue a lifelong diet. However there are other causes of temporarily abnormal small intestinal mucosa including post-gastroenteritis and cows' milk protein intolerance. Therefore children under 2 years or in whom the above conditions are not met should have a gluten challenge and re-biopsy.

Planned or unplanned gluten exposure may or may not result in the early return of symptoms. Planned challenge prior to confirmatory biopsy may have to be continued for several months before mucosal changes occur. Dietary compliance becomes an increasing problem in adolescence, particularly in those who have few symptoms. There is still some dispute as to whether chronic gluten exposure and mucosal inflammation increases the likelihood of small intestinal lymphoma.

Sugar intolerance

Sugar intolerance results from the failure to absorb particular sugars, most commonly lactose. The osmotic load of the undigested sugar results in explosive watery diarrhoea and the intraluminal fermentation produces an excess of lactic acid and carbon dioxide. The fluid stools are acid, pH less than 5.5 and contain reducing substances.

Lactose intolerance. Secondary lactose intolerance is common after gastroenteritis. It contributes to loose stools but is usually short lived and does not result in significant malabsorption or necessitate major dietary adjustment.

Severe or recurrent gastroenteritis, especially in malnourished infants, can damage the small intestinal mucosa and cause symptomatic lactase deficiency. Coeliac disease and cytotoxic therapy are other examples of gut insults that lead to secondary lactase deficiency. A diet has then to be designed which excludes lactose and replaces it with glucose or glucose polymers which are more readily absorbed. An attempt should be made to distinguish lactose intolerance which lasts a few weeks from cows' milk protein intolerance which lasts 4 or more months. Both conditions can be treated by selecting a milk free of lactose and cows' milk protein such as a soya or hydrolysate formula.

Lactose intolerance also occurs in premature infants, as a rare inherited disorder in Caucasians (autosomal recessive), and as a frequent finding in non-Caucasians after early childhood (autosomal dominant).

Sucrase-isomaltase deficiency can occur after severe mucosal damage or be inherited in an autosomal recessive mode.

Galactose-glucose malabsorption is extremely rare, and results in severe persistent diarrhoea from birth.

CHRONIC DIARRHOEA

Chronic non-specific diarrhoea

Persistent or episodic diarrhoea containing segments of undigested vegetables in a thriving preschool child is a very common complaint. The most frequent explanation is rapid intestinal transit due to an exaggerated gastrocolic reflex repeatedly provoked by small snacks and cold drinks. Simple short-term measures such as restricting fluid intake to meal times obviates the need for antidiarrhoeal preparations of dubious therapeutic value.

Cows' milk protein intolerance

This is a mainly clinical diagnosis which is made when either acute or chronic symptoms appear to be related to cows' milk ingestion. Acute reactions after small amounts of milk include excessive crying, vomiting, diarrhoea, urticaria, lip swelling, stridor and bronchospasm, and when this happens the association with milk intake is fairly readily established. It is more difficult to confirm that chronic effects such as failure to thrive, rectal bleeding, anaemia and hepatosplenomegaly are due to a reaction to milk protein. Immunological studies indicate a variety of mechanisms. Susceptible infants may have enhanced absorption of antigenic quantities of lactoglobulin in early infancy and this may in turn be related to transient IgA deficiency or follow gastroenteritis. Jejunal biopsy shows patchy partial villous flattening. The disorder is usually temporary and can be managed by dietary adjustments. Protein is given in the form of casein hydrolysate, chicken meat or soy protein.

Other food intolerance

Children may have clearly documented hypersensitivity to one or more foods, for example eggs and fish. More difficult are the claimed associations between a wide range of food substances and problems such as behavioural disturbance, headaches and even convulsions. While it is appropriate to conduct sensibly structured dietary trials, the doctor must ensure that the child is not exposed to unfounded, bizarre or deficient diets. Allergy to egg is not a contraindication to immunisation.

Acrodermatitis enteropathica

This is a rare autosomal recessive disorder linked to a defect of zinc metabolism. The infants develop severe diarrhoea and failure to thrive with a characteristic rash over the mucocutaneous junctions and pressure areas. There is also alopecia and nail dystrophy. The onset is delayed if the child is breastfed. Without zinc supplements it is a fatal condition.

Crohn disease

This is a chronic inflammation of unknown cause found anywhere from mouth to anus in which the pathognomic histological marker is non-caseating epitheloid granulomata. While uncommon in children, around 40 per million population, the incidence has increased over the last 30 years. Crohn disease and ulcerative colitis occur more often within families than would be expected by chance. Western lifestyle, lack of breastfeeding and a higher frequency of diarrhoeal illnesses in infancy appear to be predisposing factors. Research has focused on chronic infection such as atypical mycobacterium and measles virus but Koch's postulates have not been met.

Presenting features include recurrent abdominal pain, anorexia, growth failure, fever, diarrhoea, oral and perianal ulcers, and arthritis. Diagnosis is often delayed by confusion of the symptoms with functional complaints. Crohn disease should be considered in adolescents with suspected anorexia nervosa. Screening blood tests are C-reactive protein, ESR, platelet count and haemoglobin; when these are all normal Crohn disease is unlikely. The granulomatous involvement of the gut may be diffuse so that both upper and lower endoscopy with biopsy, as well as contrast studies of the bowel, play a part in assessment. The resulting malnutrition leads not only to growth failure but also aggravates the disease process. Energetic nutritional programmes based on elemental diets correct the growth failure and induce remission of active disease. This nutritional approach is as effective as corticosteroids, and avoids the hazard of iatrogenic growth impairment. There is a place for surgical resection of localised disease which either causes anatomical problems such as obstruction or which accounts for persisting growth failure.

Ulcerative colitis

Ulcerative colitis presents with diarrhoea containing visible blood and mucus. It is important to exclude an infectious cause for an initial presentation of colitis. The early episodes of ulcerative colitis may be intermittent and short lived. Others produce more systemic upset with abdominal pain, weight loss, arthritis, and liver disturbance. Skin manifestations include erythema nodosum and pyoderma gangrenosum.

Colonoscopy with multiple mucosal biopsy is the key investigation for confirming the disease and assessing its extent. Although the disease may be limited to a proctosigmoiditis at outset, approximately 60% of children will go on to have more extensive involvement of the colon.

Acute attacks of proctosigmoiditis are treated with topical corticosteroid preparations; enemas, foam or suppositories. More extensive disease requires oral corticosteroids with careful supervision because of the risks of fulminant colitis. Sulphasalazine or similar drugs are valuable for treating mild symptomatic disease and sustaining remission. Extensive refractory colitis may be an indication for immunosuppressant therapy with azathioprine or cyclosporin. The disruption of life with repeated episodes, poor nutrition, anaemia and drug side-effects may be such that colectomy is justified. There is also the cumulative risk of mucosal dysplasia and neoplasia. When colectomy is indicated, the procedure of choice is restorative proctocolectomy with ileal pouch.

Food allergy colitis

Milk protein allergy can provoke colitis in infants and cause frankly bloodstained diarrhoea.

INTESTINAL PARASITES

In the developing world these provide a further threat to children's health and result in malabsorption, anaemia and chronic diarrhoea.

Giardia lamblia

Giardiasis is caused by ingestion of food or water contaminated by the cysts of this flagellate protozoan. It is endemic in most countries and the prevalence is high in young and malnourished children. Host factors are important in determining whether the trophozoite form adheres to small intestinal mucosa and disrupts structure and absorptive function. The clinical spectrum of infection ranges from asymptomatic cyst carriage to severe diarrhoea and malabsorption. It is a differential diagnosis of 'toddler's diarrhoea'. Diagnosis can be confirmed by microscopy of fresh stool, jejunal juice or intestinal biopsy. Metronidazole is the treatment of choice but treatment failure or reinfection is common.

Enterobius (threadworm)

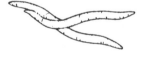

Enterobius is a frequent cause of perianal and vulval pruritis. The mobile thread-like worms are easily recognised on separating the buttocks of the sleeping child. They are difficult to eradicate and justify treatment only when symptomatic. The entire family must be treated with, for example, piperazine. Hygiene measures are also necessary to break the cycle of self-infection.

Ascaris lumbricoides

Roundworm infection follows ingestion of the eggs. The larvae migrate via the portal system to the lungs where they ascend the bronchial tree to re-enter the gut. Heavy infestation may result in pneumonitis and eosinophilia during the larval phase. Gut symptoms are rare but include pain, obstruction and appendicitis. Piperazine treats the adult phase.

Ankylostoma (hookworm)

Hookworm is a major cause of iron deficiency in hot, humid climates. Bephenium hydroxynaphthoate is an effective treatment.

Threadworm, roundworm, hookworm and toxocara

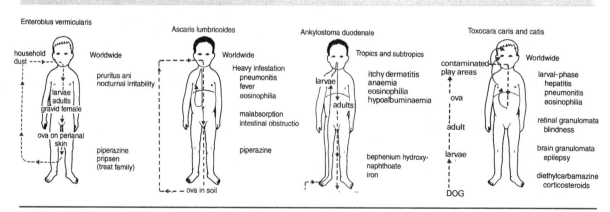

Toxocara canis **and** *catis*

Toxocara canis and *catis* may have their migratory larval phase in children who are in close contact with animal excreta. Infection produces eosinophilia, hepatomegaly and bronchospasm. The larvae may encapsulate in the eye producing retinal granulomata, or in the brain acting as potential epileptogenic foci.

Taenia

The adult worms of *Taenia saginata* (beef tapeworm) and *Taenia solium* (pork tapeworm) inhabit the intestinal canal of man. It is also possible for man to be infected by the larval phase of *T. solium* as a result of consumption of inadequately cooked pork. The larvae or cysticerci may encapsulate and calcify in the tissues. The adult tapeworms may be killed by niclosamide.

CONSTIPATION

Constipation is a frequent complaint in all age groups and reflects a common obsession with regular bowel function. It is valid to differentiate the problem of infrequent hard stools from the less worrying complaint of infrequent normal stools. Healthy infants show a considerable variation in the pattern of bowel frequency depending on their diet, and indeed mother's diet if breastfed. They may also show alarming colour changes and vigorous abdominal contractions during defaecation which may be interpreted by the mother as straining. Genuine hard stools may result from an inadequate milk intake, hunger stools, or from overstrength artificial feeds where the free water is diverted to facilitate renal solute excretion. The change from an artificial milk formula or breast milk to cows' milk is accompanied by the production of smaller, harder and less frequent stools. Their passage may require more effort and the resulting anal irritation may provoke withholding, and a pattern of behaviour which can evolve into troublesome constipation. Constipation may accompany more generalised disorders but it is seldom the chief complaint. Hypothyroidism, idiopathic hypercalcaemia and neuromuscular problems fall into this category.

In older children, acute constipation is a common accompaniment of febrile illnesses and the resulting hard stools may cause an anal tear which in turn initiates the cycle of faecal retention and chronic constipation. The prompt use of gentle laxatives and abundant fluids facilitates healing of the traumatised anal margin and helps the child to regain confidence in his toilet activities. It is sad that so many of these children are allowed to develop chronic constipation with all its attendant problems. These include abdominal pain, anorexia, vomiting, failure to thrive and a predisposition to urinary tract infections. The accumulation of hard stool in the rectal ampulla leads to an acquired megacolon. The distension of the rectum results in relaxation of the internal sphincter so that the child must continually call on the external sphincter and the levator ani, which are voluntary muscle groups, in order to resist stool passage. Eventually this effort fails and the external sphincter is no longer able to prevent constant leakage of faecal matter. The soiling is often the dominant complaint and the families become desperate in their attempts to cope with this unsocial problem. Examination confirms the presence of the indentable faecal mass, the perianal soiling and the firm stool just within the internal sphincter.

Constipation: palpation for 'rocks' in the descending colon and rectum

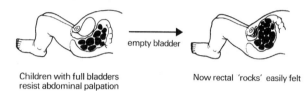

empty bladder

Children with full bladders   Now rectal 'rocks' easily felt
resist abdominal palpation

Treatment requires an enthusiastic but relatively simple approach. The main objectives are to dislodge the faecal mass, overcome withholding behaviour and promote a regular bowel habit. Success revolves around the child regaining confidence in being capable of painless easy defaecation. A short course of a powerful liquid laxative is an effective means of dislodging the faecal mass. The parents should be empowered to titrate the medication against the child's stools. More refractory cases may require a brief course of enemas but the oral approach is more satisfactory for both child and therapist. This is followed by a programme of copious fluids, a high roughage diet and Senokot at a dosage sufficient to amplify the gastrocolic reflex. The child must learn to take advantage of the latter by spending 5–10 minutes on the toilet after breakfast and the evening meal. It is worth checking that the child has firm foot support so that he can obtain the optimal mechanical advantage while sitting on the toilet. The use of laxatives may cause the soiling to be worse during the initial period of treatment and parents must be warned about this. In most children, the physical and emotional problems improve in parallel with the recovery of normal bowel function. In a minority there are more profound behavioural problems which warrant a careful psychiatric evaluation.

Chronic constipation

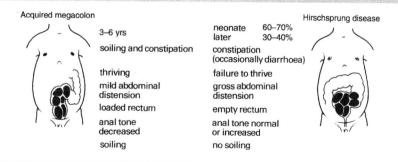

Acquired megacolon

3–6 yrs

soiling and constipation

thriving
mild abdominal
distension
loaded rectum
anal tone
decreased
soiling

neonate   60–70%
later   30–40%

constipation
(occasionally diarrhoea)

failure to thrive
gross abdominal
distension
empty rectum
anal tone normal
or increased
no soiling

Hirschsprung disease

Although chronic constipation can usually be overcome by this regimen, in some children the possibility of short segment Hirschsprung disease arises. If the problem persists and requires an anal dilatation under general anaesthetic a suction biopsy to exclude Hirschsprung disease is necessary.

Hirschsprung disease

Hirschsprung disease must be considered if constipation presents in infancy. The incidence is 1 in 4500 live births. It accounts for about 10% of neonatal intestinal obstruction, but it may also present in the older child. It results from failure of migration of ganglion cells to the submucosal and myenteric plexuses of the large bowel. The aganglionic segment, which remains tonically contracted and aperistaltic, invariably involves the internal sphincter. Sometimes there is a very short segment, but 80% involve the rectosigmoid colon and 15% extend to the more proximal colon. In one large series 85% developed difficulties in the first month of life and 95% by the end of the first year.

The typical infant fails to pass meconium within the first 24 hours of life, develops progressive abdominal distension, refuses to feed and finally has bilious vomiting. A severe form of enterocolitis with perforation and septicaemia may complicate this picture and has a high mortality rate. The older child suffers with intermittent bouts of intestinal obstruction from faecal impaction, failure to thrive, hypochromic anaemia and hypoproteinaemia. Soiling is extremely unusual but not unknown in Hirschsprung disease. On examination, the upper abdomen is distended with gas as well as faeces, the costal margin is flared and the umbilicus is displaced downward. Characteristically, the anal canal and rectum are free of faeces and may feel narrow and grip the finger. The diagnosis may be confirmed by barium enema of an unprepared colon, rectal biopsy and anorectal manometry. The latter demonstrates an absence of the normal reflex inhibition of the internal anal sphincter on rectal distension. Surgical treatment often entails an initial colostomy to relieve the obstruction. The subsequent definitive operation is designed to bypass the aganglionic segment and bring the normal bowel down to the anus.

Surgical approaches to Hirschsprung disease

Swenson — anastomosis

Duhamel — anastomosis of adjoining bowel

Soave — seromuscular cuff; no anastomosis

LIVER DISEASE

Hepatomegaly

Liver disease presents with hepatomegaly, jaundice, metabolic disturbance or haemorrhagic problems either singly or in combination. The normal liver has a soft, smooth, non-tender edge 1–2 cm below the costal margin with a span in the midclavicular line of up to 4 cm in babies and to 8 cm in older children. An enlarged liver may be a transient finding accompanying acute disorders like infectious hepatitis or glandular fever, or it may be longstanding, requiring detailed investigation.

Prolonged neonatal jaundice

Jaundice persisting beyond the second week requires investigation to exclude rare treatable conditions. A distinction must be made between conjugated and unconjugated hyperbilirubinaemia.

Breast milk jaundice

First week physiological jaundice is often more conspicuous in breastfed infants. Rarely, this is followed by prolonged unconjugated hyperbilirubinaemia in otherwise healthy thriving infants. The mechanism is not clear although in some it may be due to a complex steroid in the milk which inhibits hepatic glucuronyl transferase. There is a tendency for a breast fed sibling to show the same pattern. It is seldom necessary to advise against breastfeeding as the jaundice resolves spontaneously.

Crigler–Najjar syndrome

Crigler–Najjar syndrome is a rare, autosomal recessive condition in which hepatic glucuronyl transferase is deficient or absent. In its most severe form kernicterus can only be avoided by long periods of phototherapy and liver transplantation.

Causes of persistent neonatal jaundice

Unconjugated hyperbilirubinaemia	Conjugated hyperbilirubinaemia
Infection, e.g. urinary tract	(a) Neonatal hepatitis syndrome
Hypothyroidism	Congenital infection, e.g. rubella,
Haemolytic anaemia	cytomegalovirus, toxoplasmosis
High gastrointestinal obstruction	Metabolic
Breast-milk jaundice	α_1-antitrypsin deficiency
Transient familial hyperbilirubinaemia	Galactosaemia
Crigler–Najjar syndrome	Tyrosinosis
	Cystic fibrosis
	Storage disorders
	(b) Duct obstruction or obliteration
	Extrahepatic biliary atresia
	Intrahepatic biliary hypoplasia
	Choledochal cyst

Biliary atresia

Biliary atresia is an acquired condition of early postnatal life in which a previously patent biliary tree becomes sclerosed. Without surgical intervention to re-establish bile drainage, cirrhosis and a fatal outcome are inevitable. It affects approximately 1 in 14 000 infants and is the single most common cause of childhood liver related death in the United Kingdom. The cause of the inflammatory process remains unknown.

All infants with persistent jaundice must have their stool colour checked; pale stools suggest obstructive jaundice. The child may be thriving and without conspicuous hepatomegaly but can still be at risk of developing biliary cirrhosis unless prompt diagnosis and surgery is provided. Diagnosis is based on finding conjugated hyperbilirubinaemia, elevated transaminases, an absent gall bladder on ultrasound imaging, and a supportive needle liver biopsy. The diagnosis is excluded by demonstrating bile duct patency with a radiolabelled bile acid excreted into the bowel on gamma imaging. Tests to exclude the recognised causes of neonatal hepatitis are also performed but it is important that a decision regarding surgery is reached promptly and preferably before age 60 days. Bile drainage is created by anastomosing the porta hepatis to a Roux-en-Y loop of jejunum, a hepatic portoenterostomy or Kasai procedure. Between 60 and 70% of those operated on before 60 days become jaundice free, this figure falls to 25–35% if surgery is later. Long-term survival depends on the status of liver fibrosis and cirrhosis. An increasing proportion are having good quality survival into adult life. Others develop portal hypertension or progressive liver failure. Early liver transplantation is now a realistic option for children who fail to benefit from initial surgery.

Neonatal hepatitis syndrome

Causes of acute hepatic failure

Infective
  Hepatitis A, B, C, etc.
  Epstein–Barr
  Adenovirus
  Echo virus
Toxic or drug-related
  Paracetamol
  Halothane
  Valproate
  Amanita phalloides
Metabolic
  Galactosaemia
  Fructosaemia
  Tyrosinaemia
  Wilson disease
  Alpha-1 antitrypsin deficiency
Autoimmune
Infiltrative
Ischaemic

Neonatal hepatitis syndrome refers to conjugated jaundice with liver cell damage but without bile duct obstruction. It is not a discrete entity but is the end result of a range of injurious processes which produce a similar histological picture, hepatocellular necrosis and inflammatory cell infiltrates in the portal tracts and lobules. Investigations are directed at the known infective, genetic and metabolic causes.

Alpha-1-antitrypsin deficiency is an important cause of neonatal hepatitis. The deficiency is associated with PiZ or Pi nul phenotypes of protease inhibitor. It is unclear why deficiency in some families manifests as liver disease while in others it predisposes to emphysema in early adult life. There is a spectrum of severity of liver involvement from subclinical hepatitis through to severe cholestasis and cirrhosis. As yet there is no specific treatment; management aims to maintain growth and avoid deficiency of fat soluble vitamins A, K and D. Transplantation is indicated if the liver function is decompensating. Genetic counselling must advise heterozygote parents of a 25% risk of recurrence. Gene probing directed at a fragment of chromosome 14 is available.

Infectious hepatitis

Hepatitis A (incubation 15–50 days). Hepatitis A infection is the commonest cause of jaundice in older children. It spreads by the oral

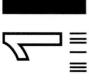

BMA Library

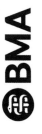

Freepost RTKJ-RKSZ-JGHG
British Medical Association
PO Box 291
LONDON
WC1H 9TG

FREE RETURN POSTAGE FOR STUDENTS & FY DOCTORS!

Use this label for the **FREE** return of books to the BMA Library

route and is usually mild or subclinical. Anorexia, fever, vomiting and abdominal pain may precede the jaundice. Elevation of serum transaminase levels is the first biochemical abnormality and they remain raised for up to 3 weeks in most cases. Passive immunisation with pooled immunoglobulin provides protection and may be indicated for family and other close contacts. Hepatitis A-specific IgM is the best single marker of recent infection.

Hepatitis B (incubation 50–180 days). Hepatitis B is uncommon in European children, but infection and chronic carrier status are frequent in developing countries. Vertical transmission from carrier mothers to newborn babies is a major route of spread, and contributes to a new generation of chronic carriers. Antenatal screening can identify the mothers with carriage, who require clear information of the risk of the infection to themselves and their baby. Infected infants are seldom symptomatic but are vulnerable to cirrhosis and hepatocellular carcinoma in adult life. Programmes to protect infants with combined passive and active immunisation schedules from birth prevent carriage in over 90% of infants.

Hepatitis C is transmitted by blood products and leads to chronic liver disease. Infectious mononucleosis and cytomegalovirus also cause acute hepatitis.

Acute hepatic failure

Acute or fulminant liver failure refers to the multisystem failure which follows severe impairement of liver function caused by hepatocellular necrosis in a patient with no recognised underlying liver disease. Resultant management challenges include encephalopathy, electrolyte and energy substrate imbalance, coagulopathy, circulatory and respiratory failure. Acute liver failure is rare in childhood but becomes an increasing threat in adolescence with the use of paracetamol in self-harm. The potential causes are diverse.

Initial management priorities are to identify the cause, assess the deterioration of liver function and organise transfer to a specialist unit able to sustain homeostasis either until spontaneous recovery or until the availability of liver transplantation.

Reye syndrome

Reye syndrome presents in a similar way but with a characteristic liver biopsy of microvesicular fatty infiltration rather than necrosis. It probably represents a variety of interactions between genetic susceptibility and environmental insults. Patients may have inherited disorders of mitochondrial function, for example errors of the urea cycle, or fatty acid transport and oxidation. Various viral illnesses have been identified as triggers. Epidemiological and experimental evidence incriminated aspirin as a causative factor, and salicylates no longer have a product licence for children. Since their withdrawal the incidence of this rare condition has dropped.

Chronic hepatitis

Chronic liver inflammation is caused by a wide range of congenital disorders and environmental insults. We have already dealt with important early disorders such as congenital infection and α_1-antitrypsin deficiency. In a worldwide context hepatitis B and possibly C generate a vast amount of chronic liver disease. In older children other causes include autoimmune chronic active hepatitis, sclerosing cholangitis usually associated with chronic inflammatory bowel disease, Wilson disease, drugs and biliary obstruction. The chronic inflammation carries the threat of progressive fibrosis, disruption of liver architecture and cirrhosis. The progress of the liver damage may be highlighted by chronic jaundice or malnutrition and ill health, but it can also be an insidious process which only comes to light when the child presents with bleeding problems, splenomegaly, ascites or growth failure.

Autoimmune chronic hepatitis

This is predominantly a disease of older children and young adults with females accounting for over 70%. Genetic susceptibility is linked to HLA antigens B8 DR3, but the environmental trigger that causes a cellular immune reaction against liver cell specific antigens has yet to be established. It may present as an apparent acute hepatitis, or more gradually with intermittent fever, acneiform rashes, colitis, arthritis and hepatosplenomegaly. Elevated liver transaminases and hypergammaglobulinaemia are characteristic, and autoantibodies are usually positive. The prothrombin time is typically prolonged. Formal diagnosis hinges on the liver biopsy which shows widening of the portal tracts with chronic inflammatory cell infiltrate, and destruction of the limiting plate at the junction of portal tracts and parenchyma together with hepatocyte necrosis.

Immunosuppressant therapy is indicated in order to relieve symptoms and to delay the progression to cirrhosis. Recommended regimens incorporate prednisolone and azathioprine, with repeat liver biopsy to determine whether remission has been achieved. Long-term follow up is necessary as there is a high risk or relapse.

Wilson disease

Wilson disease (hepatolenticular degeneration) is a rare, autosomal recessive disorder of copper metabolism which can readily escape prompt diagnosis. The classically described features of copper deposition at the peripheries of the cornea (Kayser–Fleischer rings), neurological problems, and a low caeruloplasmin may be absent in the young. Children can present with either acute or chronic hepatitis, deteriorating school performance, haemolytic anaemia, proteinuria or arthralgia. Liver problems typically present before neurological complaints, and unfortunately acute liver failure or cirrhosis may determine the prognosis. Wilson disease needs to be considered in any child with otherwise unexplained acute or chronic hepatitis. Investigations include plasma caeruloplasmin measurement, liver biopsy with copper estimation, and studies of urinary copper excretion. Diagnosis before irreversible tissue damage allows for a good response to treatment with penicillamine which promotes urinary clearance of copper ions. Liver transplantation is an option for patients who present too late to benefit from chelation therapy. Genetic counselling and screening of siblings is essential.

Childhood cirrhosis

Cirrhosis may evolve as the end stage of recognised liver disease, or may already be established at first presentation with portal hypertension or liver failure. The liver failure may lead to sudden deterioration, or may be more gradual with growth impairment, intermittent ascites and a coagulation disorder. Children can tolerate cirrhosis for years, sustaining adequate growth and a nearly normal life style. Investigations should be aimed at identifying the underlying cause but this cannot be defined in a substantial proportion of cases. The degree of liver dysfunction needs to be assessed so that steps can be taken to correct reversible problems such as malnutrition, vitamin deficiency, ascites and electrolyte imbalance. Attention to these factors can considerably delay the final liver decompensation. Liver transplantation is now a realistic option for the management of these children with 1-year survival in the region of 70–80% and promising long-term results. The difficulty is recognising when a child's quality of life has deteriorated to the extent that justifies this major step and the ensuing dependence on immunosuppressant therapy.

Causes and clinical features of cirrhosis in childhood

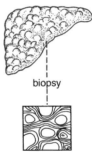

CAUSES

Genetic (metabolic/storage) cirrhosis
e.g. α_1-antitrypsin deficiency
   Wilson disease
   galactosaemia
   cystic fibrosis

Post-necrotic cirrhosis
e.g. neonatal hepatitis
   chronic aggressive hepatitis
   drugs, toxins, poisons
   venous congestion

Biliary cirrhosis
e.g. extrahepatic biliary atresia
   intrahepatic biliary hypoplasia
   choledochal cyst

biopsy

regenerating nodules
broad bands of fibrosis

CLINICAL FEATURES

Portal hypertension
   oesophageal varices
   splenomegaly
   hypersplenism
   ascites

Hepatic failure
   failure to thrive
   fatigue, anorexia
   spider naevi
   finger clubbing
   liver palms

Portal hypertension

This usually presents as intestinal bleeding and splenomegaly, but the spleen may not be palpable immediately after a severe haemorrhage. The majority of cases are due to thrombosis of the portal vein; either idiopathic or secondary to sepsis of the umbilical vein and portal system in infancy. Hepatic cirrhosis and congenital hepatic fibrosis may also cause portal hypertension. The exact cause needs to be established by detailed ultrasound imaging, selective angiography of the coeliac axis and by liver biopsy. If portal vein thrombosis is diagnosed, the long-term management should be as conservative as possible as splenorenal shunts are technically difficult and seldom successful before the age of 10 years. There is a tendency for bleeding from the oesophageal varices to improve with age.

Congenital hepatic fibrosis Congenital hepatic fibrosis may be either sporadic or familial and is diagnosed by liver biopsy which shows marked portal fibrosis but retention of the normal hepatic lobular architecture. It may be associated with polycystic disease of the kidneys.

Causes of hepatomegaly and clinical signs which may aid diagnosis

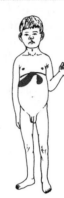

Causes

- Systemic infection
  infectious hepatitis
  glandular fever
- Primary liver disease
  chronic hepatitis
  polycystic disease
  hepatocellular carcinoma
- Other neoplasia
  leukaemia
  reticulosis
  nephroblastoma
  neuroblastoma
- Metabolic storage
  glycogenoses
  lipidoses
  mucopolysaccharidoses
- Cardiac

Signs

mental retardation
  mucopolysaccharidoses

Kayser-Fleischer rings:
  Wilson disease

spider naevi:
liver palms:
finger clubbing
  chronic liver failure

splenomegaly
collateral veins
ascites
  portal hypertension

bone lesions
  lipidoses

REFERENCE

Apley J 1975 The child with abdominal pains. Blackwell Scientific, Oxford

Kelly DA, Booth IW 1997 Pediatric gastroenterology and hepatology. Mosby-Wolfe, London

Mowat A P 1993 Liver disorders in childhood, 3rd edn. Butterworth-Heinemann, Oxford

Tripp J H, Candy D C A 1992 Manual of paediatric gastroenterology, 2nd edn. Churchill Livingstone, Edinburgh

Urinary tracts and testes

RENAL FUNCTION TESTS
URINARY TRACT MALFORMATIONS
RENAL CALCULI
URINARY TRACT INFECTIONS
ENURESIS
HAEMATURIA
ACUTE NEPHRITIC SYNDROME
NEPHROTIC SYNDROME
RENAL TUBULAR DISORDERS
ACUTE RENAL FAILURE
CHRONIC RENAL FAILURE
THE TESTES
THE PREPUCE .

Renal function undergoes a major transition with the onset of extra-uterine life and the demands of water conservation and electrolyte homeostasis. Although nephron formation is complete before birth, the newborn kidney contains less than 20% of its adult cellular component, and the total renal blood flow is reduced due to higher renal vascular resistance. The glomerular filtration rate at term averages 20 ml per minute per 1.73 m^2 with adult values of 110–120 ml per minute per 1.73 m^2 only being reached in the second year of life. The functional limitations of the newborn kidney are reflected in higher blood urea and phosphate levels, and a lower plasma bicarbonate concentration.

The higher metabolic rate of the infant in relation to body weight, greater insensible water losses and the inability to control oral intake, increase the susceptibility of young patients to dehydration and metabolic abnormalities. Acute renal failure with acidosis, uraemia and hyperkalaemia can develop very rapidly in the young infant.

RENAL FUNCTION TESTS

Urinalysis. A multiple urine test strip can be employed and it is preferable to examine a fresh morning sample of urine.

Proteinuria. This can signify renal disease but transient proteinuria is also common during febrile illnesses or after exercise. Heavy proteinuria with oedema suggests nephrotic syndrome.

Postural or orthostatic proteinuria is suggested by the absence of significant proteinuria on a first morning specimen compared to one tested after the child has been ambulant. Measurements of proteinuria on 24-hour urine collections have now been replaced by measuring protein to creatinine ratios on spot urine samples (normal ratio <20 mg/mmol).

Haematuria. Microscopic haematuria may also be a transient finding but macroscopic haematuria always required further investigation. The commonest cause is urinary tract infection. Microscopy of fresh

Urinary output (ml/day)	
infant	250–600
child	500–1000
adolescent	500–1500
adult	500–2000

urine should always be performed to confirm the presence of red blood cells rather than a false-positive test due to free haemoglobin, myoglobin, beeturia, drugs or confectionary dyes.

Glycosuria and aminoaciduria. Glycosuria and aminoaciduria may be secondary to elevated serum levels or may be the result of tubular defects.

Urine pH and osmolality. Normal urine pH is between 5 and 7 and is affected by dietary intake. Formal acidification tests may be required if renal tubular acidosis is suspected. A first morning urine sample after fasting overnight provides a useful screening test of renal concentrating ability with normal values being above 800 mOsm per kg (specific gravity above 1.020).

Nitrite and leucocyte tests. Many test strips now incorporate nitrite detection which can indicate the presence of urinary infection when nitrate is reduced to nitrite. Leucocytes may also indicate infection but false-positive and- negative tests do occur.

Urine microscopy

red blood cells

white blood cells

hyaline casts

epithelial cells

crystals

bacteria

Microscopy. This may give useful information especially in the presence of proteinuria or haematuria. Fresh urine should also be used when examining for casts. Red blood cell casts suggest glomerulonephritis. The presence of increased white blood cells, above 5 per high powered field, or motile bacteria suggest urinary tract infection. The latter needs confirmation by urine culture.

Blood tests. These will include full blood count, electrolytes including bicarbonate, urea, creatinine, calcium, phosphate, alkaline phosphatase and albumin. Urea levels can be effected by dehydration, protein meals and drug therapy, so plasma creatinine levels are favoured for monitoring renal function. However, it should be remembered that the plasma creatinine can remain within the normal range until the glomerular filtration rate is less than 50% of normal.

Glomerular filtration rate (GFR). Derived from 24-hour urine volume and measurement of plasma creatinine, this is very liable to error in young children because of the difficulty of collection techniques. The approximate GFR can be derived from the plasma creatinine using the equation: GFR/1.73 m^2 surface area = 38 × height (cm)/plasma creatinine (μmol/l). The rate of fall in the blood concentration of injected isotope, ^{51}Cr-EDTA or ^{99}Tc-DTPA is used for more precise measurement.

Radiological investigations. Ultrasound is now the investigation of choice for urinary tract problems with the intravenous urogram (IVU) being reserved for when further details of the urinary tract are required. The micturating cystourethrogram (MCUG) is still required to exclude reflux or lower urinary tract obstruction. Increasing use is made of radionuclide investigations such as DMSA (to define scars from vesicoureteric reflux and differential function) or ^{99}Tc-MAG3 or DTPA (to define obstruction and as an indirect method for following reflux).

URINARY TRACT MALFORMATIONS

Spectrum of urinary tract abnormalities detected antenatally: Nottingham 1986–96	
Pelviureteric junction obstruction	26%
Multicystic dysplastic kidney	18%
Vesicoureteric junction obstruction	8%
Vesicoureteric reflux	7%
Duplex systems	6%
Posterior urethral valves	5%
Others, e.g. renal agenesis, single kidney	16%
'Transient'	14%

These are relatively common but most are functionally insignificant, for example duplex systems. A small proportion are lethal and may have important genetic implications. The increased use of ultrasound in pregnancy has resulted in renal malformations being diagnosed more frequently in utero. Fortunately most abnormalities are unilateral. Intervention techniques to relieve fetal obstructive uropathy such as vesico-amniotic shunts are rarely required.

Renal agenesis. This results in oligohydramnios and compression of the fetus, Potter syndrome. Other urinary tract malformations such as polycystic kidneys or obstructive lesions may also cause oligohydramnios. The degree of the associated pulmonary hypoplasia is critical to early survival.

Unilateral renal hypoplasia and dysplasia. This may be an incidental finding but a large multicystic dysplastic kidney may present as an abdominal mass in a newborn infant. Differentiation from hydronephrosis is important. The function of the apparently normal contralateral kidney must be carefully assessed as part of the evaluation.

Polycystic kidneys. Infantile polycystic disease results in grossly enlarged spongy kidneys and cystic changes in the liver and other viscera. The bilateral kidney enlargement is conspicuous at birth or in early infancy. There are several varieties with an autosomal recessive inheritance. The adult form, with autosomal dominant inheritance, can also present in early life although most survive to be young adults and are therefore capable of transmitting the abnormal gene.

Simple cysts. These are very common in adults and have to be distinguished from cancers, but they are rare in childhood. They appear to be an acquired condition.

Renal tract abnomalies causing obstruction

hydronephrosis

hydroureter

bladder wall thickening

A pelvi-ureteric obstruction
B uretero-vesical obstruction
C urethral valves

Obstructive malformations   These produce unilateral or bilateral hydronephrosis.

Pelvi-ureteric junction (PUJ) obstruction is the commonest cause of hydronephrosis and may be produced by intrinsic stenosis, functional obstruction or compression from an aberrant artery or bands. Treatment for PUJ obstruction is by pyeloplasty.

Vesico-ureteric junction (VUJ) obstruction produces megaureters. Treatment is by reimplantation of the ureter which often requires tapering at its lower end.

Horseshoe kidneys produce a characteristic IVU picture—the upper poles are further from the midline than the lower poles. Hydronephrosis due to PUJ obstruction may occur.

Ureteric duplication. The bifid ureter is more common than complete duplication. Usually there is a strong family history of this abnormality. When the ureters enter the bladder separately the ureter draining the upper renal moiety is situated in a lower position or may be ectopic. Because it has a longer intravesical course it is liable to become obstructed resulting in hydronephrosis of the upper pole. The ureter draining the lower moiety has a short intravesical course and is therefore prone to vesico-ureteric reflux resulting in chronic pyelonephritis of the lower pole.

Ureterocoele. Ureterocoele is an expanded end of either a normally situated ureter or one which enters the bladder ectopically. It affects girls more than boys and the abnormality may appear as a filling defect of the bladder. Occasionally it can prolapse through the bladder neck and may appear as a mass in the vagina.

Horseshoe kidneys

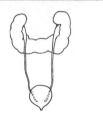

Ureteric duplications

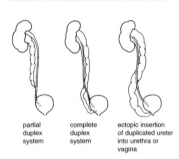

partial duplex system

complete duplex system

ectopic insertion of duplicated ureter into urethra or vagina

Urethral valves

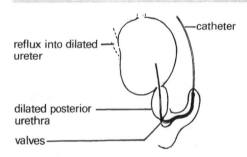

catheter

reflux into dilated ureter

dilated posterior urethra

valves

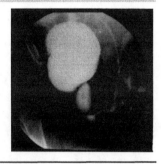

Posterior urethral valves. Posterior urethral valves are the commonest cause of lower urinary tract obstruction in the male child. The diagnosis may be made on antenatal ultrasound or postnatally on routine examination of a healthy neonate who has a distended bladder with a poor urinary stream. Otherwise infants may present with a urinary infection and septicaemia, or overflow incontinence in later years. The kidneys show secondary bilateral hydronephrosis due to obstruction and/or vesico-ureteric reflux. Diagnosis is by MCUG and treatment is by ablation of valves via endoscopy. Temporary diversion is rarely necessary. Chronic renal failure can develop at any age and reflects the degree of renal dysplasia and residual renal mass.

Bladder exstrophy. This results from failure of midline fusion of the infra-umbilical midline structures. Males are affected more commonly than females. Clinically, the bladder mucosa is present as a small contracted circular plaque in the low abdomen, the umbilicus is abnormally low, the penis up-turned and epispadic, the pubic bones unfused and the lower limbs therefore apparently externally rotated. In girls the genital tract is normal although vaginal stenosis may need surgery in early adult life. Bladder and especially bladder neck reconstruction is extremely difficult and many children are treated by urinary diversion.

Urachal remnants may persist producing blind tracts or cysts in the lower abdominal wall. Complete patency between the bladder and umbilicus is exceptionally rare.

Prune belly syndrome. This occurs almost exclusively in males and is a triad of deficiency of abdominal muscles, complex genito-urinary malformation and bilateral undescended testes. Pulmonary hypoplasia may prove fatal in the newborn period but other less affected children can survive with appropriate therapy.

RENAL CALCULI

Stones in the urinary tract (urolithiasis) are rare in children compared to adults. Most are associated with haematuria, abdominal pain and particularly urinary tract infection. Mixed stones with magnesium ammonium phosphate and calcium phosphate are often associated with proteus urinary tract infection. Deposition of calcium in the renal parenchyma (nephrocalcinosis) occurs with hypercalcaemia, hyperoxaluria and distal renal tubular acidosis. Stones in children require thorough investigation. Treatment also requires a high fluid intake and lithotripsy or direct surgical removal may be required.

URINARY TRACT INFECTIONS

This is a common and important paediatric problem because it is a significant cause of morbidity in childhood. Association with vesico-ureteric reflux may lead to renal damage (reflux nephropathy) which can give rise to hypertension and end stage renal disease in late childhood or adult life. Approximately 2–3% of girls and less than 1% of boys are at risk of asymptomatic urine infections throughout childhood. Proven bacterial infections warrant further investigation and this needs to be more comprehensive in preschool children who are most at risk of developing renal scars.

The younger the child the more non-specific the symptoms. In the newborn prolonged jaundice, excessive weight loss or a septicaemic episode may be secondary to urinary tract infection. The young child may also present with poor weight gain, irritability, fever, vomiting and diarrhoea. In any septicaemic infant suprapubic aspiration of the urine should be considered a routine part of the infection screen, along with blood cultures and lumbar puncture. Otherwise every effort should be made to obtain a proper clean catch urine. Positive urine cultures based on bag specimens are often misleading.

Organisms derived from bowel flora are the commonest infecting agents with *E. coli* predominating. Some individuals are more prone to urinary tract infections than others and this may be associated with abnormal gram-negative bacterial colonisation of the introitus and peri-urethral areas. Studies showing increased adherence to uroepithelial cells by pyelonephritogenic bacteria may allow improved preventative measures in the future.

Management. The management of acute infection includes copious fluids, mild analgesia if required, and antibacterial therapy; septicaemia or acute pyelonephritis merits intravenous co-amoxiclav, gentamicin or a cephalosporin. Oral therapy for less severe cases includes trimethoprim, co-amoxiclav, nalidixic acid, nitrofurantoin or a cephalosporin. A 7–10-day course of chemotherapy is usually sufficient and a sterile urine should be obtained following treatment. Prophylaxis with bedtime administration of antibiotics is generally continued until investigations are complete. All proven urinary tract infections require radiological evaluation. Initially this is an ultrasound which may be combined with a plain abdominal X-ray to show details of the spine and exclude renal calculi. Children under 1 year of age are investigated further with an MCUG to rule out vesico-ureteric reflux with which renal scarring and damage may be associated. The MCUG is only performed in older children if pyelonephritis is strongly suspected, or if there is a history of repeated urinary tract infections or renal problems in relatives. Reflux can be a familial problem. It is therefore justified to screen other family members (usually by ultrasound alone) when gross reflux is present in one child. If moderate to severe reflux is detected then any associated scarring of the kidneys can be documented by DMSA scanning.

Grades of vesico-ureteric reflux during micturating cystogram

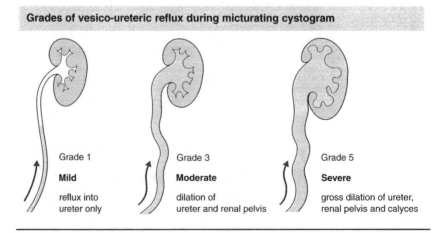

Grade 1

Mild

reflux into ureter only

Grade 3

Moderate

dilation of ureter and renal pelvis

Grade 5

Severe

gross dilation of ureter, renal pelvis and calyces

The presence of vesico-ureteric reflux warrants continuous prophylaxis with antimicrobial agents such as trimethoprim (2 mg/kg/single dose) or nitrofurantoin (1 mg/kg/single dose). Previously many of these children were subjected to surgery for reimplantation of the ureters, but because reflux will cease spontaneously in a large number of children maintained on prophylactic therapy alone, surgery is now generally restricted to cases of urinary obstruction, or to children with 'breakthrough' urinary infections while on prophylaxis.

Drugs commonly used in the treatment of urinary tract infection

Drug	Dose	Comments	Side effects
Trimethoprim	8 mg/kg/day	Useful in prophylaxis. Good compliance	Rashes, vomiting
Co-amoxiclav	20–45 mg/kg/day	Less useful in prophylaxis	Rashes, diarrhoea
Nitrofurantoin	3–5 mg/kg/day	Useful in prophylaxis	Nausea, vomiting
Nalidixic acid	50 mg/kg/day	Useful in boys with proteus infection	Rashes
Cephradine	50 mg/kg/day	Less useful in prophylaxis	Allergic reactions
Gentamicin	2 mg/kg/day	Parenteral use only	Nephrotoxic, ototoxic
Cefotaxime	100 mg/kg/day	Parenteral use only	Rashes, diarrhoea

It is important to emphasise general preventive measures in all children with urinary tract infection. These include a regular bowel habit, adequate fluids, proper voiding techniques and double micturition, good hygiene and the avoidance of irritants such as bubble baths and nylon underwear.

Older children may complain of a urethral syndrome with frequency and dysuria and no bacteriological confirmation of urine infection. Viral infections may play a role but acute vulvitis or balanitis may be associated with poor hygiene, perineal candidiasis or contact sensitivity to nylon pants.

Sexual abuse should also be borne in mind in a child with recurrent urinary tract symptoms, especially with genital signs.

Screening. Extensive surveys have attempted to monitor the impact of detection, investigation and treatment of asymptomatic bacteriuria in schoolgirls aged 5–12 years. The results suggest that such screening is not worthwhile and that kidney damage associated with infection generally occurs before 5 years. Screening the preschool child is time consuming and the yield of treatable abnormalities is small.

ENURESIS

Wetting is a common symptom which can cause much distress and anxiety to child and family. It may be referred to as enuresis which can be defined as the involuntary voiding of urine in a child over 5 years of age with a normal urinary tract, whereas incontinence is the leakage of urine when a structural or neurological disease of the bladder or urinary tract is present. Nocturnal enuresis is considered in Chapter 21.

Causes of wetting in children

Diagnosis	Clinical pointers
Urinary tract infection	Other urinary tract symptoms, secondary onset wetting
Detrusor instability	Daytime symptoms of urinary frequency, urgency and urge incontinence usually with a minor degree of wetness and worse in the afternoons
Neuropathic bladder	Constant severe daytime wetting, soiling, lumbosacral dimple or naevus, abnormal gait, abnormal peri-anal or lower limb neurology, palpable bladder
Ectopic ureter	Constant dribble of urine between voidings
Chronic renal disease	Chronic ill health, hypertension, palpable kidneys or bladder, anaemia, polydipsia
Diabetes mellitus	Recent illness with weight loss, thirst and polydipsia

HAEMATURIA

Haematuria may occur as an isolated symptom or may be accompanied by signs of a systemic disorder, for example Henoch–Schönlein purpura or acute glomerulonephritis. It may be associated with renal colic due to clot, calculus or obstructive malformation, or a loin mass, for example Wilms tumour or hydronephrosis. Red cell casts and significant proteinuria establish glomerular lesions while pyuria and bacteriuria point to infection, the latter being the commonest cause for haematuria in childhood. An abdominal ultrasound or IVU is indicated if renal tract pathology is suspected. Cystoscopy is seldom required unless the bloodstaining is prominent at the start or finish of the stream. Renal biopsy is reserved for children whose haematuria is persistent, and accompanied by significant proteinuria, hypertension or impaired renal function. Fictitious haematuria may be part of the syndrome of Münchhausen by proxy where blood is added to the child's urine by a close relative.

Causes of haematuria with examples

Causes	Examples
Infection	Bacteria, viruses, tuberculosis, schistosomiasis
Glomerulonephritis	Post-streptococcal, mesangial IgA nephropathy
Trauma	
Calculus	
Congenital abnormality	Hydronephrosis due to pelvi-ureteric obstruction
Tumour	Wilms tumour
Vascular	Arteritis, infarction
Bleeding disorder	
Drug induced	Cyclophosphamide
Exercise induced	
Fictitious	

Recurrent or persistent haematuria

Recurrent macroscopic haematuria exacerbated by upper respiratory tract infections suggests IgA nephropathy or Berger disease. Some healthy children with persistent microscopic haematuria and similar findings in other family members fall into the category of benign familial haematuria. A positive family history of nephritis in association with sensorineural nerve deafness suggests Alport syndrome which is X-linked, and boys with this condition tend to be affected more severely than girls. Longer-term follow up of patients with recurrent haematuria suggests that there may be more morbidity than previously suspected.

Acute haemorrhagic cystitis

This may occur with viral infection, notably adenovirus 11, or as a complication of cyclophosphamide therapy.

ACUTE NEPHRITIC SYNDROME

Poststreptococcal glomerulonephritis

Acute glomerulonephritis occurs predominantly in schoolchildren. Although it characteristically occurs 7–14 days after a group A β-haemolytic streptococcal throat infection, an increasing percentage appear to have another, possibly viral explanation. In areas of the world with poor hygiene, glomerulonephritis following streptococcal skin infection with pyoderma is relatively common. Only certain serotypes of streptococcus are responsible and the detection of streptococcal antigen in the glomerular mesangium supports the concept of acute soluble complex injury. Reduced serum complement levels also indicate an immunological pathogenesis. Many affected children are asymptomatic. Typical complaints include malaise, headache, and vague loin discomfort but it may be the smoky urine which at first causes alarm. Oedema tends to collect around the orbits and on the backs of the hands and feet. Urine microscopy shows gross haematuria with granular and red cell casts. Proteinuria is also present. In the majority of cases oliguria is only mild but severe fluid retention can occasionally produce acute hypertension, with encephalopathy and seizures, or heart failure.

Management. The confirmation of post-streptococcal glomerulonephritis establishes an excellent prognosis in most instances, and therefore all cases should have an antistreptolysin titre determination as well as a throat swab. The remainder of the family should also have throat swabs.

Treatment includes eradication of streptococcal infection with a 10-day course of phenoxymethyl penicillin. Hospital admission is required if there is any suggestion of oliguria, fluid overload or hypertension. The reduced glomerular filtration rate (GFR) should be assessed by a plasma creatinine estimation and serial progress monitored by daily weight and fluid balance. Oliguria requires salt restriction and water intake balanced against insensible loss, 400 ml per m² surface area per day, plus the previous day's urine output. More aggressive management with diuretics and hypotensive drugs may be needed to control hypertension. Acute peritoneal dialysis is necessary to treat severe fluid overload, hyperkalaemia and a deteriorating clinical state.

The normal course is for the creatinine to return to normal in 10–14 days. If oliguria persists or progresses, a renal biopsy is justified to define the nature of the glomerular lesion. Rapidly progressive glomerulonephritis with scarring and deteriorating renal function is fortunately rare in the young.

The long-term prognosis of post-streptococcal glomerulonephritis is assumed to be excellent, 92–98% achieving resolution. There is still some caution about the eventual status of the non-streptococcal group.

Henoch–Schönlein purpura Although approximately 70% of children with Henoch–Schönlein purpura (HSP) have haematuria and or proteinuria, the glomerulonephritis is usually asymptomatic and non-progressive. However, children with HSP presenting with an acute nephritic syndrome or rapidly progressing to a nephrotic syndrome have an ominous future. Normal renal function 2 years after the initial insult is unlikely to deteriorate but there are exceptions. Renal histology is some guide to prognosis, the glomerular lesions varying from minimal change to focal or diffuse mesangial proliferation with crescents, and in the most advanced stages, sclerosis. There is no specific therapy for this nephritis and management is symptomatic. Children with urinary abnormalities after HSP should continue to have urine examinations and blood pressure measurements at periodic intervals in order to detect the late development of hypertension and renal impairment.

NEPHROTIC SYNDROME

Oedema

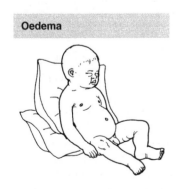

The nephrotic syndrome occurs when there is gross urinary protein loss resulting in hypoalbuminaemia and oedema. It is uncommon, with an incidence of 2 per 100 000 children (9–16 per 100 000 in Asian population) and a peak incidence between 1 and 5 years. Males are more commonly affected than females, 2.5 : 1. The cause is unknown. Approximately 85% of Caucasian children with nephrotic syndrome have the so-called 'minimal change' type.

Peri-orbital or dependent oedema and abdominal ascites are usually noticed first. There may also be abdominal pain, vomiting and diarrhoea. Hypovolaemia and circulatory collapse is a danger in the early phase of the illness, because fluid shifts from the intravascular to the extracellular space, and it may be exacerbated by vomiting and diarrhoea. A careful review of pulse, blood pressure and haematocrit must be maintained until the situation stabilises. Intravenous albumin infusions may be necessary. These children are also susceptible to infection, particularly penumococcal peritonitis and urinary tract infection. Fever in the presence of ascites justifies a diagnostic ascitic fluid tap for microscopy and culture.

Pathology. The term minimal change nephrotic syndrome is derived from light microscopy appearance. Electron microscopy shows fusion of the epithelial cell foot processes, a non-specific consequence of proteinuria. Although the pathogenesis of the renal insult leading to proteinuria is uncertain, it is thought to be a reduction in the fixed negative charge on the glomerular capillary wall. Renal biopsy is not required if the clinical picture matches minimal change nephrotic syndrome and there is a definite response to corticosteroids. Other pathological conditions such as focal segmental glomerulosclerosis and membrano-proliferative glomerulonephritis carry a more guarded prognosis.

Management. Diuretics should be used with care as they promote hyponatraemia and may further reduce the intravascular volume. Salt poor albumin infusion temporarily restores the circulating volume but is required in only a minority of children. Rest is normally guided by the patient's behaviour, and moderate fluid restriction is necessary only while the child is oedematous. Prophylactic penicillin should be given during the oedematous phase. The recovery is monitored by daily weights and proteinuria. Ninety per cent of children with minimal change disease will respond to corticosteroids within 8 weeks.

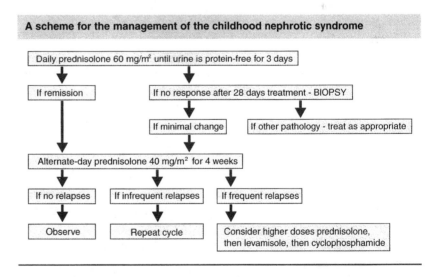

Frequent relapses may be controlled by alternate-day prednisolone, but if corticosteroid toxicity occurs there may be a case for a course of cyclophosphamide. Concern about the long-term gonadal effects of cytotoxic therapy restricts its usage.

Congenital nephrotic syndrome. Congenital nephrotic syndrome is very rare and either presents at birth with placental oedema or develops in the first year. It may be familial with autosomal recessive inheritance, and is more common in Scandinavia. Dialysis and transplantation can now be offered to children with this previously fatal condition.

Systemic causes of nephrotic syndrome. These include infections (e.g. malaria), poisons (e.g. mercurials), allergies (e.g. bee sting) and collagen vascular disorders (e.g. SLE).

RENAL TUBULAR DISORDERS

It is essential to consider these disorders when urine analysis reveals glycosuria, aminoaciduria or impaired ability to concentrate or acidify urine.

Renal tubular disorders: a schematic representation of the renal tubule indicating defects, associated conditions and clinical manifestations

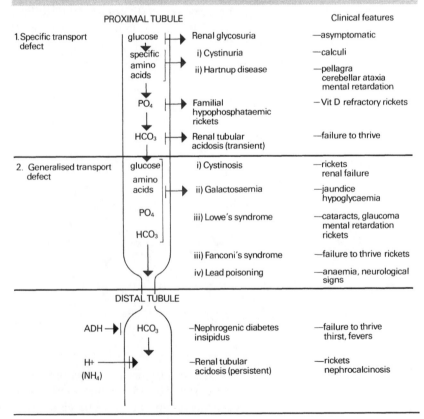

	PROXIMAL TUBULE		Clinical features
1. Specific transport defect	glucose	Renal glycosuria	—asymptomatic
	specific amino acids	i) Cystinuria	—calculi
		ii) Hartnup disease	—pellagra cerebellar ataxia mental retardation
	PO₄	Familial hypophosphataemic rickets	—Vit D refractory rickets
	HCO₃	Renal tubular acidosis (transient)	—failure to thrive
2. Generalised transport defect	glucose amino acids PO₄ HCO₃	i) Cystinosis	—rickets renal failure
		ii) Galactosaemia	—jaundice hypoglycaemia
		iii) Lowe's syndrome	—cataracts, glaucoma mental retardation rickets
		iii) Fanconi's syndrome	—failure to thrive rickets
		iv) Lead poisoning	—anaemia, neurological signs
	DISTAL TUBULE		
ADH →	HCO₃	—Nephrogenic diabetes insipidus	—failure to thrive thirst, fevers
H+ (NH₄)		—Renal tubular acidosis (persistent)	—rickets nephrocalcinosis

ACUTE RENAL FAILURE

Acute renal failure is an uncommon but important problem in which the kidneys are no longer able to maintain biochemical homeostasis. Oliguria, less than 300 ml per m² surface area per day, is usually present but polyuria may be present especially with relief of obstructive lesions. The possible causes fall into three main groups: pre-renal, renal, and post-renal.

Management. In practical terms the priorities are to distinguish pre-renal from established renal failure, and to exclude obstruction and preexisting renal disease (acute on chronic renal failure). The presenting illness, gastroenteritis or septicaemic shock, may be very suggestive of circulatory failure and a pre-renal cause, but if oliguria has developed there is a risk that tubular nephropathy has already occurred. The examination of urine and plasma makes the distinction, as normal kidneys will concentrate urinary urea and reabsorb sodium. Proteinuria, cells and casts also suggest a renal lesion.

Pre-renal failure demands urgent vascular volume expansion and careful monitoring of fluid and electrolyte replacement. Renal failure may respond to intravenous, high-dosage frusemide but preparations should be made for peritoneal or haemodialysis, especially if the picture is complicated by hypertension, pulmonary oedema or worsening biochemistry. Gentamicin and other drugs with a primarily renal excretion should be used with caution. Potentially reversible obstruction must not be overlooked and an early ultrasound examination is advocated. Acute renal failure of childhood has in general a good outlook if dealt with expertly. However the survival is less good for acute renal failure accompanying multiorgan failure or following surgery for complex congenital heart disease.

Manifestations and management of acute renal failure

	Complication	Therapy	
water overload	hyponatraemia	fluid restriction, twice daily weight	**D**
sodium overload	hypertension, oedema	salt restriction	**I**
potassium overload	cardiac arrhythmias	salbutamol cation exchange resin dietary restriction	**A** **L**
metabolic acidosis		cautious administration of sodium bicarbonate	**Y**
nitrogen retention		high calorie intake protein restriction	**S**
hypercatabolic metabolism			**I**
burns, sepsis			**S**

pre-renal→
renal→
post-renal→

Haemolytic uraemic syndrome (HUS)

This triad of acute renal failure, haemolytic anaemia with fragmented erythrocytes and thrombocytopenia is the commonest cause of acute renal failure in infants and children. Small outbreaks occasionally occur in the United Kingdom. Typically an episode of vomiting and diarrhoea is followed by pallor, haematuria and oliguria as acute renal failure supervenes. Seizures may reflect hypertension or direct central nervous system involvement. Other organs such as the gut, liver and heart can also be affected.

The epidemic form of HUS has been associated with a variety of bacterial and viral agents, with the predominant infection being with verotoxin producing *E. coli* 0157. While the pathophysiological mechanisms in HUS are still unclear it is suggested that an initial toxic insult to vascular endothelial cells may disturb the balance between prostacyclin production in endothelial cells and thromboxane synthesis by platelets.

The epidemic form of HUS generally has a good prognosis with supportive treatment alone, but sporadic cases in older children with no clear prodromal illness often result in residual renal impairment.

CHRONIC RENAL FAILURE

The incidence of chronic renal failure in children is much less than in the adult population but the effects on growth and development can be profound. Symptoms do not usually develop until 60–80% of renal function is lost. There may be an insidious onset with growth failure, anorexia and nocturia, or an acute on chronic crisis may be precipitated by superimposed infection. Urinary tract infection or salt wasting can cause a rapid deterioration in renal function, while extrarenal infection with increased catabolic demands and vomiting may cause an acute decline in GFR.

Manifestations and management of chronic renal failure

	Effect	Cause	Therapy
chronic renal failure	growth failure	poor caloric intake deranged biochemistry -acidosis anaemia salt and fluid loss	calorie and vitamin B, C supplements balanced first class protein sodium bicarbonate and salt supplements growth hormone early dialysis
	renal osteodystrophy	phosphate retention defective vit D metabolism secondary hyperparathyroidism	dietary phosphate restriction calcium carbonate phosphate binders vit D supplements
	anaemia	nutritional reduced erythropoeitin blood loss	erythropoietin iron supplements only if iron-deficient folic acid
	hypertension	sodium retention renal disease / renin release	sodium restriction, diuretics antihypertensives nephrectomy

These children should be supervised by a paediatric nephrology unit which can provide the optimal care consisting of specialist dietary advice, surgical liaison and psychosocial preparation if dialysis and transplantation become imminent. Growth impairment in chronic renal failure is a multifactorial problem but aggressive feeding regimens with supplements in older children, and nasogastric or gastrostomy feeding in the first 2 years of life may help to prevent the short stature which has been a feature of such children.

Children develop end-stage renal disease requiring dialysis and transplantation at the rate of approximately 8–10 per million child population. Dialysis is seen only as an interim measure before transplantation which offers the best overall form of rehabilitation with growth potential. Recent experience with erythropoietin and growth hormone suggests that both the chronic anaemia and growth failure associated with chronic renal failure can be ameliorated by the use of these synthetic hormones.

Haemodialysis can be technically difficult in any child because of problems with vascular access and is most readily achieved using jugular venous catheters. For most children the favoured method for chronic dialysis is continuous ambulatory peritoneal dialysis (CAPD) or continuous cycling peritoneal dialysis (CCPD). These provide opportunities for children of all sizes to be treated at home with generally freer diets and improved wellbeing. Dialysis and transplantation are now feasible at any age, but such patients place considerable demands on family and treatment resources which can only be met by a fully integrated team approach that can decide the best treatment options for each individual.

THE TESTES

The testes develop as intra-abdominal structures, entering the inguinal canal during the seventh month of fetal life. At birth the testes are usually in the scrotum but in about 10% of children they are undescended at birth and it is not uncommon for descent to be completed during the first 2 weeks of life. Descent is unlikely to take place after 1 year of age. The endocrine control of testicular descent is complex, involving gonadotrophins, androgens and müllerian inhibitory factor.

Retractile testes

Normal testes in young boys are readily elevated to the upper scrotum by the cremasteric muscle. This commonly causes confusion and anxiety at routine medical checks. Careful, preferably parent-held records, should confirm that the testes were both descended at the time of the newborn check. Retractile testes will descend if the boy is examined in a warm and relaxed atmosphere, and if he is asked to adopt a squatting position.

Undescended testes

Testes which fail to reach the scrotum may be classified into the following categories:

Incompletely descended testes (20%). Incompletely descended testes lie along the path of descent but fail to reach the scrotum. They may be intra-abdominal or within the canal and hence impalpable.

An emergent or high scrotal testis is easily palpable. These testes often appear grossly abnormal at operation, being small, soft and with a disassociated epididymis. Most are accompanied by a large hernial sac.

Spermatogenesis is poor and is probably not significantly altered by operation. Orchidopexy may be difficult as the vessels are usually short. Sometimes no testicular tissue can be found and this is either the result of intra-uterine torsion or true agenesis. In the latter case abdominal ultrasound should be performed to determine whether there is associated renal agenesis.

Maldescent and undescent of the testes

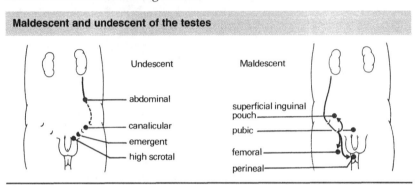

Ectopic or maldescended testes (80%). Ectopic or maldescended testes pass through the inguinal canal and emerge from the superficial inguinal ring, thereafter following an abnormal course. Ectopic sites include the superficial inguinal pouch, perineal, femoral and pubic positions. Most ectopic testes are easily palpable. The testis is usually normal in appearance and a hernial sac is only occasionally present. Orchidopexy is easy because of adequate cord length. Spermatogenesis is almost normal with or without operation. The main indication for orchidopexy is to achieve optimal gonadal function. This is temperature dependent, the temperature of the scrotum being 1°C less than the intra-abdominal temperature. Previously orchidopexy was performed late in childhood but now most paediatric surgeons operate

Features which distinguish maldescent from undescent of the testes

	Maldescent	Undescent
Frequency of occurrence	80% of cases	20% of cases
Presence of hernia	Some cases	100% of cases
Prognosis for fertility	Good	Poor
Technique of orchidopexy	Inguinal approach	Abdominal approach
Likelihood of getting testis into scrotum	Easy in all cases	Unpredictable
Normality of testis: naked eye and histology	Normal	Abnormal
Risk of torsion	Increased	Slightly increased
Risk of malignancy (both sides in unilateral presentation)	Slightly increased	Increased

at the age of 2–3 years. The other indications for orchidopexy are cosmetic, psychological, and to reduce the risks of torsion, trauma and unrecognised malignancy.

Testicular malignancy in the fourth decade of life is known to occur more frequently in individuals born with their testes outside the scrotum. Orchidopexy does not diminish the incidence of malignancy but it does bring a previous impalpable testis into a palpable position.

Torsion of the testis

Approximately 20% occur in the perinatal period and present as a discoloured scrotum. Unfortunately the diagnosis is often delayed and orchidectomy inevitable. However the opposite testis must be fixed in a stable position. The majority of torsions occur around puberty and present acutely as abdominal pain radiating to the testis or as intermittent testicular pain. There may be associated anomalies; a clapper bell testis due to high attachment of the tunica vaginalis or a long meso-orchium. The twist usually occurs in the spermatic cord. The undescended testis is also at risk of torsion. Urgent surgery is indicated when torsion is suspected.

Torsion of the hydatid of Morgagni. This is very common and can usually be distinguished from torsion of the testis because the pain is less severe, and as a consequence the history is usually longer than 6 hours. Sometimes it is possible to feel the torted hydatid and to demonstrate it by transillumination.

Varicoceles

Varicoceles occur infrequently in children. They do not usually need treatment during childhood.

Inguinal hernias and hydroceles

During its descent into the scrotum the testis is accompanied by a pouch of peritoneum, the processus vaginalis. The processus begins to close at birth and is normally obliterated during the first year of life. Both inguinal hernias and hydroceles are due to persistent patency of the processus. Where the processus remains very narrow, it allows peritoneal fluid to enter its cavity creating a hydrocele. If the hydrocele is present at birth and does not vary in size, it is called a non-communicating hydrocele and will usually resolve within 4–6 months of birth. Beyond this age it is more common for the hydrocele to vary in size, a communicating hydrocele, and spontaneous closure is unlikely.

Inguinal hernia and hydrocele

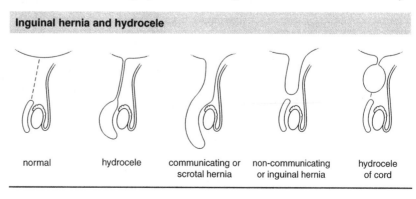

| normal | hydrocele | communicating or scrotal hernia | non-communicating or inguinal hernia | hydrocele of cord |

In these children ligation of the patent processus is performed at the internal ring. In an older child sudden development of a hydrocele without a history of trauma may be a feature of a testicular tumour.

Where the processus remains sufficiently wide in part or all of its course, the bowel may enter the cavity resulting in an inguinal or scrotal hernia. Spontaneous resolution does not occur and an operation is essential. In children there is no underlying muscular weakness and therefore excision of the sac, a herniotomy, is all that is necessary. The younger the child the more urgent the operative procedure. Irreducibility is more common in young babies and it not only puts them at risk of bowel ischaemia but also of testicular necrosis.

The child with a hernia may present with a history of swelling which comes and goes and the only clinical evidence of the hernial sac may be thickening of the spermatic cord on the affected side. Almost as commonly, however, the swelling appears suddenly and is apparently irreducible, thus requiring emergency admission. If the history is of less than 12 hours and there is no reddening of the skin over the hernia, gallows traction is applied to the legs and the child sedated with diamorphine. In 99% of children undisturbed sleep will result in the hernia reducing spontaneously or as a result of easy manipulation. Following such an episode the child should be kept in hospital and a herniotomy performed within days as the oedema subsides. If the hernia does not reduce with conservative means, or if the bowel within the hernial sac is clearly strangulated, emergency operation is essential. This can be one of the most difficult operations in paediatric practice. All infants noted to have a hernia should be referred to a surgeon promptly for elective surgery.

THE PREPUCE

The prepuce is closely adherent to the glans penis during the first year of life and any attempt at retraction must be avoided until spontaneous separation occurs. This is usually in the second year but may be delayed until 4 years of age. Ammoniacal dermatitis of the prepuce is common, and often confused with balanitis. Because of this, circumcision should never be performed until a child is out of nappies.

Phimosis

Phimosis refers to a scarring and stenosis of the apex of the foreskin. It is acquired as the result of recurrent balanitis or after traumatic attempts at foreskin retraction. It leads to ballooning and a poor stream during urination. Treatment is by circumcision. It should be differentiated from a tight foreskin which is amenable to gentle dilatation and retraction. The skin may be made more elastic by topical application of a corticosteroid and antimicrobial preparation.

Circumcision using Plastibell

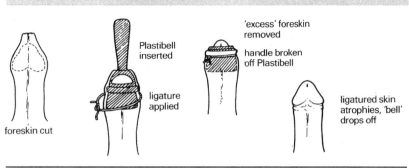

foreskin cut

Plastibell inserted

ligature applied

'excess' foreskin removed

handle broken off Plastibell

ligatured skin atrophies, 'bell' drops off

Paraphimosis

This can only occur in a child with a moderate phimosis, a preputial aperture slightly less than the size of the coronal sulcus. Following forcible retraction the foreskin is trapped in the retracted position. Treatment is by reduction under anaesthesia, with or without a dorsal slit, followed 6 weeks later by circumcision.

Hypospadias

Hyospadias/epispadias: incidence

Year	Numbers (England)	Rate per 10 000 births
1986	959	15.4
1991	691	10.5
1995	470	7.7
1996	483	7.9

The urethra opening on to the ventral aspect of the penis, at a point proximal to a normal site, is one of the commonest congenital abnormalities of the male genitalia, occurring in 1 in 350. The severity varies from a glandular orifice to scrotal and perineal types. There may also be a ventral curvature or chordee of the penis distal to the abnormal urethral meatus which becomes more conspicuous during erection. Failure of fusion of the ventral part of the foreskin results in a redundant dorsal hood. Until recently surgical repair was offered only if the hypospadias was likely to produce a functional problem, for example a socially unacceptable urinary stream or potential sexual difficulties. Nowadays cosmetic indications also prevail. Corrective techniques include meatal advancement and glanuloplasty.

Hypospadias

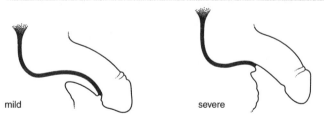

mild

severe

BIBLIOGRAPHY
Edleman C M 1992 Pediatric kidney disease. Little Brown & Co, Boston
Holliday M A, Barratt M T, Avner E D (eds) 1994 Pediatric nephrology. Williams & Wilkins, Baltimore
Postlethwaite R J (ed) 1994 Clinical paediatric nephrology. Wright, Bristol

12 Blood

IRON DEFICIENCY ANAEMIA
APLASTIC ANAEMIA
HAEMOLYTIC ANAEMIAS
DISORDERS OF HAEMOGLOBIN
  SYNTHESIS
BLEEDING DISORDERS

Interpretation of haemoglobin concentrations and white blood counts during infancy and childhood demands some knowledge of the physiological adjustments occurring during this period. The polycythaemia present at birth is followed by a progressive fall in haemoglobin concentration, reaching its minimum at 2–3 months. This fall is paralleled by relative erythroid hypoplasia in the marrow; the haemoglobin concentration of healthy infants seldom falls below 10 g/ 100 ml. During the fourth and fifth months, iron deficiency contributes to the anaemia and may be corrected by oral iron supplements. Folate deficiency may also occur particularly in infants born before term. Premature infants are also liable to develop anaemia during the first 4 months of life simply because the blood volume, in line with body size, increases rapidly at a time when the bone marrow is relatively hypoplastic.

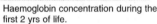

Age-related changes in haemoglobin concentration during the first 2 yr of life

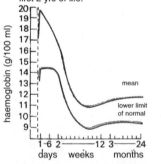

Haemoglobin concentration during the first 2 yrs of life.

Age-related changes in white cell count

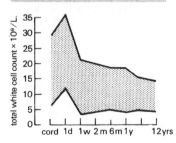

Causes of anaemia in childhood			
	Neonatal	Infancy	Childhood
Haemorrhage	Feto-maternal Twin-to-twin Placental Subaponeurotic Cephalhaematoma	Hiatus hernia	Hiatus hernia Meckel diverticulum Epistaxis
Haemolysis	Rhesus incompatibility ABO incompatibility Spherocytosis G6PD deficiency	Sickle cell Thalassaemia Spherocytosis	Sickle cell Thalassaemia Spherocytosis
Infection	Intrauterine (CMV, rubella) Septicaemia Urinary tract infection	Urinary tract	Chronic infection Chronic disease
Bleeding disorders	Haemorrhagic disease of the newborn	Haemophilia Christmas disease	Haemophilia Christmas disease
Deficiency		Physiological Prematurity Iron Folate Bone marrow depression	Iron Folate Bone marrow depression

The white cell count, which is high at birth, rapidly falls to normal adult levels. During the first 4 years of life lymphocytes predominate rather than neutrophils.

IRON DEFICIENCY ANAEMIA

Anaemia in children may be suggested by tiredness, lethargy or pallor, but it is often only discovered during investigation for other conditions, particularly infection and poor weight gain. Overt gastrointestinal bleeding is rare in childhood. Although it is important to exclude serious underlying problems, the majority of childhood anaemia is due to dietary iron deficiency.

Three-quarters of the total body iron of a newborn infant is found in circulating haemoglobin. In the full-term infant this reserve is adequate to meet requirements for the first 4–6 months but probably lasts only 6 weeks in the premature. The dietary requirements of a normal infant for elemental iron are 1 mg/kg/day. Although breast milk has a relatively low iron content, it is probably unnecessary to give iron supplements, particularly if mixed feeding is introduced at 4–6 months. Oral iron supplements are contraindicated during early breastfeeding because the iron binding globulin of breast milk, lactoferrin, has bactericidal properties which are reduced by iron saturation.

Depending on a community's dietary and social habits between 10 and 60% of children may be iron deficient. The higher figures occur in children of immigrant populations or those who live in impoverished inner city areas. It is recommended that unmodified cows' milk should not be given before 1 year; earlier introduction increases the incidence of iron deficiency unless iron supplements are provided. Cows' milk and tea reduce the absorption of iron, vitamin C increases it. Iron deficiency develops in a staged way, storage iron measured by serum ferritin levels is depleted first and only later do haemoglobin and red cell indices fall. As there is insufficient iron to combine with the protoporphyrin to form haem there is a rise in the free erythrocyte protoporphyrin.

Iron balance in infancy

birth
total iron = 75 mg/kg.
75% circulating in blood

requirements
1.0 mg/kg/day

breast milk contains	1.5 mg/l
cows' milk	0.5 mg/l
fortified milk formula	5–9 mg/l
mixed diet	4–9 mg/l

Iron preparations

	Total daily dose (age 1m–12yr)
sodium iron edetate (Sytron)	
10 ml = 55 mg iron	5–10 ml
ferrous glycine sulphate (Plesmet)	
5 ml = 25 mg iron	5–15 ml

Investigation of suspected iron deficiency anaemia

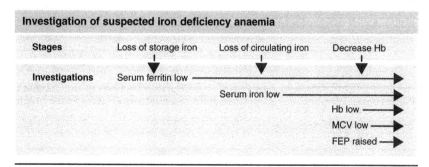

A hypochromic microcytic blood film is usually sufficient evidence to justify a trial of oral iron therapy. The history may provide clues to alternative diagnoses, for example recurrent vomiting indicating reflux oesophagitis or pica suggesting lead poisoning. If oral iron is given for 1 month and the haemoglobin rises by 1.0 g/dl or more then iron deficiency was present. Children who fail to respond to an adequate course of iron warrant more detailed investigation including serum ferritin and haemoglobin electrophoresis, radiological studies of the gastrointestinal tract, and renal and thyroid function tests. Intestinal malabsorption may present with iron deficient anaemia, and there may be associated folate deficiency. There is some evidence that severe iron deficiency may itself impair the integrity and function of the intestinal mucosa. Iron treatment should be continued for 3 months to replenish iron stores as well as to correct haemoglobin concentrations.

APLASTIC ANAEMIA

A pancytopenia necessitates marrow examination which may show either reduced cellularity without infiltration, aplasia, or invasion by malignant cells. Aplastic anaemia may be inherited or acquired.

Inherited aplastic anaemia Fanconi anaemia, an autosomal recessive condition, is the most common of the inherited types, and presents in boys at 4–7 years of age and in girls between 6 and 10 years of age. Bruising and purpura are the usual presenting complaints with anaemia appearing more insidiously. Associated features include abnormal pigmentation, short stature, skeletal and renal malformations and there may be chromosomal breakages and a high Hb F. The condition is progressive but the deterioration may be delayed with androgens and corticosteroids. Most children with Fanconi anaemia die within a few years of diagnosis due to complications of pancytopenia, and some develop acute leukaemia. Bone marrow transplantation from a compatible sibling or donor offers the main hope of therapy.

Acquired aplastic anaemias These may occur at any age. Some cases follow the ingestion of drugs such as chloramphenicol; others follow hepatitis A, B or C and several other virus infections, though there is frequently no obvious precipitating cause. If the bone marrow is moderately cellular at diagnosis there is a greater chance that spontaneous remission may occur. The majority with severe pancytopenia respond poorly to corticosteroids and androgens, and are at risk of dying of infection. Compatible bone marrow transplantation is now the treatment of choice. Transplantation is more successful in those patients who have had the fewest blood transfusions and it is important therefore to explore the availability of suitable donors early in the course of the illness. Recently antilymphocyte globulin or antithymocyte globulin have brought about a prolonged remission in up to 40% of children with aplastic anaemia; both deplete the T-cell population. With developments in bone marrow transplantation the prognosis has improved greatly.

HAEMOLYTIC ANAEMIAS

Haemolytic anaemias may be congenital or acquired. Some of the acquired group produce problems in the first days of life and are due to maternal antibodies haemolysing the infant's cells. The diagnostic feature of haemolytic anaemias is a normal or low haemoglobin and a raised reticulocyte count.

The pathogenesis of haemolytic anaemias

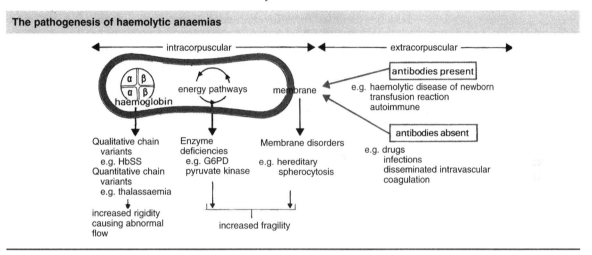

Hereditary haemolytic anaemia

The majority of haemolytic anaemias encountered in infancy and childhood are due to intrinsic disorders of the red cells. They are characterised by anaemia, an increased reticulocyte count, an unconjugated hyperbilirubinaemia and, if severe, skeletal changes secondary to compensatory marrow hyperplasia.

Hereditary spherocytosis

This is predominantly an autosomal dominant condition, with a high new mutation rate, in which defects of the complex sandwich structure of the red cell membrane result in abnormal permeability to sodium; the resulting fragile spherocytes are more readily destroyed in the spleen. The disorder may present as neonatal jaundice and has been confused with ABO incompatibility, as spherocytes may also be seen in this condition. In later childhood hereditary spherocytosis may cause anaemia, chronic malaise and splenomegaly. Mild variants may only come to light on detailed fragility studies of family members. The continuous high rate of bilirubin excretion can lead to pigment gall stones. The haemoglobin concentration generally runs in the range of 9–11 g/100 ml, but may drop during an infection because of an increased rate of haemolysis and relative bone marrow hypoplasia. Jaundice may also become conspicuous in these episodes. The diagnosis is confirmed by demonstrating increased osmotic fragility. Splenectomy is indicated if symptoms are severe but is usually delayed until later childhood because of the risk of overwhelming septicaemia in young splenectomised children.

Continuous prophylactic penicillin and vaccination against *Streptococcus pneumoniae, Haemophilus, influenzae* and *Neisseria meningitidis* are recommended. Following splenectomy the red cell survival is returned to normal although spherocytosis persists.

Hereditary red cell enzyme deficiencies

Two important pathways are essential for the normal function of the mature red cell. The hexose-monophosphate pathway provides a supply of reduced nicotinamide adenine-dinucleotide phosphate ($NADPH_2$) which is essential for protection against oxidative damage. The glycolytic or Embden–Meyerhof pathway provides the majority of energy for the cell. Deficiency of many of the enzymes in these two pathways has been described but the most important deficiencies are those of glucose-6-phosphate dehydrogenase (G6PD) and pyruvate kinase.

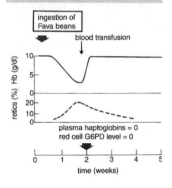

Typical timing of a toxin-induced episode

Metabolic pathways of the red blood cell

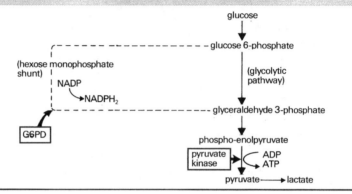

An abbreviated list of drugs to be avoided in glucose-6-phosphate dehydrogenase deficiency

antimalarials	primaquine chloroquine
sulphonamides	
nitrofurans	nitrofurantoin
antipyretics	acetylsalicylic acid
Vitamin K (water soluble analogues)	

Glucose-6-phosphate dehydrogenase deficiency. There are many variants of this enzyme, each having a different geographical distribution. The form seen in black Americans results in haemolysis when the person is exposed to antimalarial and other drugs. The Mediterranean and Oriental variants often present in the newborn period with jaundice due to excess haemolysis and they may require an exchange transfusion. These conditions are also 'drug sensitive'. Ingestion of Fava beans is a well recognised hazard in affected children. Patients with glucose-6-phosphate dehydrogenase deficiency should be given a list of drugs to avoid. The condition is X-linked, but females may have minimal symptoms, demonstrating the Lyon hypothesis, whereby the normal X chromosome gene compensates for the abnormal gene.

Pyruvate kinase deficiency. This is considerably less common and affects mainly north European populations. It causes neonatal jaundice, anaemia and splenomegaly. Splenectomy may be beneficial.

DISORDERS OF HAEMOGLOBIN SYNTHESIS

These fall into two main categories: those in which there is an amino acid substitution in the globin portion of haemoglobin, the haemoglobinopathies; and those in which there is relative failure of globin chain synthesis, the thalassaemia syndromes. It is unusual for these conditions to present in the newborn period when fetal haemoglobin is the predominant haemoglobin type.

Changes in haemoglobins during development

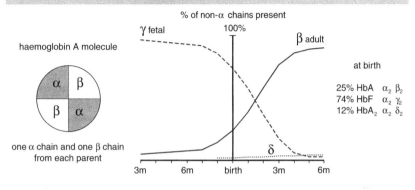

Sickle cell anaemia

Sickle cell anaemia is by far the most common of the haemoglobinopathies; 15% of all black people carry the gene that causes valine to replace glutamine in the sixth position of the beta chain. The homozygous condition is referred to as sickle cell anaemia or disease, and the heterozygote as sickle cell trait. There are also compound heterozygous states linking the sickle cell gene and those for HbC or beta-thalassaemia. The disease is a potentially serious condition not so much because of the chronic anaemia, but because of associated occlusive and sequestration events (crises). Painful swelling of the hands and feet, dactylitis, is a common presentation in young children due to distal vascular occlusion. In later life bone involvement may lead to aseptic necrosis of humeral and femoral heads. There is also an increased risk of osteomyelitis sometimes due to atypical organisms such as *Salmonella typhi*. The splenomegaly of the younger child becomes less prominent as repeated painful or asymptomatic infarctions produce 'autosplenectomy'.

Features of sickle cell disease

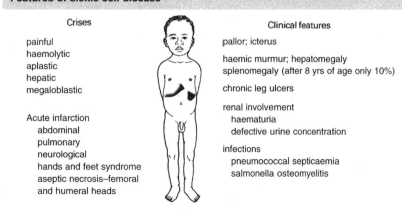

Crises are usually precipitated by infection and further aggravated by dehydration, poor tissue perfusion, hypoxia and acidosis. They may escalate to life-threatening massive sequestration of red cells in the liver and spleen, and sickling with occlusion within pulmonary and cerebral circulations.

Treatment of crises is largely symptomatic with analgesia, antibiotics, warmth and adequate fluids. Transfusion or exchange transfusion is needed for more severe episodes. Anaemia may be exacerbated by temporary marrow failure secondary to parvovirus infection.

In developed countries the prognosis for a normal life is moderately good. Unfortunately children in the developing world still suffer considerable mortality and morbidity due to the additional health burdens of infection and malnutrition. The heterozygote with sickle cell trait is asymptomatic except under conditions of low oxygen tension as might occur at high altitude or under general anaesthesia. Maternal and neonatal screening programmes identify infants with HbSS, HbSC and sickle cell beta-thalassaemia. Protective measures include education, prophylaxis with daily penicillin, and a full immunisation programme including vaccines against *S. pneumoniae*, *H. influenzae* and *N. meningitides*.

Thalassaemia

Thalassaemia syndromes are most common among Asian and Mediterranean races, and are subdivided into alpha- and beta-thalassaemia depending on the chain affected by the synthetic failure. Beta-thalassaemias are more common resulting from over 150 mutations of beta-globin genes.

Beta-thalassaemia major, the homozygous state, results in severe haemolytic anaemia with hypochromic microcytic cells, target cells and circulating nucleated red cells. The compensatory bone marrow hyperplasia produces a characteristic overgrowth of the facial and skull bones. Although a more acceptable life may be sustained by repeated transfusion, this resource is unavailable to the majority of the world's affected children. Repeated transfusion also introduces the hazards of blood-borne infections, chronic iron overload and tissue

Features of thalassaemia major

anaemia
growth failure

skull bossing
maxillary overgrowth

hepatomegaly

brittle long bones

repeated transfusions
haemosiderosis
cardiomyopath
cirrhosis
skin pigmentation
eindocrine failure

world distribution of thalassaemia

damage, including cardiomyopathy, diabetes and skin pigmentation. Continuous nocturnal desferrioxamine subcutaneous infusion is moderately effective in reducing the positive iron balance. Bone marrow transplantation is being explored as definitive therapy and, if there is an HLA compatible sibling, may be the treatment of choice.

In the first trimester fetal diagnosis for haemoglobinopathies is now available based on the techniques of trophoblast biopsy and restriction endonuclease analysis of fetal DNA.

Heterozygous beta-thalassaemia produces a mild anaemia, haemoglobin 9–11 g/dl with hypochromic, microcytic red cells and may be confused with iron deficiency. Haemoglobin electrophoresis confirms the elevated HbA2 ($\alpha2\delta2$).

Alpha-thalassaemias are a spectrum reflecting deletion of one, two, three or four of the alpha-chain genes. A single gene deletion is asymptomatic while a four gene deletion results in Hb Barts based on mainly γ tetramers and incompatible with life.

BLEEDING DISORDERS

A variety of disorders may lead to excessive bleeding in childhood. A detailed history is important for distinguishing congenital from acquired problems. Previous surgery, including dental extractions, without undue bleeding provides good evidence against an inherited disorder. Tonsillectomy is notorious for putting a considerable strain on coagulation systems and may uncover mild haemophilia. A family history is often helpful in diagnosing sex-linked recessive disorders such as haemophilia or Christmas disease, but may be absent in up to a third of new cases. Von Willebrand disease and hereditary telangiectasia have a dominant pattern of inheritance.

Classification of bleeding disorders

Presentation	Mechanism	Diagnosis
injury provoked	defective blood vessels	hereditary haemorrhagic telangiectasia allergic or post-infectious vasculitis vit C deficiency - scurvy
skin and mucosal bleeding	thrombo-cytopenia	immune
		drug induced
	platelet function defect	thrombasthenia
Spontaneous and injury provoked	coagulation disorder	haemophillia A, B von Willebrand disease vit K deficiency liver disease
deep haematomas haemarthrosis		

The character of the bleeding problem together with four basic tests of coagulation should make it possible to decide from which group of disorders a patient is suffering. These tests also serve as screening

Characteristic laboratory results

Test	ITP	von W.	Haemo- philia	Vit K def.
platelets	↓	N	N	N
bleeding time	↑	↑	N	N
PT	N	N	N	↑
PTT	N	N	↑	↑/N

procedures in cases of suspected child abuse or before liver or jejunal biopsy. Normal results in the four tests exclude all deficiencies other than factor XIII (fibrin stabilising factor) deficiency, and some rare platelet functional abnormalities. Inherited deficiencies of each of the coagulation factors have been described; they are all rare with the exceptions of haemophilia A and B, and von Willebrand disease.

Coagulation pathways

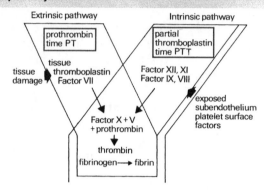

Haemophilia A and B (Christmas disease)

Classic haemophilia A or factor VIII deficiency occurs in approximately 1 in 14 000 males and is six times more common than haemophilia B, otherwise known as Christmas disease and due to factor IX deficiency. Haemophilia A is transmitted as a sex-linked recessive, and carrier females are asymptomatic but may be detected because of an excess of immunoreactive factor VIII over that which is biologically active. The severity of haemophilia is linked to the degree of deficiency of factor VIII; concentrations of factor VIII less than 1% of normal causes severe problems, 1–5% causes moderate problems and 5–20% only mild symptoms. Spontaneous bleeding into joints and muscles with resulting orthopaedic problems is the main hazard. Haemophilia management is based on prompt infusion of the appropriate factor either derived from human plasma by fractionation or synthesised by recombinant techniques. Many families have now been trained to treat bleeding episodes at home. In general, the aim of replacement is to increase the factor VIII level to a biologically effective concentration of 10–20%. Activity up to 50% may be necessary in severe trauma or as preparation for surgery. Analgesia but not by intramuscular injection may be required. Physiotherapy is needed to preserve the strength of muscles which might otherwise become weakened during periods of immobilisation, therefore increasing the likelihood of the joint bleeding again, as muscles are important in providing joint stability.

von Willebrand disease

This is an autosomal dominant disorder in which reduced factor VIII activity is linked to impaired platelet adhesiveness. The latter results in prolonged bleeding time which differentiates the condition from haemophilia A. Apart from bruising the main bleeding occurs into gut, urinary tract or uterus and there is less joint involvement. As in haemophilia, minor bleeding may respond to local measures (pressure, cold compresses) or tranexamic acid. Factor VIII fraction infusion is required for major episodes. Bleeding severity improves with age.

Thrombocytopenia

Idiopathic thrombocytopenic purpura (ITP) is the most common of the thrombocytopenias in childhood. It is presumed to have an immunological basis triggered by viral infections, and there is a relationship with rubella. Platelet associated IgG antibodies are sometimes detectable. ITP is not usually apparent unless platelet counts fall below $40 \times 10^9/l$, and severe bruising and mucosal bleeding suggest counts below $5 \times 10^9/l$. It is very rare for haemorrhage to occur in the brain or viscera. Increasing awareness that ITP is usually a benign and self-limiting disease, with over 90% recovering within 3 months, justifies non-interventional management with minimal hospitalisation or enforced rest. For the minority who present with very low counts, mucosal bleeding or threatening bleeds either prednisolone or intravenous human immunoglobulin can produce a useful elevation of platelets.

The differential diagnosis includes acute leukaemia, aplastic anaemia, systemic lupus erythematosis (especially in adolescent girls) and rare congenital syndromes. It is recommended that a bone marrow examination be performed before prednisolone or immunoglobulin treatment. In ITP the marrow confirms an active marrow with normal or increased numbers of megakaryocytes. Chronic thrombocytopenia, persisting beyond 6 months, does not necessarily require treatment and splenectomy is seldom justified.

Drug-induced thrombocytopenia is unusual in childhood.

Neonatal thrombocytopenia may arise by mechanisms which parallel maternofetal blood group incompatibility, for example mother being platelet antibody negative (PLA –ve) while the baby is PLA +ve. This is called neonatal isoimmune thrombocytopenia. Intrauterine infection, maternal drug ingestion and idiopathic thrombocytopenia in the mother may also cause thrombocytopenia in the neonatal period. There is also a group of rare hereditary thrombocytopenias.

Wiscott–Aldrich syndrome

This is a X-linked familial disorder in which boys present with early thrombocytopenia, eczema and susceptibility to infection, probably due to immunoglobulin abnormalities. Regular gammaglobulin administration reduces infection, but it remains a severe and potentially fatal disease. It may be amenable to bone marrow transplantation from an HLA compatible sibling.

Disseminated intravascular coagulation

Severe disturbances such as septicaemia, shock and acidosis may promote simultaneous activation of both the coagulant and the fibrinolytic pathways, with a resulting consumption of platelets, fibrinogen, factors V and VIII but without the formation of insoluble fibrin. Soluble complexes of fibrin monomers circulate as fibrin degradation products and their detection is a further indication of consumptive coagulopathy. Disseminated intravascular coagulation (DIC) should be suspected in a gravely ill child with both shock and generalised bleeding. Every attempt should be made to determine and treat the underlying cause. In the neonatal period this may be asphyxia, infection or profound hypothermia. In childhood meningococcal infection, severe trauma and burns are leading causes. The mainstay of treatment is fluid replacement, circulatory support and antibiotics. The tools of molecular biology are being used to study the pathways which link tissue damage and coagulation, and these may lead to better focused therapeutic agents.

BIBLIOGRAPHY

Hann I, Lake B, Lilleyman J, Pritchard J, Weatherall D 1996 Colour atlas of paediatric haematology, 3rd edn. Oxford University Press, Oxford

13 Malignancy

MANAGEMENT OF CHILDREN WITH
  CANCER
ACUTE LEUKAEMIA
LYMPHOMAS
BRAIN AND SPINAL TUMOURS
NEUROBLASTOMA
SOFT TISSUE SARCOMAS
RENAL TUMOURS
GERM CELL TUMOURS
BONE TUMOURS
OTHER TUMOURS
HISTIOCYTIC DISORDERS

Causes of death 1–14 years

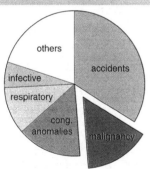

Organ growth curves

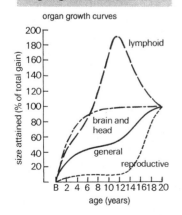

In purely numerical terms childhood malignancies are relatively uncommon with approximately 1500 new cases presenting in the United Kingdom each year. This equates to an incidence of 1 in 600 under age 15 years. Successful management and improved survival have resulted in a substantial number of these young people facing the dual challenge of prolonged, threatening illness and demanding treatment regimens. Paediatric malignancies differ from adult tumours in that they arise mainly from the embryonal mesoderm, whereas adult tumours usually arise from the endoderm and ectoderm. Paediatric tumours often contain embryonal cell lines and clearly arise from cells undergoing rapid proliferation during normal growth and development.

Like all tumours, the aetiology of childhood cancers is complex and probably multifactorial. Their development at such an early age suggests that genetic factors make a significant contribution. It was from the observation of a paediatric malignancy—retinoblastoma—that Knudson postulated a mutational basis for some cancers. The subsequent identification of tumour suppressor genes by molecular biologists was confirmation of Knudson's 'double hit' theory. Further evidence of the genetic basis for many paediatric tumours arose from their association with previously recognised childhood syndromes. Some of these are listed in the following table.

Examples of conditions associated with malignancy in childhood	
General	Beckwith–Weidemann syndrome
	Hemihypertrophy
	Multiple exostosis
	Neurofibromatosis
DNA repair defects	Ataxia telangectasia
	Fanconi anaemia
	Xeroderma pigmentosa
Immune deficiency syndromes	Common variable immune deficiency
	Severe combined immune deficiency
	Wiskott–Aldrich syndrome
Chromosomal abnormalities	11p13 deletion
	13q14 deletion
	Trisomy 21
Family cancer syndromes	Familial adenomatous polyposis
	Familial Hodgkin disease
	and there are many others

THE MANAGEMENT OF CHILDREN WITH CANCER

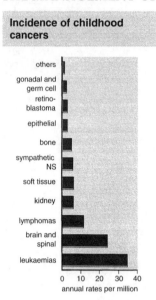

Incidence of childhood cancers

others
gonadal and germ cell
retino-blastoma
epithelial
bone
sympathetic NS
soft tissue
kidney
lymphomas
brain and spinal
leukaemias

0   10   20   30   40
annual rates per million

Children with cancer need complex and disciplined management programmes to achieve the best chance of a cure and to minimise the pain and distress of the disease and its treatments. A comprehensive service includes ready access to specialist diagnostic facilities and experts in the planning, delivery and coordination of chemotherapy, surgery and radiotherapy. The management programme involves many health professionals whose clinical skills must be complemented by an awareness of the psychosocial aspects of the care of each individual child. Cancer in children is relatively rare, and therefore multicentre, national and international cooperation is required to evaluate new treatment techniques. In the United Kingdom, the Medical Research Council (MRC) coordinates childhood leukaemia (UK Acute Lymphatic Leukaemia trials—UKALL) and bone tumour trials, while the UK Childhood Cancer Study Group (UKCCSG) and the European paediatric oncology group (SIOP) coordinates the majority of trials for other solid tumours.

Support for child and family

If cancer is suspected the management must be prompt and thorough. The child and family initially need support in coming to terms with the diagnosis and, as soon as it is possible, should be told of the nature of the cancer, its prognosis and its treatment. Anxieties should be anticipated at all stages—from the initial diagnosis, through treatment and on to the long-term follow up, where fears of subsequent relapse can become intense. Sound emotional and financial support are invariably needed for the family. Relationships within the family become disturbed and siblings may be forgotten. Good care includes support of the whole family as well as the child with cancer. In the United Kingdom, Sargent Cancer Care for Children and a number of local charities run by parents provide invaluable support by funding dedicated social workers and counsellors as well as offering financial assistance.

Symptom management

Pain, distress and discomfort can be the results of the primary malignancy, its investigation and its treatment. The team should have expertise in the management of such disabling symptoms. The dying child should, wherever possible, receive care at home with the support of the community paediatric nursing service. As a back up, there should be ready and easy access to a familiar ward.

There are three established treatment modalities that can be directed against cancer: surgery, radiotherapy and chemotherapy.

Surgery

In earlier years, surgery was the first-line treatment for most solid tumours. With the success of modern chemotherapy, however, primary surgical resection is becoming a rare event. Instead, tumour biopsy (open or closed) is followed by chemotherapy-induced tumour shrinkage and subsequent tumour resection. This approach has reduced the extent of local surgical damage and increased the chance of complete resection. Surgery, however, is required to insert permanent indwelling central venous catheters to facilitate the delivery of intensive chemotherapy, intravenous fluids and blood sampling. The use of these catheters is not without risk as they can become infected both within the lumen and in the soft tissues around them. They are also prone to blockage and displacement. These risks can be reduced by adopting meticulous techniques.

Radiotherapy

Radiotherapy is effective against most malignancies. External beam radiotherapy can be delivered precisely and safely to any area of the body. The delivery of radiotherapy does require an immobilised patient, which in younger children can be achieved by careful preparation with the help of videos and specially directed play therapy. Sedation or anaesthesia is necessary for those in whom this approach fails. Radiotherapy is only effective in the region where it is

Distortion of growth in the pelvis following irradiation

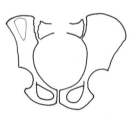 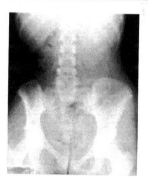

applied and so it is mainly used to treat areas of known disease, although total body irradiation can be used in conjunction with bone marrow transplant. Radiotherapy does, however, damage the growing tissue and its use in the paediatric population can lead to local disfigurement in later life.

Cranial irradiation has been used extensively to treat 'sanctuary sites' of leukaemia in the brain. The side effects of such treatment include short-term memory defects, difficulties with mental arithmetic and poor attention span. These symptoms are more severe in those children who were irradiated at a younger age. Repeated irradiation for CNS relapse of leukaemia or high dose radiotherapy for intracranial malignancies may damage the hypothalamic–pituitary axis leading to a variety of endocrine disturbances such as growth hormone deficiency, hypothyroidism and precocious puberty. Attempts are being made to target radiotherapy more specifically by injecting radioisotopes attached to antibodies or chemicals taken up by the tumour.

Chemotherapy

The majority of chemotherapy agents kill cancer cells by interfering with the replication and division of DNA during cell division. They are

Central venous line

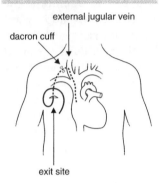

external jugular vein

dacron cuff

exit site

most commonly given intravenously, although some individual agents are given orally, topically, intrathecally and even directly into pleural or abdominal cavities. Their effectiveness depends upon the cytotoxicity to the cancer cells being greater than the cytotoxicity to normal dividing cells. This may relate to the higher rate of cell division by cancer cells or their reduced ability to recover between courses of treatment. The concurrent use of several agents reduces the likelihood of chemoresistance developing in the malignant cells.

Toxicity. Some drug doses are limited by the toxicity of the drug on normal tissues. The common toxicities are nausea, vomiting, hair loss and bone marrow suppression. Emesis occurs during administration of chemotherapy and up to 2–3 days afterwards. Anaemia, neutropenia and thrombocytopenia occur about 10 days after and hair loss over the following weeks. During the severe and prolonged neutropenic episodes any fever is treated with broad spectrum antibiotics until an infecting agent has been identified or excluded. Mucosal and systemic fungal infections are common. Immunosuppression exposes the child to the risk of suffering severe forms of common infections like measles and chicken pox. Such risks can be reduced by previous active immunisation of the child, good community immunisation rates and antiviral drugs. The gut, brain, liver, kidney and heart are also affected by specific chemotherapy agents in either a dose-related or idiosyncratic fashion. Management is simplified by the use of permanent indwelling central venous catheters for the delivery of intravenous drugs, blood products and parenteral nutrition.

Bone marrow transplantation and stem cell rescue. Higher doses of chemotherapy can be used if stem cells are available for re-infusion after the drugs have been cleared from the circulation, thus 'rescuing' the patient from prolonged myelosuppression. These stem cells may have been previously 'harvested' from the patient (from bone marrow or stimulated peripheral blood) or 'harvested' from a matched related or unrelated donor. These methods of stem cell 'rescue' are hazardous due to the profound immunosuppression and the severity of associated organ toxicities caused by high doses of chemotherapy and radiotherapy. Donor transplantation has the added risk of graft versus host disease (GvHD) where the foreign marrow does not recognise its host as 'self' and mounts an immune response against it. Patients with GvHD then develop skin rashes, gut desquamation and liver toxicities and will require immunosuppressive drugs for their control.

Bone marrow growth factors. Recent research has identified bone marrow growth factors (colony stimulating factors) which stimulate white blood cell production. These growth factors can reduce the duration of chemotherapy-induced neutropenia, which may limit the duration of chemotherapy-induced bone marrow suppression for patients with curable disease and permit a safe increase in dose intensity for patients with more resistant disease.

Long-term follow up

Long-term follow up is essential to monitor patients for signs of early relapse and the secondary effects of their treatment. Secondary effects include specific organ toxicities such as cardiomyopathy after anthracyclines (e.g. doxorubicin), sterility after the use of alkylating agents (e.g. cyclophosphamide) and renal toxicity after the use of platinum compounds (e.g. cisplatin). Second primary malignancies do occur with an increased frequency compared to the rest of the population. This is probably due to a combination of circumstances, including the underlying genetic predisposition and the carcinogenic effects of radiotherapy and certain chemotherapeutic agents.

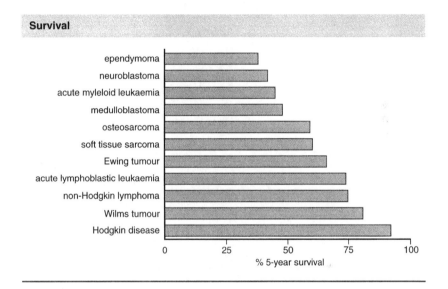

Survival

Prognosis

The overall long-term survival rates have now reached 65% with many children cured and looking forward to adult life. It has been estimated that by the year 2000, 1 in 650 people aged 20 years will have been cured of cancer. The quality of life for these survivors and the consequences for the adult medical services must be a high priority in future health planning.

ACUTE LEUKAEMIA

This is characterised by a malignant clonal proliferation of white cell precursors (blast cells) which occupy and inhibit the function of the bone marrow. They may circulate in the blood and form leukaemic deposits in many tissues, such as the spleen, lymph nodes, meninges and eye. There are two main categories of acute leukaemia, lymphoblastic and myeloblastic. In acute lymphoblastic leukaemia (ALL), the blast cells resemble primitive precursors of lymphoid origin while in acute myeloid leukaemia (AML) they resemble the myeloid precursors.

Acute lymphoblastic leukaemia:

ALL accounts for 85% of childhood leukaemias. It can occur at any age, although the peak incidence is around 5 years of age. It is equally common in both sexes.

Aetiology. A variety of causes for the development of ALL have been proposed. ALL is more common in Down syndrome and in syndromes involving chromosomal instability like Fanconi anaemia. Development of ALL has also been associated with exposure to excessive radiation, seen in survivors of radiation from nuclear devices. A viral aetiology has also been proposed although no specific virus has been identified.

Clinical features of acute leukaemia

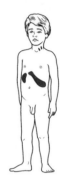

Symptoms
anorexia / lethargy
fever / infection
bleeding
gum hypertrophy
bone / joint pain
symptoms of raised intracranial pressure

Physical signs
pallor
ecchymoses / petechial haemorrhages
hepatosplenomegaly
papilloedema
cranial nerve palsies
testicular enlargement
superior vena cava obstruction

Clinical presentation. The onset is usually insidious although acute presentations, over a few days, occur in about 15%. Examination of the blood or bone marrow will show an excess of lymphoblasts in conjunction with the depressed production of red cells, other white cells and platelets. White cells will express different surface proteins depending upon their degree of maturity or their ultimate cell lineage (T-cell lymphoid, B-cell lymphoid or myeloid). The majority of children with acute lymphoblastic leukaemia are typed either as 'common' or 'pre B' according to these surface marker proteins. The CSF should be examined for evidence of CNS disease.

Prognostic features. Multifactorial analysis of large numbers of children with leukaemia has identified a variety of clinical and cellular characteristics which predict prognosis and those justifying changes to standard treatment approaches are indicated on page 219.

Treatment. Multi-agent chemotherapy and high dose steroids are the mainstay of treatment which is initially directed at inducing a bone marrow remission. The early stages of such treatment may be associated with life-threatening disturbances of fluid and electrolytes due to rapid lysis of tumour cells (tumour lysis syndrome). The rapid release of intracellular contents (potassium, phosphate, purines) can lead to hyperkalaemia, hypocalcaemia, urate nephropathy and, finally, renal failure. These possibilities must be anticipated and treated.

Prognostic features in acute lymphoblastic leukaemia

Patient features	Therapeutic action
Age < 1 year	Intensify systemic treatment, delay/omit radiotherapy
Sex	Girls do better than boys: no change to treatment approach
White cell count > $50 \times 10^9/l$	Intensify systemic and CNS treatment
CSF involvement	Intensity CNS directed therapy
Cellular features	
Cell morphology (L3)/cytochemistry B cell	Intensify treatment systemic treatment
T-cell type	Risk linked to blast count
B-cell type	
mature B cell	Intensify chemotherapy
common ALL antigen	Standard risk
pre B cell	Standard risk
Null cell (commonly infant leukaemia)	Intensify chemotherapy
Cytogenetics	
t(8:14)(q24: q32) commonly mature B cell	Intensify treatment
t(4: 11)(q21: q23) (congenital leukaemia)	Intensify treatment
t(9: 22) Philadelphia chromosome	Intensify treatment

Subsequent therapy is directed at eradicating residual leukaemic cells which may be present in the bone marrow or the CNS and involves the use of blocks of intensive systemic treatment (consolidation therapy). One of the most significant changes in the treatment of children has been the selection of CNS-directed therapy to prevent CNS relapse. Cranial irradiation was the initial modality used to protect children from such relapse but, as the long-term sequelae have proved to be significant, most children now receive intrathecal methotrexate or high dose methotrexate. Only a small number of high risk patients still receive cranial radiotherapy. Daily, low dose, oral chemotherapy forms the basis of the last 18 months of 'maintenance' treatment and makes the whole programme some 2 years in duration.

Prognosis. These complex treatment schedules have evolved over a number of years and have resulted in dramatic, successive improvements in survival rates, such that overall there is now a greater than 70% chance of long-term survival. Further improvements are expected with recent developments in treatment. Intensification of chemotherapy with bone marrow transplantation from a matched related donor may be performed in children with adverse features in first remission or after relapse in other groups. However, only a minority of children have suitable donors, so this form of therapy is not widely applicable. The risks for unrelated donor transplants are considerably greater and are justifiable only when the prognosis is extremely poor.

Age of survivors of cancer in childhood: numbers are increasing year on year

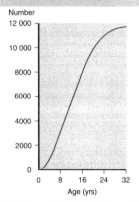

Age of survivors of childhood cancer 1994

Acute myeloid leukaemia

AML accounts for 15% of childhood leukaemias, it occurs equally in both sexes and is evenly distributed throughout the paediatric age range. Its aetiology in children is largely unknown, although previous exposure to radiation or chemotherapeutic agents is known to be a precipitating factor. Its clinical presentation closely mirrors that of ALL. Favourable prognostic features have only recently been recognised and include specific cytogenetic abnormalities in the leukaemic cells (t(8:21); t(15:17)) and a good response to the initial course of chemotherapy. Intensive, high dose, chemotherapy of often shorter duration is used in AML and has recently produced encouraging improvements in survival (50%). CNS disease is a rare event and CNS directed treatment does not need to be as intensive. Matched, related, bone marrow transplantation is performed in patients with poor risk factors.

Chronic leukaemias

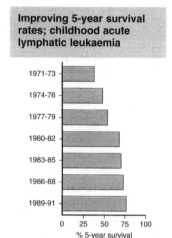

Improving 5-year survival rates; childhood acute lymphatic leukaemia

The most common is chronic myeloid leukaemia (CML), presenting in either adult (ACML) or juvenile (JCML) form. Both are characterised by an excessive production of mature white cells. ACML presents with symptoms of anaemia, massive splenomegaly and a very high white cell count which consists of predominantly mature granulocytes. Cytogenetic studies of bone marrow commonly identify the Philadelphia chromosome t(9:22) in the leukaemia clone. There is a high incidence of malignant transformation to acute leukaemia at a median of 4–5 years from diagnosis. JCML, on the other hand, is characterised by skin rashes, lymphadenopathy, fevers, bleeding and an elevated HbF. The white count is mildly elevated with a marked monocytic component. Children die from infection or progressive marrow failure. ACML can be controlled in the short term with oral chemotherapy, but JCML cannot. Both conditions can be treated with donor bone marrow transplantation.

Myelodysplastic disorders

These disorders represent a poorly defined collection of bone marrow diseases where there is disordered blood cell production, often with malformed, disordered or suppressed cell production. They are associated with a variety of characteristic chromosomal abnormalities and a variable predisposition to malignant transformation into acute leukaemia.

LYMPHOMAS

Malignant lymphomas are a group of lymph system tumours which can be broadly classified into the Hodgkin and non-Hodgkin types.

Hodgkin disease

This is characterised by areas of lymph tissue hyperplasia, containing giant multinucleate Reed–Sternberg cells, reactive inflammatory infiltrate and granulomata. The patients have clinical and laboratory evidence of a predominantly cellular immune deficiency which may be instrumental in the development of the disease. They present mainly in later childhood, adolescence and young adulthood with enlarged lymph nodes and systemic upset. Diagnosis is dependent upon lymph node biopsy and thorough staging investigations to look for evidence of disease in the rest of the lymph system, adjacent non-lymphoid structures and the bone marrow. Treatment with multi-agent chemotherapy results in a very favourable prognosis for most cases (90% chance of long-term cure). Some Stage I patients may be treated with local radiotherapy. Relapse many years after treatment is a cause for continued review.

Clinical features of Hodgkin disease

Presentation

night sweats
persistent fever
pruritus
lymph node enlargement
      cervical 70%
      axillary 20%
      inguinal 10%
hepatosplenomegaly
weight loss >10% body weight

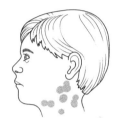

Non-Hodgkin lymphoma

This group of disorders is characterised by a malignant clonal proliferation of lymph tissue which can be subclassified both histologically and immunologically. The majority of NHL in children are highly malignant tumours which are either undifferentiated and mainly T-cell type (40–50%), or lymphoblastic and B-cell type (30–35%). T-cell lymphomas more commonly arise in the mediastinum while B-cell lymphomas may arise within the cervical region or abdomen.

Clinical features of non-Hodgkin lymphoma

Presentation

fever
malaise
lymph node enlargement
multifocal signs

Investigations

tumour biopsy
bone marrow
CSF sample
pleural/ascitic fluid for cytology
renal function tests

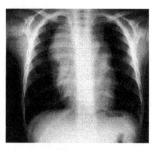

mediastinal mass

Clinical presentation is commonly with fever, malaise and symptoms of lymph node enlargement in any part of the body. The disease may present with dramatic enlargement of lymph nodes, or it may be insidious in onset. In some patients there is obstruction of major airways or vessels such as the superior vena cava, leading to a 'superior mediastinal syndrome' which constitutes an oncological emergency! It is not uncommon for the disease to be multifocal including the CNS, yet with no apparent primary tumour. Treatment uses multi-agent chemotherapy with the lymphoblastic lymphomas responding well to ALL treatment and having a similar prognosis. The undifferentiated tumours require more intensive chemotherapy and the consideration of bone marrow transplantation, if the disease is extensive. The outlook is improving and there is now up to a 75% chance of long-term survival even in patients with extensive disease.

BRAIN AND SPINAL TUMOURS

Brain and spinal tumours are the second commonest group of malignant disorders. Their aetiology is largely unknown, although they may be associated with family cancer syndromes, pre-existing brain malformations and previous treatment for other malignancies.

Brain tumours

These may occur throughout infancy and childhood and present with signs and symptoms related to raised intracranial pressure, focal neurological defects and endocrine disturbances. Classically their presentation is late, as the initial symptoms are often attributed to a variety of non-specific clinical and psychological disorders. Computerised tomography (CT) and magnetic resonance imaging (MRI) have revolutionised the investigation of suspected brain and spinal tumours while CT/MRI guided stereotactic biopsy and neuroendoscopic biopsy has allowed accurate histological diagnosis of conventionally inaccessible lesions. Two-thirds of the tumours present infratentorially with cerebellar or brain stem dysfunction. Astrocytic,

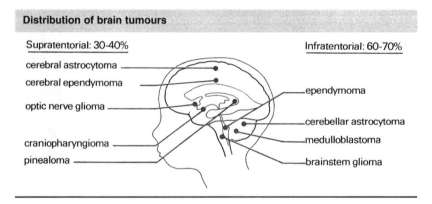

Distribution of brain tumours

Supratentorial: 30-40%

cerebral astrocytoma
cerebral ependymoma
optic nerve glioma
craniopharyngioma
pinealoma

Infratentorial: 60-70%

ependymoma
cerebellar astrocytoma
medulloblastoma
brainstem glioma

embryonal and ependymal tumours predominate. Posterior fossa tumours, in particular the embryonal lesions, can metastasise down the spinal column and formal imaging of the spine is mandatory. Metastasis outside the CNS does rarely occur. Supratentorial tumours may either be located within the hypothalamic–pituitary axis (producing endocrine or visual disturbances), or distant from this axis (producing symptoms of epilepsy or spasticity). Supratentorial tumours are most commonly astrocytic or ependymal with varying degrees of malignant potential.

Clinical features of brain tumours

Raised intracranial pressure
headache (early morning)
vomiting
mood changes
papilloedema
VI cranial nerve palsy
head tilt

Focal neurological signs
cerebral-seizures, spasticity, focal fits
cerebellar-ataxia, nystagmus, diplopia
brain stem-facial weakness, dysphagia, ocular palsies

Endocrine
short stature
hypogonadism
precocious puberty
diabetes insipidus

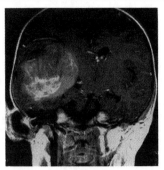

MRI scan of parietal lobe astrocytoma

Spinal tumours

These are rare, but require prompt recognition if irreversible cord damage is to be avoided. They most commonly present with back pain or disturbances of gait or sphincter control. Back pain, particularly at night, almost always has a sinister significance in childhood and adolescence and should be extensively investigated. Spinal tumours may arise from neural tissue within the spinal cord, astrocytomas and ependymomas being the most common. Alternatively, cord compression may be caused by extrinsic, non-neural tumours such as neuroblastoma, lymphoma and Ewing tumour.

Treatment. Successful treatment of CNS tumours relies heavily upon the control of raised intracranial pressure, primary tumour resection and subsequent chemo/radiotherapy. Chemotherapy is currently being explored more widely for the younger age group, where CNS radiotherapy is particularly damaging and difficult to deliver. The prognosis for these tumours is dictated both by the location of the tumour and its potential for local growth and metastatic spread. Overall, there is a 50% chance for long-term survival although this figure hides the degree of disability in the survivors.

NEUROBLASTOMA

Neuroblastoma is a malignant tumour of sympathetic neuroblasts which may arise in any part of the sympathetic nervous system. It is a puzzling tumour in that prognosis is better in the youngest infants and in some children there may even be spontaneous tumour regression. As the tissue has the ability to produce adrenaline and noradrenaline, most patients (90–95%) will excrete precursors or breakdown products of these compounds in the urine. These urinary catecholamines—dopamine, vanillylmandelic acid (VMA) and homovanillic acid (HVA)—provide a reliable marker for diagnosis and monitoring during treatment. VMA has also been used as the basis for population screening in infancy, although the impact of this procedure for reducing later presentations has yet to be determined. Half the children present in the first 2 years of life and it is rare after the age of 5. Clinical presentation is dependent on the site of the primary tumour (80% in the abdomen) and the extent of tumour metastasis. Seventy-five per cent of the tumours have metastasised at the time of presentation. The children are frequently miserable, fail to thrive and may have extensive bruising, mimicking the appearance of a physically abused child. Diagnosis is dependent on the presence of a typical mass, elevation of urinary catecholamines and identification of tumour cells in the marrow or biopsy of a tumour mass.

Clinical features of neuroblastoma

Presentation

pallor, weight loss, irritability
limb pains, hypertension
proptosis, periorbital bruising
neck mass, mediastinal compression
paraplegia
abdominal mass (midline deep nodular)
hepatomegaly
skin nodules

Investigation

blood count
24 hr urine VMA, HVA
chest X-ray, intravenous pyelogram
biopsy, bone marrow
ultrasound, CT and MRI scans
bone scan and mIBG scan

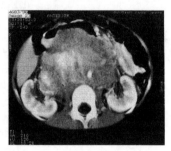

Central mass encasing IVC

Presentation in the newborn period is remarkable for its rapid progression and potential for spontaneous resolution. Treatment is dictated by stage at presentation, with localised tumours resected and adjuvant chemotherapy given to eradicate residual disease. Infants with widespread disease to specific sites (stage 4s) are treated conservatively and chemotherapy given if tumour progression is relentless or potentially life threatening. More disseminated disease, however, requires high dose multi-agent chemotherapy. Despite this, the over 1 year age group is associated with a poor prognosis (< 15% survival). Novel treatment approaches are being explored, including targeted radiotherapy using mono-iodobenzyl-guanidine (mIBG), a breakdown product of noradrenaline, specifically taken up by neuroblasts.

Neuroepithelial tumour

Peripheral neuroepitheliomas or malignant peripheral neuro-sectodermal tumours (PNET) are a collection of malignant tumours which are thought to arise from the embryonic neural crest and may be located within soft tissues or bone. They are small round cell neoplasms, clinically distinct from neuroblastoma, and most commonly presenting in the thoracopulmonary region. Treatment, in the majority of cases, is with primary chemotherapy followed by surgical resection and subsequent irradiation of residual disease. Outcome is dictated by the presence or absence of metastatic disease at the beginning of treatment and the amenability of the primary lesion to complete surgical resection or high dose irradiation.

SOFT TISSUE SARCOMAS

The most common of these is rhabdomyosarcoma, a highly malignant tumour thought to arise from the primitive mesenchyme and showing characteristics of striated muscle. Such tumours can arise anywhere in the body but they are most common in three regions: (1) head and neck; (2) genitourinary tract; (3) limb extremities. Their presenting features are dictated by the location of the tumour and they may metastasise widely. Treatment is with primary chemotherapy, followed by consideration of surgical resection and radiotherapy depending on the consequences of such treatment in the anatomical location. Other soft tissue sarcomas may have features of smooth muscle (leiomyosarcoma), adipose tissue (liposarcoma), fibrous tissue (fibrosarcoma), synovium (synovial cell sarcoma) and blood vessels (angio-/lymphangiosarcoma).

RENAL TUMOURS

The commonest renal tumour is the nephroblastoma (Wilms tumour). It is a tumour of embryonic kidney tissue which may arise from

Clinical features of Wilms tumour

Presentation
fever, poor appetite, vomiting
abdominal mass 90% (lateral, superficial)
haematuria 30%
abdominal pain 20%

Investigations
urine analysis, blood count
chest X-ray, PA and lateral
renal ultrasound and/or CT scan
chromosomes

Staging
1. encapsulated tumours completely removed
2. microscopic invasion of capsule
3. involvement of regional lymph nodes
   or tumour rupture
4. metastatic tumour
5. bilateral renal tumour

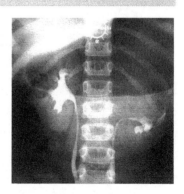

large mess arising from L kidney

primitive metanephric blastema (nephroblastomatosis). It presents most commonly from birth to 5 years of age and 10% of cases are bilateral. It is most notable for its association with a number of congenital anomalies as well as cytogenetic abnormalities on chromosome 11p. Although predicted in the 1970s, it was not until 1990 that the Wilms tumour suppressor gene (WT1) was finally identified at 11p13. The genetic pattern of the tumour is most commonly sporadic, although about 2% of all patients have a family member with the disease. Use of the staging system has permitted tailoring of treatment to the requirements of individual patients, thereby minimising the duration and consequences of therapy.

A number of other renal tumour types are recognised in childhood, including mesoblastic nephroma, an almost universally benign tumour of infancy, rhabdoid tumour, clear cell sarcoma and renal cell carcinoma.

GERM CELL TUMOURS

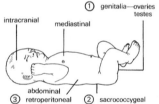

Germ cell tumours

Germ cell tumours may be malignant or benign. They arise from precursors of sperm and ova but retain the potential to produce tissues resembling any somatic or supporting structure. They can occur either within the gonads or extragonadally; in the latter case they are found predominantly in the midline, particularly in the pineal gland and hypothalamus. There are two age incidence peaks—under 3 years and around puberty.

The commonest presentation is a congenital sacrococcygeal teratoma. The tumours often secrete alpha-fetoprotein (AFP) or beta human chorionic gonadotrophin (βHCG) which can be used as tumour markers to monitor response to treatment and detection of early relapse. Disseminated tumours and those incompletely resected are treated with chemotherapy and a greater than 90% chance of cure is possible in most cases.

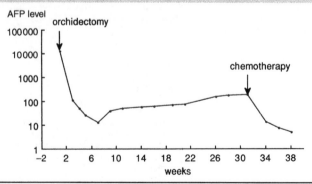

Use of AFP measurements to monitor for early relapse in a presumed stage 1 testicular germ cell

BONE TUMOURS

Osteosarcoma and Ewing tumour are the two most common malignant bone tumours. Clinical presentation is with local swelling, pain and occasional pathological fractures. Osteosarcomas arise more commonly in the femur around the knee or in the proximal humerus of adolescents and young adults. Ewing tumours present commonly in flat bones of the axial skeleton and the midshaft of long bones and usually in children under 10 years of age. Osteosarcoma exhibits strong evidence of a genetic predisposition as there are frequent reports of familial cases as well as an association with a previous history of retinoblastoma. Ewing sarcoma cells are characterised by (11:22) translocation corresponding to the cytogenetic abnormality in neuroepithelioma.

Osteogenic sarcoma

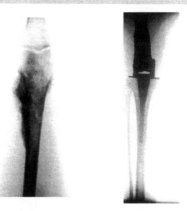

Treatment is dictated by the bone involved and tumour responsiveness to chemotherapy. Axial tumours are often difficult to resect. Tumours of long bones are more amenable to surgery and recent techniques have increased the likelihood of salvaging the limb. Initial chemotherapy is used to reduce tumour bulk and allow resection followed by prosthetic bone replacement. With such approaches there is an overall 60% chance of cure in these tumours.

Ewing sarcoma

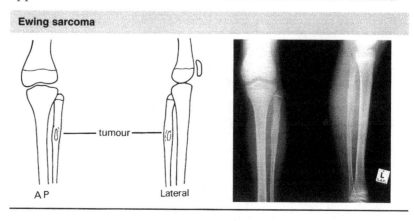

AP   tumour   Lateral

OTHER TUMOURS

Hepatic tumours

Hepatoblastoma is an embryonic tumour affecting children less than 3 years of age and is associated with hemihypertrophy and family cancer syndromes. Hepatocellular carcinoma occurs later in childhood and is associated with pre-existing cirrhosis brought about by infection (hepatitis B), longstanding biliary obstruction, α_1-antitrypsin deficiency or some inborn errors of metabolism, for example hereditary tyrosinaemia. A combination of primary chemotherapy and surgical resection has resulted in improved success rates, while liver transplantation should be considered in tumours unsuitable for resection.

Retinoblastoma

This retinal tumour is the best known hereditary tumour. Sixty per cent of tumours arise as a result of sporadic mutations and are almost always unilateral. The remaining 40% are bilateral tumours which are thought to be hereditary and associated with deletions of the retinoblastoma gene at 13q14. Only 10% of these cases have a positive family history. Those with the hereditary form are at increased risk of subsequently developing osteosarcoma in their thirties, particularly within irradiation fields. Presentation is most commonly before 2 years of age with a white pupil (leukokoria), strabismus, a painful red eye or poor vision. Prognosis for survival is determined by the extent of local spread and for vision, by the location of tumours and treatment necessary for their control. The risk of continued tumour formation persists until around 4–5 years of age.

Carcinomas and other tumours

There are many other rarer tumours of childhood including adrenal, thyroid and nasopharyngeal carcinoma. Adrenal carcinoma is important for its association with family cancer syndromes and hemihypertrophy. Differentiated thyroid cancer is notable for its increased incidence in patients after therapeutic irradiation and the medullary cell tumours of the thyroid for their association with the multiple endocrine neoplasia syndrome type II. Nasopharyngeal carcinoma is the the most common of these three and the Epstein–Barr virus is implicated in its aetiology.

HISTIOCYTIC DISORDERS

This group of disorders includes a variety of conditions which may be life threatening but are not thought to be true malignancies. The commonest condition is Langerhans cell histiocytosis (Class I histiocytosis) which may present in many ways, depending on the system within which the disease process is active. Symptoms at presentation result from proliferation of components of the histiocyte-macrophage system which may occur anywhere in the body. Such proliferations may take a variety of forms including skin rashes, bony lesions, lymphadenopathy, diabetes insipidus, a variety of organ dysfunctions due to histiocytic infiltrates and associated systemic upset with fever. It is thought to be a disorder of immune regulation. The natural history is for the disease to burn itself out during childhood and adolescence so treatment approaches must be tailored to cause minimal long-term damage.

Familial erythrophagocytic lymphohistiocytosis (Class II histiocytosis) presents with pancytopenia and splenomegaly in the first year of life and a family history of children dying with similar conditions. Other related syndromes are thought to be precipitated by previous viral infections. Malignant histiocytosis (Class III histiocytosis) has recently been recognised as a large cell anaplastic lymphoma which is clearly malignant. These conditions are usually managed by paediatric oncologists because of their multisystem nature and the potential value of cytotoxic treatments in their management.

BIBLIOGRAPHY

Pizzo P A, Poplack D G 1997 Principles and practice of paediatric oncology, 3rd edn. Lippincott-Raven, Philadelphia
Plowman P N, Pinkerton C R 1992 Paediatric oncology. Chapman & Hall, London

14 Growth

HEAD GROWTH
HEIGHT AND WEIGHT
SHORT STATURE
EXCESSIVE HEIGHT

Serial accurate measurements of height, weight and head circumference plotted on record charts provide an invaluable illustration of growth and development. Growth reflects not only general health but also the nutritional and emotional environment of a child, and disordered growth may be the only obvious manifestation of disease or deprivation.

HEAD GROWTH

At term head circumference, 32–37 cm, is three-quarters of its adult value, 52–57 cm, and the majority of postnatal growth occurs in infancy. The anterior fontanelle, which normally measures approximately 2.5 by 2.5 cm at birth, may no longer be palpable by 6 months but often remains patent until 18 months.

Head circumference chart (after Nellhaus)

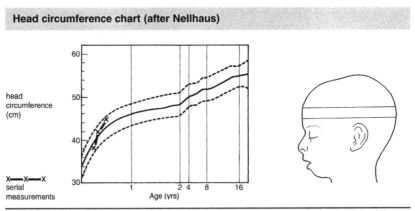

Microcephaly is commonly associated with brain hypoplasia or fetal brain damage, for example that caused by intrauterine infection.

Macrocephaly refers to a large head from whatever cause. With hydrocephalus the increased volume is due to accumulation of CSF within the ventricular system. In megalencephaly the brain tissue is bulkier than usual. Megalencephaly is commonly benign and often familial but is occasionally associated with mental handicap.

Hydrocephalus must be considered when serial head circumferences deviate away from a normal growth curve, and with proper measurement it should be detected before there are signs of raised intracranial pressure. This condition more than any other emphasises the need for accurate measurement and careful plotting on an appropriate chart. Cranial ultrasound through the window provided by the anterior fontanelle will clarify whether there is ventricular dilatation.

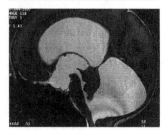

MRI hydrocephalus

Asymmetrical skulls are caused by inequality of growth rates at the coronal, sagittal and lambdoid sutures. The inequality may be due to an innocent cause like the postural effect which leads to mild plagiocephaly or rarely it may be due to premature fusion of the sutures, craniosynostosis.

Asymmetrical skulls and craniosynostosis

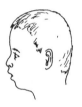
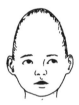
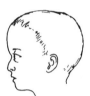

plagiocephaly   brachycephaly   oxycephaly (turricephaly, acrocephaly)   scaphocephaly

Premature craniosynostosis occurs as an isolated congenital deformity or as a component of certain inherited syndromes. Localised forms of craniosynostosis produce characteristic skull shapes and there may be potentially damaging pressure effects upon the brain, eyes and cranial nerves. Infants suspected of having this condition require prompt referral to a neurosurgical centre experienced in assessing and treating these problems. Craniectomy or reconstruction of the sutures is usually performed in the first months of life, and may have to be followed by additional cosmetic procedures.

HEIGHT AND WEIGHT

Height and weight are interpreted by plotting accurate measurements against population standards for age. A child's position on the chart is described in terms of centile. This is a useful illustration of the child's size compared to normal but it is an approximation. There are secular

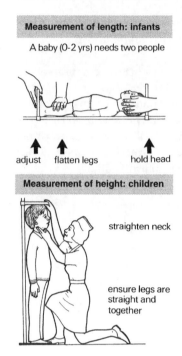

Measurement of length: infants

A baby (0-2 yrs) needs two people

adjust   flatten legs   hold head

Measurement of height: children

straighten neck

ensure legs are
straight and
together

trends which reduce the relevance of standards derived decades earlier, and standards cannot readily accommodate a multiracial society. It is important therefore to follow the rate of a child's growth to determine whether he remains parallel to or deviates away from population centiles. A deviating height or low height velocity is more indicative of pathology than a low but stable height centile.

Height velocity for age charts show three main components of growth: infancy, childhood and puberty. Height velocity in infancy starts high, above 15 cm per year, and decelerates rapidly. This rapid growth is a continuation of fetal growth in which nutrition is the dominant influence.

Childhood growth is a phase of slow decline in height velocity, although it should not fall below 5 cm per year. There are many factors involved in childhood growth with the growth hormone axis playing a pivotal role.

Puberty paralleled by increased sex hormone release results in height acceleration, peaking at 7–10 cm per year. This change in the tempo of growth has a very variable timing with respect to chronological age and is more closely linked to sexual maturation and bone age. The tempo of puberty alters the rate at which an individual reaches adult height but does not alter genetically programmed final height.

SHORT STATURE

Statistical definitions of short stature as a height below the 2nd or 0.4th centile are useful for population screening but for the individual child and family the issue is whether height presents a problem. Tall parents or those whose child attends a school with a bias towards above average stature may well consider their 10th centile son or daughter to be short. The challenge for health professionals is to determine whether height is a real or perceived problem, and to recognise children with genuine growth failure. Ideally growth failure should be recognised before the child falls below the 2nd or 0.4th centiles.

The population below the 2nd centile, 1 in 50, includes many healthy children and it is usually sufficient for their assessment to be conducted by primary care or community staff trained to recognise growth failure by serial measurement, and height which is inconsistent with the child's family. A child with height below the 0.4th centile, 1 in 250, is more likely to have underlying organic disease including hormone deficiency and requires specialist assessment. Many of these children will already be known because of already recognised problems, for example low birth weight with persisting infancy growth failure or syndromatic growth failure such as Down syndrome. Special growth charts are available to clarify whether children with disorders like Down syndrome or achondroplasia are growing at rates consistent with other effected children.

Growth charts (after Tanner and Whitehouse)

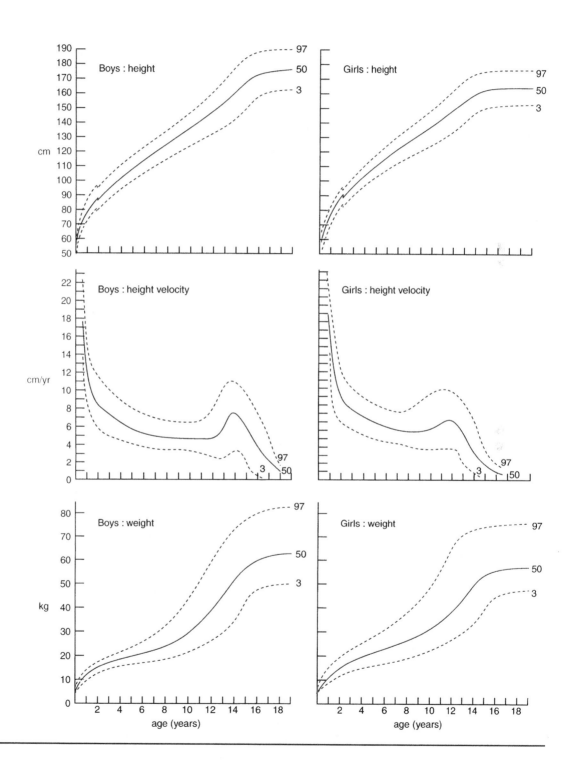

Longitudinal growth assessment

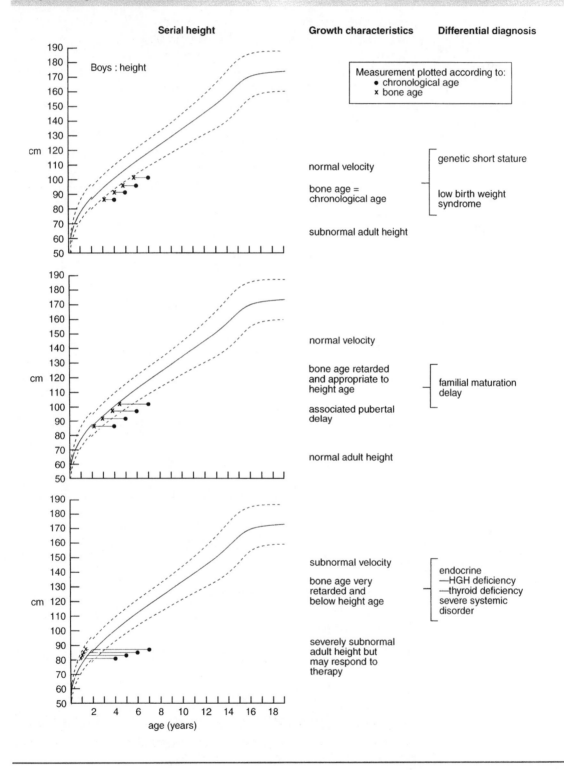

Serial height

Boys : height

cm

age (years)

Growth characteristics

Measurement plotted according to:
- • chronological age
- × bone age

normal velocity

bone age =
chronological age

subnormal adult height

normal velocity

bone age retarded
and appropriate to
height age

associated pubertal
delay

normal adult height

subnormal velocity

bone age very
retarded and
below height age

severely subnormal
adult height but
may respond to
therapy

Differential diagnosis

genetic short stature

low birth weight
syndrome

familial maturation
delay

endocrine
—HGH deficiency
—thyroid deficiency
severe systemic
disorder

Genetic and environmental causes of short stature

Familial short stature. Adult height is subject to polygenic inheritance and has a normal distribution. In assessing a child's stature it is useful to plot the parents' height centiles on the child's growth chart. In calculating the midparental height for a boy add 12 cm to his mother's height; for a girl subtract 12 cm from her father's height. It must be remembered that parental short stature may have resulted from inherited disease, for example skeletal dysplasia, or from a recurrent cycle of deprivation.

Constitutional delay of growth and puberty (CDGP). Delayed maturation and a delay in the pubertal phase of growth is a common cause of late childhood growth failure and short stature, especially in boys. These youngsters remain prepubertal and in the decelerating phase of childhood growth, while their contemporaries are developing sexually and accelerating in height. The problem is magnified if it is superimposed on familial short stature. CDGP is often genetically determined and hence the importance of enquiring about patterns of puberty in close relatives. In the absence of a positive family history it is important to exclude environmental or health factors which have either restrained growth in the past or may still be active. Bone age estimation typically shows approximately 2 years' delay and when height is adjusted for this delay it falls into a range which matches the target height predicted from parental stature.

For most affected youngsters explanation and reassurance about their acceptable final height is sufficient. Boys tend to be more vulnerable to psychological problems associated with CDGP given that physical stature is a more conspicuous asset in the male. Girls have height acceleration as an early component of puberty whereas boys have to wait until the second half of puberty, equating to testicular volumes of above 8 ml. When behavioural problems and social isolation blight a teenage boy's passage through what is already a turbulent period, then there is justification for artificially altering the tempo of puberty and height acceleration with a short course of either low dose testosterone depot injections or the weak orally active androgen, oxandrolone.

Intrauterine growth failure persisting into childhood. The majority of preterm and small-for-gestational age infants achieve catch-up growth in the first 2 years and reach normal adult size, but approximately 10% have permanently restricted growth. This is a heterogeneous group consisting of infants exposed to adverse environmental influences such as congenital infection or maternal drugs, or having intrinsic disorders, for example chromosomal anomalies or metabolic disease. Many have no obvious explanation but are presumed to have had suboptimal nutrition during critical phases of organogenesis and tissue programming. The latter produces end-organ resistance to endocrine control from insulin and the growth hormone–growth factor axis. These disturbances of tissue programming and endocrine regulation limit growth, and also appears to determine adult vulnerability to ischaemic heart disease, cerebrovascular disease and non-insulin dependent diabetes.

small face
short stature.
low birth weight
asymmetry (50%)
short 5th finger (75%)
mental retardation (20%)

Russell–Silver syndrome refers to small-for-gestational age infants who also have typical dysmorphic features including triangular facies, small mandible, body asymmetry and clinodactyly (incurved fifth fingers).

Social deprivation. Short stature is most prevalent in the lower social classes and reflects the superimposition of environment on genetic potential. It is not easy to define the latter as successive generations have usually been exposed to the same adverse factors. Maternal health during her own fetal life may be a key factor determining her ability to nourish the next generation. The normal pulsatile pattern of growth hormone release is depressed in emotionally deprived children but rapidly reverts to normal when they are provided with love and reasonable care. These disturbed children may also show bizarre, compulsive eating behaviour, to the extent that they develop distended abdomens and bouts of vomiting. Nutritional starvation produces a different response with exaggerated growth hormone secretion but a block at tissue level where there is diminished synthesis of the growth factors which mediate in the peripheral anabolic effects of growth hormone.

Chronic diseases sufficient to restrict growth are usually severe and can be diagnosed by careful history and examination. Exceptions which may remain undetected include malabsorption and inflammatory bowel disease. Coeliac disease is a particular problem in that it may mimic growth hormone deficiency producing subnormal height velocity, delayed bone age and suppressed growth hormone responses to provocative tests. Gliadin and endomysial antibody tests together with inflammatory markers such as C-reactive protein are therefore valuable in the investigation of growth failure.

Endocrine causes

Growth hormone physiology. The mechanisms responsible for the release and action of growth hormone (GH) are complex and are only gradually being unravelled. At the hypothalamic level a cascade of neurotransmitters modulates the balance between growth hormone releasing factor (GRF), and growth hormone releasing inhibitory factor or somatostatin. This sequence controls the pulsatile pattern of GH release from the anterior pituitary. GH acts indirectly on chondrocytes to promote linear growth via insulin-like growth factor-1 (IGF-1) which is released in response to GH mainly in the liver. Nutritional status and insulin levels also influence IGF-1 synthesis. The action of IGF-1 on cartilage growth plates is in turn dependent on binding proteins and the status of cell receptors which are also regulated by thyroxine, cortisol and paracrine growth factors. The concept of GH deficiency is therefore simplistic and the modern emphasis is increasingly directed at defining the precise level at which the axis is defective.

Growth hormone deficiency may be congenital or acquired, and it may be isolated or part of a generalised pituitary failure. Familial disorders account for less than 10%. Congenital abnormalities vary from isolated failure of neuronal migration in the pituitary stalk to more profound

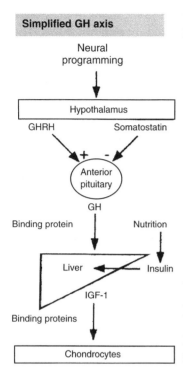

Simplified GH axis

Neural programming

↓

Hypothalamus

GHRH   Somatostatin

+ −

Anterior pituitary

GH

Binding protein   Nutrition

Liver ← Insulin

IGF-1

Binding proteins

↓

Chondrocytes

gh = growth hormone,
ghrh = growth hormone
releasing hormone,
igf-1 = insulin-like growth factor 1

midline malformation involving hypothalamus, pituitary and optic nerves. High definition MRI imaging is now an essential tool for classifying these conditions. Many children who qualify for GH therapy have no detectable anatomical lesion and are classified as having isolated GH deficiency. This may represent the extreme lower end of the normal distribution of GH secretory capacity in the population. The challenge which faces growth specialists, and the health service which has to finance GH prescription, is where to draw the line between those who qualify and those who do not qualify for treatment.

Acquired hypopituitarism occurs as a result of a range of hypothalamic–pituitary axis insults including tumours or infiltration, following basal meningitis and after severe head injuries. Cranial radiotherapy used to treat intracranial malignancy or in acute leukaemia protocols may also result in pituitary deficiency.

The diagnosis of GH deficiency depends on demonstrating that a child has a subnormal growth rate, a delayed bone age, and a clinical picture compatible with subnormal GH production rather than other identifiable health restraints. In a minority of patients, associated pituitary hormone deficiencies or imaging evidence of an anatomical abnormality in the pituitary region will help to confirm the diagnosis. It is impractical to perform the frequency of blood testing that is necessary to properly assess physiological GH secretion. A compromise approach is to measure end products of GH secretion, for example plasma IGF-1 and its main binding protein IGFBP3 or urinary GH. Unfortunately these measures have poor predictive value in selecting children who will benefit from GH therapy. Potential candidates for GH therapy are usually selected on the basis of their GH response to provocation tests using clonidine, glucagon and arginine. A clearly subnormal GH response is diagnostically useful, but many short children produce borderline levels and there is considerable intra-individual variation in the response. Height acceleration after starting GH treatment is a further useful step in consolidating the diagnosis. Children with severe GH deficiency and subnormal pretreatment height velocities have a striking response to modest dosage GH and, if diagnosed sufficiently early, can be restored to a trajectory which takes them to an acceptable adult height. Short children with intermediate GH secretory capacity and near normal height velocities require higher dosage GH therapy to gain significant height acceleration, and it is still uncertain whether they can achieve final height advantage which justifies long-term, costly therapy.

GH used in treatment is derived from biotechnology and has an excellent safety profile. The main concerns are cost and the uncertainty that altered metabolism and tissue programming during growth may have unpredicted morbidity in later life. The latter is unlikely to reduce the justification for treatment in children whose growth failure is a real disability, but it should moderate the enthusiasm for intervention in children whose short stature is more modest.

Craniopharyngioma. This is a rare but important condition to exclude whenever there is a possibility of acquired hypopituitarism. The tumour is composed of expanding cystic remnants of Rathke's pouch, a dorsal protrusion of the embryonic foregut, and its strategic location results in life threatening pressure effects. Headache and defective vision are more common initial complaints than short stature so that visual field assessment and fundoscopy are essential in the assessment of short children. Plain skull X-rays may reveal calcification in the cyst, but when there is a likelihood of intracranial pathology the appropriate imaging is either CT scan or MRI. Treatment aims for complete excision but not at the expense of causing further damage to the hypothalamus. Patients are likely to have lifelong panhypopituitarism and it is important to avoid the additional hypothalamic morbidity of disturbed behaviour, polyphagia and escalating obesity.

Other examples of tumour related hypopituitarism include germinoma and optic nerve glioma associated with neurofibromatosis.

Pressure effects and clinical features of craniopharygioma

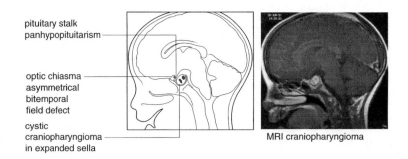

pituitary stalk
panhypopituitarism

optic chiasma
asymmetrical
bitemporal
field defect

cystic
craniopharyngioma
in expanded sella

MRI craniopharyngioma

Juvenile hypothyroidism, usually secondary to autoimmune thyroiditis, may present as progressive growth failure. A goitre may be present but the other manifestations are often insidious and readily overlooked. Fortunately, hypothyroidism is readily confirmed by finding a low plasma thyroxine and an elevated TSH, and it responds to thyroxine replacement. It is important to recognise that a low thyroxine level paralleled by a low TSH points to hypothalamic-pituitary disease rather than primary hypothyroidism.

Adrenal insufficiency and hypoparathyroidism account for a small number of children with short stature. Corticosteroid therapy at a dosage in excess of prednisolone 5 mg per day or its equivalent interferes with linear growth. Alternate-day single dose oral corticosteroid regimens permit more normal growth, and the success of inhaled corticosteroid regimens in asthma prevention has substantially reduced the number of children faced with potential growth suppressing treatment.

Investigation of short stature

In the majority of short children a careful history and examination will reveal a genetic or environmental basis for their stature, or will identify health disorders likely to suppress growth. It is important to document dysmorphic features which may favour a syndromatic cause such as Turner or Noonan syndrome. Disproportionate shortening of limbs or spine may be obvious but should be confirmed by measurement of sitting height or crown–rump length. Pubertal staging, optic fundi and visual field assessment are also essential parts of the physical examination.

Laboratory investigations are guided by the clinical findings and where appropriate the preliminary screen is limited to full blood count, inflammatory markers (ESR, CRP), plasma electrolytes, creatinine, calcium, phosphate, alkaline phosphatase and thyroid function. Gliadin and endomysial antibody titres help to exclude coeliac disease.

A karyotype is indicated in short girls even when dysmorphic features do not provide compelling evidence for Turner syndrome. Boys with dysmorphic features or hypogonadism are also candidates for chromosome analysis. An X-ray of the left wrist and hand for bone age determination is a valuable tool. A child is unlikely to have an endocrine basis for short stature unless the bone age is substantially delayed. Cranial imaging, preferably an MRI scan, is reserved for children with neurological or ophthalmic signs and it is also useful to define the anatomy of the pituitary and its stalk if there is endocrine evidence of hypopituitarism. Plain skull X-rays have a poor yield for the detection of pituitary pathology.

The pulsatile nature of GH secretion, and its wide variability in normally growing children presents a challenge to investigation. A single random blood GH level cannot be used to diagnose deficiency. Ideally GH levels should be measured at 20-minute intervals during sleep but this is impractical, and a number of provocative tests have been developed in an attempt to measure peak GH production. Currently glucagon, arginine and clonidine provocative tests are in regular use but research is being directed at alternative assays within the GH–IGF-1 axis so as to avoid subjecting children to these arduous investigations. It is important that short children are not subjected to these tests before at least 6 months of careful measurement has confirmed that they have genuine growth failure, that is a low height velocity.

The selection of children for biosynthetic GH treatment and their subsequent monitoring requires specialist involvement. While it is relatively straightforward to recognise that a child with congenital or acquired panhypopituitarism requires GH as part of their total hormone replacement programme, it is difficult to distinguish the child with partial isolated GH deficiency from the larger population of short children who have relative GH insufficiency compared to their taller peers.

A scheme for investigating short stature

Growth surveillance	Preliminary assessment	Features of hypothalamic pituitary disorder
• Abnormal growth pattern • Severe or inappropriate short stature • Subnormal growth rate	• Familial stature • Familial growth rate • Intrauterine and infancy growth failure • Dysmorphic features • Disproportionate body • Nutrition and environment • General health-symptomatic • General health-unrecognised • Hypothyroidism	• Neurological-symptoms of raised intracranial pressure • Visual loss of acuity of field • Neurocutaneous, neurofibromatosis • Endocrine-diabetes insipidus, hypogonadism

		Specialist assessment
		• Cranial and pituitary imaging • Endocrine evaluation and GH provocation test

Disproportionate short stature

Skeletal disorders account for the majority of this group and may be classified into those where abnormality originates in the skeleton, or has a systemic metabolic basis, for example the mucopolysaccharidoses. They may also be divided into those with short limbs or short trunks, the latter usually having kyphoscoliosis.

Achondroplasia serves as an example of a conspicuous disorder with an incidence of 1 in 15 000 live births. It has been linked to a mutation of chromosome 4 which controls the structure of the fibroblast growth factor receptor 3 associated with transmembrane tyrosine kinase. It is inherited as an autosomal dominant but many arise as new mutations and there is an association with more advanced paternal age.

Achondroplasia

Adult: male—mean 131 + 6 cm   female—mean 127 + 6 cm

large square head

small foramen magnum

lordosis

trident hands

bow legs

Hypochondroplasia is a distinct and milder dysplasia which may be quite a common cause of familial short stature in which affected members have relatively short broad limbs. It is debatable whether they benefit from having this label applied to them but the diagnosis needs to be considered if they present their children as candidates for possible GH therapy. It is also uncertain whether GH therapy has a useful role in enhancing the final height of children with skeletal dysplasias. Surgical limb lengthening requires a major investment in time and discomfort but does add useful length to legs and possibly arms.

The wide spectrum and variability of skeletal dysplasias is such that patients and parents need the combined expertise of paediatricians, geneticists, radiologists and orthopaedic surgeons for precise diagnosis, counselling and optimal management.

EXCESSIVE HEIGHT

The great majority of exceptionally tall children come from tall families and accept their stature as normal although sometimes inconvenient. Society tends to favour tall individuals and clothing manufacturers are beginning to cater for this end of the market. Occasionally, girls destined to have an adult height above 5 feet 10 inches (178 cm) are referred for advice and possible medical intervention. This hinges on the reliability of final height prediction in late childhood or early adolescence, and has to take account of the variable tempo of and height contribution from puberty.

Prediction tables are liable to errors of approximately 5 cm either way, and this figure is not dissimilar to the claimed improvement from intervention. The usual intervention is oestrogen therapy at a dose which accelerates skeletal maturation but minimises the potential side effects including nausea and weight gain. The girl and family must share in the decision, given that the treatment aims are primarily cosmetic and social.

Pathological causes of excessive stature are uncommon but there is an overlap between children with long slender limbs and those who meet the criteria of Marfan syndrome.

Marfan syndrome is suggested by a family history and major features in skeletal, ocular and cardiovascular systems. Key clinical features include joint laxity, chest deformity and scoliosis. Around one-third have echocardiographic evidence of aortic root enlargement or mitral valve prolapse. The basis is an autosomal dominant fibrillin gene mutation on chromosome 15, but 25% represent new mutations.

Homocystinuria is a rare, 1 in 50 000, recessive disorder of methionine metabolism in which children have a marfanoid appearance. Diagnostic features include high myopia accompanied by lens dislocation, learning delay and early onset thromboembolic events.

Pathological causes of excessive height	
Endocrine disorders	Other disorders
Pituitary—eosinophilic adenoma	Cerebral gigantism (Soto syndrome)
Thyrotoxicosis	Marfan syndrome
Precocious puberty (early stages)	Homocystinuria

BIBLIOGRAPHY

Barker D J P 1994 Mothers, babies and disease in later life. BMJ Publishing Group, London

Brook C G D 1995 Clinical paediatric endocrinology, 3rd edn. Blackwell Science, Oxford

Buckler J M H 1994 Growth disorders in children. BMJ Publishing Group, London

15

Endocrine

PUBERTY
DISORDERS OF SEXUAL
  DIFFERENTIATION
ADRENAL GLANDS
THYROID
PARATHYROID GLANDS
DIABETES

Although the fetus is totally dependent on a maternally regulated environment, endocrine systems differentiate and commence autonomous activity in the first trimester. The placenta is relatively impermeable to peptide hormones so that most fetal hypothalamic-pituitary-endocrine gland circuits evolve independently of direct interference from maternal hormone levels. The adrenal cortex is an exception in that the placenta actively participates in steroid metabolism and this is reflected in the major transition from fetal to adult cortex activity with birth.

Trophic hormones are first detectable in the anterior pituitary between 5 and 8 weeks' gestation, and serum levels of thyroid stimulating hormone (TSH) and the gonadotrophins (LH and FSH) reach adult levels by 16–20 weeks. This early surge of trophic hormone activity may relate to endocrine gland differentiation prior to the establishment of sensitive feedback mechanisms.

Although the conventional endocrine system is the key to understanding control of growth and development in postnatal life, it is less directly involved with fetal organisation. Fetal life is dominated by cellular division and differentiation, events which are controlled by local or paracrine systems in which populations of cells release and respond to local growth factors. This paracrine system is a complex interplay of multiple peptide growth factors modified by transport proteins and cell receptor mechanisms. Growth factors may have a broad specificity, acting on a wide variety of cells in many tissues, for example insulin-like growth factors (IGF-1, IGF-2), or may be tissue specific, for example nerve growth factor (NGF).

Molecular biology allows us to explore the control of gene expression which, in a cascade of intracellular and extracellular signalling pathways, determines tissue differentiation and function. Disorders such as congenital hypothyroidism and incomplete virilisation can now be partially explained in terms of failure of gene expression of key transcription factors. Increasingly the variability of conditions such as congenital adrenal hyperplasia can be correlated with genome analysis. The era of attempting to explore endocrine function with plasma or urine hormone levels is gradually being replaced by molecular tools which focus on individual steps in hormone pathways.

The conductor

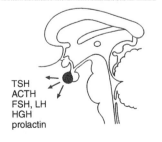

TSH
ACTH
FSH, LH
HGH
prolactin

PUBERTY

Puberty is the series of physical and physiological events which convert a child into an adult capable of reproduction. Although it is conventionally regarded as a phase of life dominated by increasing gonadal activity and the appearance of secondary sexual characteristics, it is better to regard it as part of the continuum of growth and maturation regulated by still ill defined brain-mediated programming. There is considerable variation in the tempo of growth and development. In part this variation is genetically determined, but there is also an environmental component and the secular trend towards earlier puberty and taller adult stature parallels increased childhood nutrition.

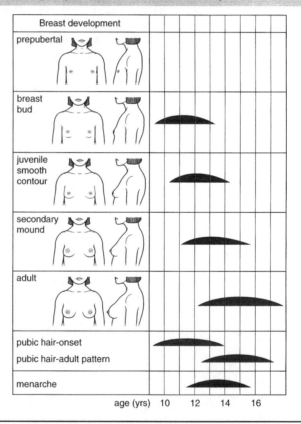

Normal breast stages, girls (after Marshall and Tanner)

As a rule girls have earlier puberty, and their growth acceleration is one of the first components, often preceding breast bud enlargement. Ninety-five per cent start puberty between the ages 9 and 13 years, and have onset of periods, menarche, between 11 and 13 years. Height growth is largely completed at menarche. Boys tend to have later puberty but this is partly because the initial stage of testicular enlargement is less obvious. Normal male puberty commences as early as age 9 years or may be delayed until 14 years. It is important for counselling purposes to appreciate that height acceleration occurs in the second half of male puberty. The 12.5-cm sex difference in mean adult heights arises from the more prolonged male prepubertal growth period and also from greater pubertal height gain particularly in trunk growth.

A standardised system for staging secondary sexual characteristics has been provided by Marshall and Tanner. Testicular volume can also be calibrated using a Prader orchidometer, the prepubertal testis being no more than 3 ml rising to between 12 and 20 ml in the adult. Other valuable tools in the assessment of pubertal problems are hand and wrist X-rays for bone age estimation, and pelvic ultrasound imaging of the ovaries and uterus.

Normal genital stages, boys (after Marshall and Tanner)

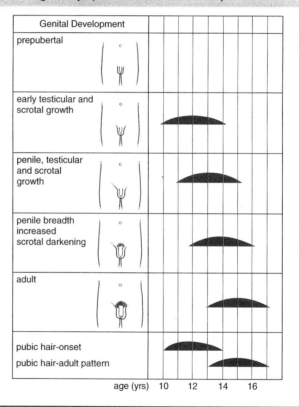

Physiology of puberty

The newborn infant is capable of releasing high levels of gonadotrophins (LH and FSH) and sex steroids but this surge of hormonal activity is subsequently inhibited during early childhood by brain mediated programming. The hypothalamic gonadotrophin releasing-hormone (GnRH) pulse generator remains largely dormant through early childhood and then, from age 6 to 8 years onwards, signals a gradual increase in the amplitude and pulse frequency of LH and FSH. Ovarian ultrasound examination reflects this emerging phase with evidence of increasing follicular activity. Clinical evidence of gonadal maturation is referred to as the gonadarche.

Delayed puberty

A convenient definition of delayed puberty is absence of early signs by age 13 years in girls and 14 years in boys. However attention should also be paid to youngsters who fail to complete puberty within an acceptable timescale of 4–5 years. Assessment of delay must also take into account the whole tempo of growth and maturation. Pubertal delay may be the most conspicuous problem, but there is often an established pattern of downward height deviation. Commonly a family history of late puberty confirms the clinical impression of constitutional delay of growth and puberty (CDGP) but it is important to recognise when the delay has been imposed by environmental or chronic health restraints. If the delay cannot be explained by family history or an identifiable restraint, then investigations need to be directed at establishing whether there is a fault in the hypothalamo–pituitary regulation of gonadotrophin release or in the gonadal response to adequate levels of LH and FSH.

Hypogonadotrophic hypogonadism. Failure of LH and FSH release may be inherited either in isolation or together with deficient smell sensation, Kallmann syndrome. Clues at birth include micropenis and cryptorchidism, but there is a wide spectrum of severity and it may not be recognised until adult life. Acquired causes include tumours in the hypothalamo-pituitary region and cranial MRI imaging may be indicated. In paediatric practice the difficulty is to differentiate delayed maturation of LH, FSH release from partial but permanent deficiency.

Hypergonadotrophic hypogonadism. High plasma LH and FSH levels indicate that the gonadal response is impaired. In girls an important cause is ovarian dysgenesis linked to Turner syndrome, but it may occur as a separate entity. Ovarian ultrasound examination and chromosome analysis are key investigations. Boys may have congenital faults of testicular differentiation, or can lose the testes as a result of intrauterine torsion and infarction.

Precocious puberty

Precocious puberty is termed 'true' or intracranial when it is activated by the hypothalamic–pituitary axis, and 'false' when an extracranial or exogenous source of hormones is responsible.

Early puberty in girls is relatively common and there is often a family history of early menarche. Detailed investigation is unnecessary unless puberty commences exceptionally early, for example before the age of 6 years, or shows an abnormal sequence of events such as disproportionate virilisation. Other warning features are neurological or visual symptoms, hypertension and abnormal growth. Of girls commencing puberty early, 90% have no demonstrable abnormality. Detailed ultrasound imaging of the ovaries and uterus is useful in confirming diagnosis and monitoring progress. Cranial imaging is less of a priority in girls than it is in boys.

Causes of precocious puberty

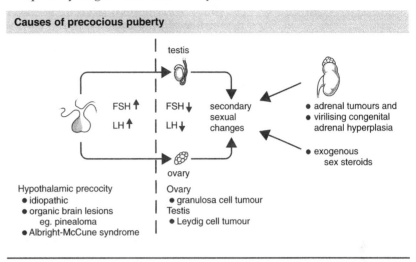

Hypothalamic precocity
- idiopathic
- organic brain lesions
  eg. pinealoma
- Albright-McCune syndrome

Ovary
- granulosa cell tumour

Testis
- Leydig cell tumour

- adrenal tumours and
- virilising congenital adrenal hyperplasia

- exogenous sex steroids

Precocious puberty in boys, starting before age 9 years, is almost always pathological and requires detailed investigation. Testicular palpation is a useful guide; infantile testes in a rapidly growing pubertal boy point to an adrenal pathology. Symmetrically enlarging testes favour an intracranial problem, and a single large testis suggests a gonadal tumour. Cranial MRI is essential to exclude hypothalamic or pineal area tumours as a cause of male precocious true puberty.

The selection of treatment is determined by the underlying cause, and by the potential disruption to the child's life from an unwanted puberty. In the majority of patients, who have lost neurohypothalamic restraint on puberty, control may be regained by using depot injection formulations of an LHRH superagonist which suppress LH, FSH release. Although this can be successful in halting and reversing sexual maturation, it fails to restore the growth potential lost because of advanced bone age, a constant feature of precocious puberty.

Premature thelarche. Infant and young girls may have transient breast development without growth acceleration or other pubertal features. Ovarian ultrasound examination shows parallel follicular development confirming that there is temporary activation of the FSH–oestradiol axis but the uterus remains small. Premature or isolated thelarche is usually self limiting and innocent so that reassurance is appropriate. In a minority of affected girls the breast development slowly merges with complete early puberty.

Premature adrenarche or pubarche. There is a normal increase in adrenal androgen release in midchildhood reflecting the maturation of the zona reticularis. This hormonal activity is thought to account for the modest growth spurt which occurs around age 6–8 years. The adrenal androgens may reach a level sufficient to produce early pubic hair as well as more pronounced growth acceleration and bone age advance. This is more commonly recognised in girls and is seldom indicative of progression into full early puberty. If pubic hair or height acceleration becomes increasingly conspicuous, or occurs in a child of less than age 6 years, then steps should be taken to exclude congenital adrenal hyperplasia or an adrenal tumour.

Disordered puberty after cranial radiotherapy. A growing population of children are survivors of leukaemia and intracranial tumour therapy regimens incorporating cranial radiotherapy. A delayed side-effect is disruption of the neural programming of growth and puberty. Girls are especially at risk of inappropriately early puberty often combined with relative growth hormone deficiency. The end result may be substantial loss of final height, further aggravated by irradiation induced spinal shortening and hypothyroidism. Cancer services need to continue longterm monitoring of growth so that these potential problems can be recognised and treated.

McCune–Albright syndrome. This curious entity links irregular skin pigmentation, fibrous dysplasia of bones and autonomy of endocrine glands. The molecular basis is a mutation of the G protein intracellular signalling mechanism which results in certain cell lines having autonomy from peptide hormone control. In the ovaries this autonomy results in oestrogen producing cysts and an atypical pattern in which menarche occurs earlier than predicted from breast changes. It may also present with pathological bone fractures or overactivity of other endocrine glands.

DISORDERS OF SEXUAL DIFFERENTIATION

Gender results from a sequence of gonadal determination and differentiation which in turn dictates internal and external genital differentiation. The primordial gonad is bipotential and will progress to an ovarian structure unless directed by genes on the Y chromosome. In mammals, female is the constitutive or default sex and the male the induced sex. The sex-determining region of Y (SRY), in concert with other genes, acts as a switch and generates DNA-binding transcription factors which regulate gonadal tissue gene expression. Sertoli and Leydig cell populations appear in the emerging testis. Sertoli cells encode a protein called anti-müllerian hormone (AMH) which diffuses locally to suppress paramesonephric ducts which would otherwise lead to the formation of female internal organs including fallopian ducts, uterus and upper vagina. Leydig cells and their production of testosterone and dihydrotestosterone are responsible for masculinisation of internal and external genitalia.

The relative complexity of male differentiation makes it more vulnerable to mutation, and a wide spectrum of incomplete masculinisation. Clinical presentation ranges from male infants with hypospadias, through severe sexual ambiguity to apparent females. This spectrum is exemplified by the heterogeneity of genetic and gonadal males with disorders of androgen receptors.

Androgen insensitivity syndromes. Mutations of androgen receptors cause XY individuals with functioning testes to have absent or incomplete virilisation of the external genitalia. In the complete form of androgen insensitivity, otherwise termed testicular feminisation syndrome, the external appearance is entirely female but the vagina is shortened with absent uterus and fallopian ducts. The diagnosis may be revealed when an inguinal hernia is found to contain a testis or when a young woman presents with primary amenorrhoea. The testes continue to secrete high levels of testosterone which undergo peripheral conversion to oestrogen and therefore stimulate adequate breast development.

Partial androgen insensitivity results in the spectrum of incomplete virilisation. The more severe forms present at birth as problems of ambiguous genitalia requiring specialist investigation. Phallic unresponsiveness to exogenous testosterone makes the allocation of a male gender inappropriate and the majority of infants are raised as girls with a strategy of gonadectomy, genital plastic surgery and oestrogen substitution in later childhood.

Female sexual differentiation is more robust and the usual cause of masculinisation is excessive exposure to endogenous or exogenous androgens. Congenital adrenal hyperplasia is the commonest cause of masculinised females.

The highly emotive nature of sexual ambiguity presents a major management challenge, and prompt specialist advice is needed to select appropriate investigations. As a general guide investigations include chromosome analysis, adrenal and gonadal steroid measurements, and imaging of the internal genitalia. The priorities are to define the basic fault at sex chromosome, gonadal, adrenal or end-organ level; to ensure that no life-threatening implications such as adrenal failure arise; and to select the gender most likely to provide an acceptable life. Reconstructive surgery is successful in correcting a virilised girl, but it can do little to convert a genetic male with a minute and hormone unresponsive phallus into an acceptable boy. The latter child is better reared as a girl but the final decision must be shared with parents who may hold strong cultural beliefs.

ADRENAL GLANDS

During intra-uterine development the adrenal cortex is considerably enlarged due to an inner fetal zone. This zone, which accounts for 80% of the cortex at full term, involutes rapidly after birth leaving the outer adult zone to synthesise essential mineralocorticoids and glucocorticoids. The fetal cortex acts in a mutually dependent relationship with the placenta to synthesise oestriol and dehydroepiandrosterone. The measurement of these steroids in the maternal serum or urine provides an index of feto-placental health. The increasing development of the adult zone at term may be a factor in initiating the onset of labour.

Congenital adrenal hyperplasia

This group of inherited, autosomal recessive disorders is caused by the absence of essential enzymes in the pathway of cortisol and aldosterone synthesis. The resulting interruption of the adreno-hypothalamic feedback stimulates excessive corticotrophin (ACTH) release and overactivity of the biosynthetic steps prior to the block, with an accumulation of androgenic steroids.

Congenital adrenal hyperplasia

21-hydroxylase deficiency is the commonest variety and the majority recognised in infancy have the salt-losing type. Female infants are virilised at birth with clitoral hypertrophy and variable fusion of the labia minor. The most masculinised girls may be confused for boys with severe hypospadias and cryptorchidism. Prompt recognition is less easy in males and they are at risk of an adrenal crisis in the second week of life. The crisis, often preceded by vomiting and poor weight gain, is biochemically characterised by low plasma sodium and high potassium. Grossly elevated serum ACTH and 17-hydroxyproges-terone levels suggest 21-hydroxylase deficiency and this may be confirmed by demonstrating elevated concentrations of urinary pregnanetriol and 17-oxosteroids. A salt-losing crisis demands urgent therapy with intravenous saline, glucose and hydrocortisone.

Long-term management aims to suppress the hyperplastic adrenal glands and provide replacement hydrocortisone and a salt-retaining steroid, fludrocortisone. Correct replacement is that which permits a healthy life style, maintains normal linear growth and in due course enables acceptable sexual maturation. Surgical correction of the masculinised female perineum is commenced in infancy, starting with a reduction clitoroplasty and staged procedures to convert the urogenital sinus to an adequate vagina.

Modern management is more successful in ensuring that adult women have the potential for heterosexual relationships and fertility. Adult men, especially those without salt loss, have few symptoms and may lack the motivation to continue treatment.

11-beta-hydroxylase deficiency is the second most common variety and results in virilisation and salt retention with hypertension.

Cushing syndrome

This is due to sustained high circulating cortisol levels of either exogenous or endogenous origin. Iatrogenic disease is now less common with the introduction of effective alternatives to systemic corticosteroid therapy in for example asthma. Endogenous Cushing syndrome is fortunately rare in childhood but is likely to be due to a potentially malignant adrenocortical tumour. It should be considered when acne and masculinisation accompany the usual signs of cortisol excess. Distinction must be made between these potentially malignant unilateral tumours and the rarer problem of bilateral adrenal hyperplasia due to pituitary microadenomata. In the majority of cases the nature of the adrenal pathology will be demonstrated by CT scans. Adrenal tumours require unilateral adrenalectomy and additional radiotherapy if there is histological evidence of capsule invasion. In acquired bilateral adrenal hyperplasia, management is directed against the pituitary adenomata using high voltage irradiation or trans-sphenoidal microsurgery.

Not infrequently obese girls with lower abdominal and thigh striae are referred with the query 'hormonal problem?'. The vast majority are healthy apart from dietary based obesity. A useful guide is to appreciate that nutritional obesity is generally accompanied by above average stature. Cushingoid features linked to growth failure are suspicious.

Adrenal cortical failure (Addison disease) is an uncommon disorder, usually with an autoimmune basis, and may occur in association with diabetes mellitus, thyroiditis and hypoparathyroidism. Children either present with an insidious onset of weakness, weight loss and increased pigmentation or become acutely ill following a brief episode of diarrhoea and vomiting. An adrenal crisis demands urgent therapy with intravenous glucose and saline together with hydrocortisone. Long-term replacement consists of hydrocortisone ($15-20 \text{ mg/m}^2$ surface area/day) and fludrocortisone (0.1–0.2 mg daily). All patients on corticosteroid replacement therapy must be provided with a steroid warning card and the parents advised of the necessity of increasing the dosage during times of illness.

Cushing syndrome: clinical features

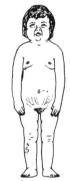

arrested growth

face and trunk obesity
heightened facial colour
hirsutism
hypertension
mood changes
muscle wasting

osteoporosis

striae

bruising

androgen effects suggest an adrenal tumour

   eg. acne and clitoral hypertrophy

THYROID

The thyroid originates from a ventral extension of the endoderm foregut which migrates to lie at the level of the upper trachea. Developmental failures may be classified as due to hypoplasia or maldescent.

Hypoplasia varies from absence of detectable thyroid and early severe hypothyroidism, to lesser degrees which, without screening, would remain asymptomatic until later childhood. An ectopic gland may account for a lingual mass or produce a thyroglossal cyst.

Physiology

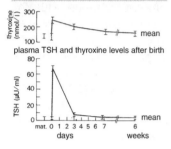

Neonatal thyroid function

plasma TSH and thyroxine levels after birth

The fetal thyroid contains colloid and iodoproteins by 10 weeks' gestation; plasma thyroid stimulating hormone (TSH) is detectable at this stage and there is evidence for early activity of the pituitary–thyroid axis. The fetal thyroid preferentially releases 'reverse T3', a molecule which differs from tri-iodothyronine (T3) by the location of a single iodine atom. Reverse T3 is thought to be inactive and its place in physiology has not been established. There is minimal transplacental passage of maternal thyroxine (T4) to the fetus.

Following birth there is a surge of TSH release later paralleled by increased T4 and T3. TSH levels return to the normal adult range by 1 week but T4 and especially T3 show a slower decline to adult values. The definition of normal neonatal thyroid function is essential for the development of screening programmes to detect congenital hypothyroidism.

Hypothyroidism

Congenital hypothyroidism is relatively common, 1 in 3000 live births. It is usually a sporadic condition and it is uncommon for there to be recurrence in siblings. Central nervous system development is critically dependent on T4 and T3, especially in late pregnancy and early infancy, and hypothyroidism is an important cause of preventable mental handicap. The hypothyroid fetus partially compensates for deficiency by diverting the minimal transplacental supply of T4 to the brain where it is converted to T3 by a specific cerebral deiodinase. Delivery interrupts this tenuous source of T4 and the natural history of the undetected infant depends on the amount of residual thyroid. The signs of hypothyroidism, notably prolonged jaundice, are usually present by age 2 weeks but are often overlooked. Fortunately screening for elevated TSH levels at age 1 week has proved to be very successful. Thyroxine therapy introduced by age 3 weeks and titrated to parallel growth enables the majority of children to achieve development closely resembling normal.

Endemic goitre and hypothyroidism. In global terms iodine deficiency remains the commonest cause of thyroid disease. It results in a spectrum of severity including profound neurological cretinism, deaf-mutism, myxoedema with dwarfism and goitres. Genetic variation and diet, notably cassava consumption, influence susceptibility to iodine deficiency. Iodination programmes and iodine depot injection in early pregnancy can dramatically reduce the prevalence of these disorders.

Goitrous hypothyroidism is rare outside of endemic regions. A group of inborn errors of thyroid metabolism may present in the newborn period or more commonly come to light in later childhood with the

Congenital hypothyroidism

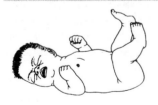

course facies   TSH ↑↑
dry skin   thyroxine ↓
hoarse cry
hypotonia
umbilical hernia
constipation
prolonged jaundice

emergence of a goitre. Antithyroid drugs given to control maternal hyperthyroidism in pregnancy can also result in a fetal goitre. Iodine containing drugs can also induce fetal hypothyroidism, and topical iodine should be avoided in preterm infants particularly as they are already at risk of borderline hypothyroidism.

Juvenile hypothyroidism. Current neonatal hypothyroid screening programmes detect the majority of congenitally hypoplastic and ectopic glands that previously resulted in presentation after infancy. Autoimmune thyroiditis is the usual cause in children and adolescents, usually girls. Features include goitre, progressive growth failure with marked bone age delay, lethargy and constipation. Secondary epiphyseal dysgenesis can produce orthopaedic problems, notably slipped upper femoral epiphyses. Intellectual development does not usually suffer because the thyroid deficiency occurs after the critical phase of brain development; paradoxically parents may complain when thyroxine treatment transforms patients from hypothyroid induced docility into normal teenagers! Thyroxine therapy is straightforward as long as compliance is adequate and plasma TSH levels are kept in the normal range. The main challenge is to recognise the relatively high requirement of infants and to adjust dosage during rapid infancy growth.

Hyperthyroidism

Neonatal hyperthyroidism is an uncommon disorder but must be anticipated in all infants of mothers with current or past hyperthyroidism. Maternal thyroid stimulating immunoglobulins may traverse the placenta to overstimulate the thyroid, producing fetal tachycardia or neonatal irritability, fever, diarrhoea and poor weight gain. Although transient the condition is potentially serious and may require antithyroid therapy.

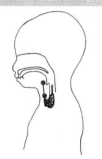

Ectopic sites of the thyroid gland

Juvenile hyperthyroidism is uncommon but the features are similar to those seen in adults with the addition of excessive growth and occasional abnormal choreiform movements. The diagnosis is confirmed by elevated plasma thyroxine levels. Medical management using carbimazole is the treatment of choice. An initial 2-year course may result in spontaneous remission in 25–75% of cases, and a further course should be completed before considering surgery or radioactive iodine.

Isolated thyroid nodules must be carefully investigated by ultrasound, isotope scans and biopsy to exclude carcinoma.

PARATHYROID GLANDS

Hypoparathyroidism

Transient hypoparathyroidism is a potential problem in very premature or sick newborn infants and the resulting hypocalcaemia may cause convulsions or apnoeic episodes. Permanent hypoparathyroidism is rare and has to be distinguished from conditions in which there is receptor insensitivity to circulating parathyroid hormone (PTH), pseudohypoparathyroidism

Features of hypoparathyroidism

Acute hypocalcaemia	Chronic hypocalcaemia	
convulsions	convulsions	
neuromuscular excitability	calcification of basal ganglia	
Chvostek sign	headache, vomiting (raised intracranial pressure)	
Trousseau sign	photophobia	
carpopedal spasm	cataracts	
	poor dentition	
	chronic diarrhoea	
	plasma calcium	down
	plasma phosphate	up
	alkaline phosphatase	normal

Hypoparathyroidism is confirmed by demonstrating inappropriately low plasma PTH levels in the context of hypocalcaemia. Parathyroid hypoplasia may be an isolated disorder or part of Di George syndrome associated with thymic hypoplasia and cardiac outflow tract defects. The syndrome results from disordered cervical neural crest migration into derivatives of the pharyngeal arches and pouches, and is linked to deletion of chromosome 22.

Pseudohypoparathyroidism is suggested by hypocalcaemia despite normal or elevated PTH levels. The biochemical defect can be further defined by demonstrating that PTH infusion fails to stimulate the normal increase in plasma cyclic AMP levels or urinary phosphate excretion. Pseudohypoparathyroidism is an example of receptor insensitivity linked to the G protein pathway. Some families have a typical phenotype with short stature, round facies, short metacarpals, ectopic calcification and mental retardation.

Pseudopseudohypoparathyroidism is the rather clumsy term applied to patients in whom the somatic features are not accompanied by biochemical derangement. There is however phenotypic and biochemical variation within families.

Treatment of hypoparathyroidism. Acute symptomatic hypocalcaemia requires urgent correction with intravenous calcium infusion. Permanent hypoparathyroidism and pseudohypoparathyroidism are treated with supraphysiological doses of vitamin D analogues which act by promoting intestinal calcium absorption and by mobilising bone calcium. The dose of vitamin D is adjusted to maintain the plasma calcium level in the low normal range (2.15–2.40 mmol/l). Chronic overdose carries the risk of nephrocalcinosis.

Classification of hypoparathyroidism

Transient neonatal
  Prematurity, cerebral injury
  Maternal diabetes
  Maternal hyperparathyroidism

Permanent life-long
  Isolated hypoplasia
  Di George syndrome

Acquired
  Autoimmune
  Post-thyroidectomy

DIABETES

Insulin dependent diabetes mellitus (IDDM) results from immune-mediated destruction of beta-cells, a process which precedes the recognition of clinical diabetes by years. Although diabetes is rarely recognised in infancy there is increasing evidence that the immune damage may be triggered by late fetal or infancy events. The incidence of recognised disease increases through childhood to reach a peak in adolescence, so that by age 16 years the prevalence is around 2 per 1000. Children account for around 5% of the total diabetic population but the life-long implications of the disease and the challenge posed to families and health professionals gives them a high priority.

Aetiology. Susceptibility to IDDM is inherited as a polygenic condition with major linkage to the MHC HLA region, notable types DR3 and DR4, but at least 12 other loci also contribute. Although 95% of diabetic children have DR3 and/or DR4, the majority of individuals with DR3 and DR4 do not develop IDDM. Identical twins share genetic predisposition but the twin of a diabetic has only a 30% risk of developing IDDM. This and other epidemiological evidence confirms a substantial role for environmental factors in triggering the activation of T cells directed against beta cell antigens. The nature of these factors remains elusive but there are grounds to suspect dietary and infective exposure in early life. Prolonged breastfeeding appears to be partially protective and there is experimental data of cross-reactivity between components of cows' milk protein and beta cell antigens. A combination of gene and immune markers can be used to select a population at substantially increased risk from IDDM. Current trials are exploring the validity of protective immune manipulation with for example nicotinamide.

Clinical features of diabetes	
Early	**Late**
polyuria	vomiting
(secondary	abdominal pain
nocturnal	hyperventilation
enuresis)	(metabolic
thirst	acidosis)
lethargy	shock
weight loss	coma
anorexia	
(increased	
appetite unusual)	
constipation	

Clinical features. The symptoms are characteristic and the diagnosis is seldom in doubt if hyperglycaemia, glycosuria and ketonuria are detected. Clinical suspicion must be matched by immediate blood glucose confirmation, the levels are usually unequivocally high and it is exceptional to have to rely on a glucose tolerance test. A better informed public and diligent health professionals have reduced the incidence of ketoacidosis in newly diagnosed IDDM. Children require same-day referral to a specialist centre so that explanation and an introduction to insulin management can be initiated with minimal delay. It is difficult to anticipate the rate of deterioration of an untreated child and it is always preferable to initiate care without the threat of ketoacidosis.

A minority of children have atypical presentations with hyperventilation mimicking pneumonia, abdominal pain suggesting an 'acute abdomen', or impaired consciousness and circulatory collapse from unrecognised ketoacidosis.

A scheme for the management of diabetic ketoacidosis

Initial management
Admit to high dependency/intensive care unit
Assess airway and circulatory status, provide 100% oxygen, attach ECG monitor
Insert intravenous line and send samples to laboratory, stop oral intake and insert nasogastric tube
Weigh

Identify provoking factors e.g. infection

Treat shock Intravenous plasma protein solution

Fluid, electrolyte, food and insulin management
Calculate total fluid requirement (deficit + maintenance + losses)
Replace over 24–48 hours

Extracellular replacement: 0.9% sodium chloride + KCl until blood U/kg/h glucose < 12 mmol/l
Insulin Short-acting insulin infusion 0.1 guided by rate of blood glucose fall until blood glucose < 12 mmol/l

Intracellular replacement: 0.18% sodium chloride in 4% glucose + KCl
Insulin Short-acting insulin infusion 0.05 U/kg/h guided by blood glucose levels

Graded introduction of drinks and snacks
Insulin Start subcutaneous insulin injections e.g. short-acting insulin × 3–4/day or premixed insulin × 2/day

Main meals and snacks
Insulin Premixed insulin × 2/day

Discharge home
Insulin Adjust insulin dose

Diabetic ketoacidosis. The basic principles of treatment consist of insulin therapy, fluid and electrolyte replacement and the correction of provoking factors. Low dose insulin infusion provides for more predictable and gradual control of blood sugar, and largely avoids hypoglycaemia and hypokalaemia. A particular hazard of diabetic ketoacidosis in the young is cerebral oedema which may evolve despite improving blood glucose levels. This threat reinforces the need to adhere to treatment protocols which pay close attention to the rate of fluid correction.

Early management. The initial encounter between family and health professionals is of key importance. A skilled and sensitive introduction to the principles of insulin injection, healthy nutrition and blood glucose monitoring can equip child and parents to cope in their own home, and should kindle the interest and motivation which will sustain them through the many challenges of a diabetic's life. It is important to emphasise the positive aspects of modern diabetes management which enables the great majority of youngsters to achieve a full and successful life style. Although the threat of complications looms in the future, these have to be seen in the context of major advances in the control of diabetes with reduced blindness due to retinopathy and a falling incidence of nephropathy.

Insulin treatment. Pen injection devices and premixed insulin formulations have greatly simplified the practical management of diabetes. The majority of children are managed on twice daily insulin regimens. In adolescence there is the option for conversion to a more intensive scheme based on short-acting insulin before main meals with medium or long-acting insulin at bedtime.

Diet. Nutritional guidance emphasises healthy eating habits for the whole family. The energy content is tailored to match individual energy expenditure and growth. Carbohydrate, principally from unrefined fibre-rich sources, should provide 50–60% of the daily energy requirement. Fat should not provide more than 40% of energy and in older children there should be a move away from saturated fats. It requires skill and imagination to persuade youngsters to break away from their dependence on chips and crisps! An eating plan based on three meals and buffer snacks provides the substrate for insulin treatment and has to be adjusted to avoid the extremes of hyperglycaemia and hypoglycaemia. Each age group provides its own demands on the expertise of dietitians. Very young diabetics raise issues of tantrums at mealtimes and fussy eating habits. The older child will need to be negotiated through school meals and the temptations provided by friends. Adolescent girls are susceptible to obesity and eating disorders.

Home monitoring. Capillary blood glucose measurement is a potentially valuable tool in childhood diabetes. Relatively pain-free finger pricking gadgets and user friendly rapid response measuring devices have revolutionised the process but for most patients it still remains an unpopular activity. The aim is that children and families should collect enough reliable information to assist them with their own management decisions, guided by the diabetes team. The resultant profiles can be used to change insulin dose or formulation, and modify diet. Erratic profiles may suggest recurrent hypoglycaemia which in turn can provoke hyperglycaemia and instability. There are also many pitfalls in the interpretation of profiles, not least the fact that they may be falsified.

The Diabetes Team. Chronic health disorders which intrude into everyday life benefit from the attention of an expert team capable of guiding patients in home, school and the workplace. Such a team is a requirement in childhood diabetes and as a minimum comprises paediatrician, specialist nurse and dietitian. There should also be seamless transfer arrangements to the adult service.

Long-term management. Diabetes management is a compromise between the goal of optimal metabolic control which is protective for late complications and an acceptable life style without the disruption of recurrent hypoglycaemia. The variable nature of childhood and the particular physiological and emotional pressures of adolescence make the target of near normal glycosylated haemoglobin (HbA1c) levels difficult to sustain. Despite advances in insulin manufacture and administration, we are still far short of matching the physiology of intact beta cells. A large part of diabetes control is not amenable to insulin adjustments but hinges on personality, family support and social fabric. Whereas a near normal HbA1c may be a reasonable goal for some youngsters, it may be an unrealistic target for others who have a daily struggle with domestic adversity as well as diabetes. A realistic objective is to work towards as good control as is possible for each individual. It should be possible to ensure freedom from troublesome symptoms such as thirst, disturbed sleep and frequent hypoglycaemia. Normal physical and emotional growth, and the avoidance of obvious risk factors such as smoking or unplanned pregnancies, are also priorities. An overriding aim is to retain a working relationship with even the most recalcitrant young person. Young adults who are lost from supervision have a depressingly poor prognosis.

Factors which influence diabetic control

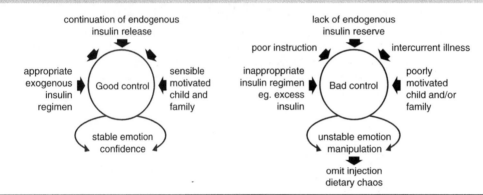

The clinic process incorporates annual checks including eye examination, blood pressure measurement and detection of microproteinuria. Other relevant screening tests include the detection of autoimmune thyroid disease and coeliac disease which have a higher incidence in patients with IDDM.

Hypoglycaemia

Hypoglycaemia is rare after the newborn period but must be considered in the assessment of non-febrile seizures or impaired consciousness, particularly after overnight fasts or coincidental with infection related poor food intake. A true, laboratory confirmed, blood glucose of less than 2.6 mmol/l is indicative. The urine should also be tested for ketones, a helpful step in distinguishing the two main categories of disorders which cause recurrent hypoglycaemia: substrate or hormone deficiency (ketones usually present) and hyperinsulinism (ketones absent). In children in whom there is no obvious explanation, a carefully monitored period of starvation with serial determinations of plasma glucose, insulin, cortisol, growth hormone, β-hydroxybutyrate and lactic acid is the most useful investigation.

Causes of hypoglycaemia

Substrate deficiency (ketones usually present)
- ketotic hypoglycaemia
- hepatic enzyme deficiencies
    glycogen storage diseases
    galactosaemia
    hereditary fructose intolerance
- exogenous hepatotoxins and poisons
    Reye syndrome
    alcohol, aspirin
    unripe Akee fruit
- endogenous hepatotoxins
    tyrosinosis
    maple syrup urine disease
- endocrine deficiencies
    pituitary, adrenal

Hyperinsulinism (ketones absent)
- pancreatic
    nesidioblastosis
    insulinoma
    mesenchymal tumours
- prediabetes mellitus
- insulin administration

Ketotic hypoglycaemia. This is the commonest cause of hypoglycaemia after infancy and before age 6–7 years. Affected children are usually small, slim and susceptible to early morning attacks comprising lethargy, vomiting and fits during coincidental illness or the day after intense exercise. Monitored starvation results in lower blood glucose and more prominent ketone production than normal, but insulin levels are very low. Limited gluconeogenic reserves probably account for this disorder and a better title may be 'accelerated starvation'. Hypoglycaemia can be avoided by high carbohydrate, high protein bedtime snacks and additional glucose drinks during illness. The problem resolves spontaneously in later childhood.

Nesidioblastosis is a rare problem of young infants in which developmental disorganisation of the islet cells and inappropriate insulin release results in persistent and brain threatening hypoglycaemia. The hypoglycaemia may be partially controlled using continuous infusion of high strength glucose combined with beta-cell suppression drugs including diazoxide and somatostatin. In patients where this fails the next option is subtotal resection of the pancreas which creates potential problems of diabetes and exocrine pancreatic insufficiency.

Hypoglycaemia is an important feature of metabolic disorders (see Ch. 16).

BIBLIOGRAPHY

Brook C G D 1995 Clinical paediatric endocrinology, 3rd edn. Blackwell Science, Oxford
Kelnar C J H 1995 Childhood and adolescent diabetes. Chapman and Hall Medical, London

16 Metabolism

ENZYME BLOCKS
ENERGY PATHWAY BLOCKS
MACROMOLECULAR CATABOLISM
  BLOCKS
MIXED MOLECULAR ANABOLISM
  AND CATABOLISM BLOCKS

When genetic faults occur and enzymes go missing it is usually not difficult to work out, by using those wall charts of the metabolic pathways which sustain life, what disorders of chemistry might result, but just how and why they cause illness is often more puzzling. In 1909 Garrod originally described the clinical features of a handful of inborn errors of metabolism, now over 300 disorders have been identified. They usually present in childhood, following the metabolic challenge of independent life, or the need to digest milk and new foods, or the stress of infective illness, all against the demands of continuing physical growth and neurological maturation.

Clinical and laboratory features suggestive of a metabolic disorder

Family history
Parental consanguinity
Unexplained infant death
Unexplained neurodevelopmental disorder

Feeding
Problems after onset of feeding
Problems after change of diet, e.g. introduction of sucrose
Apparent recovery with interruption of feeds

Presenting problem
Apparent life-threatening event
Multiple fits
Encephalopathy
Developmental deterioration
Prolonged jaundice
Haemorrhagic disease (underlying liver disease)

Examination finding
Dysmorphic, abnormal facies or bone deformity
Abnormal muscle tone
Cloudy cornea, cataracts or abnormal fundoscopy
Hepatosplenomegaly
Unexplained cardiac disease
Unusual smell

Laboratory finding
Hypoglycaemia
Metabolic acidosis, severe ketoacidosis
Abnormal LFTs, elevated NH_3
Positive metabolic screen (blood, urine)

The majority are inherited as autosomal recessive. Individually they are rare, but taken together they are not. They present in many strange and unexpected ways. Few pediatricians have not been saddened because they did not consider the possibility of an underlying metabolic disorder soon enough. Metabolic diseases are too readily demoted to the bottom of differential diagnostic lists and are only considered by a process of exclusion. The penalties of this time-consuming approach are that children may be denied life-saving or brain-protecting treatment. Overlooking a metabolic cause for infant deaths or for apparent cerebral palsy may also place siblings at risk of preventable catastrophic illnesses.

The complexity of metabolic diseases is daunting, the key for most of us is to recognise the clinical scenarios which trigger necessary investigation. That means knowing which investigations confirm or refute the diagnosis, and being familiar with the national network of clinical and laboratory based specialists available to advise on investigation and management. There are protocols for the temporary rescue of children with acute metabolic decompensation and these will usually provide a window of opportunity for making the diagnosis and introducing focused treatment. In children with slowly emerging metabolic disorders, the challenge is to appreciate the varied and multi-organ manifestations, and/or to identify the early signs of developmental delay or regression.

Biochemical screening in infancy

Test	Disease	Incidence
Phenylalanine Bacterial inhibition assay (Guthrie test)	Phenylketonuria	1 in 10 000
Chromatography	Potential for detecting other aminoacidopathies and organic acidurias	
TSH	Congenital hypothyroidism	1 in 3000
Immunoreactive trypsin (IRT) linked to DNA technology ΔF508	Cystic fibrosis	1 in 2500
Haemoglobin analysis	HbS, C and others	Common in selected populations
Electrophoresis, isoelectric focusing, chromatography, monoclonal antibody	Thalassaemias	

Mechanisms. Metabolic defects may be classified into four main groups, although there is overlap:

- Enzyme blocks with accumulation of toxic intermediate metabolites.
- Energy pathway blocks, usually mitochondrial, with secondary generalised or specific tissue failure.

- Macromolecular catabolism blocks with abnormal storage, usually in lysosomes.
- Mixed macromolecular anabolism and catabolism blocks due to peroxisomal defects.

ENZYME BLOCKS WITH ACCUMULATION OF TOXIC INTERMEDIATE METABOLITES

Enzyme blocks with accumulation of toxic metabolites

Aminoacidopathies
phenylketonuria, maple syrup urine disease (MSUD), tyrosinaemia

Organic acidurias
methylmalonic, proprionic and isovaleric aciduria

Urea cycle defects
ornithine carbamyl transferase (OCT) deficiency

Monosaccharide intolerance
galactosaemia, hereditary fructose intolerance

Certain glycogen storage disease
glucose-6-phosphatase deficiency

These inborn errors of metabolism result in acute or progressive illness depending on the severity of the block, the supply of metabolic fuel to the abnormal pathway from either diet or the breakdown of endogenous reserves, and the toxicity of the circulating intermediates. The majority present in early infancy, but partial enzyme deficiencies may only manifest when an older infant or child is exposed to additional catabolic stress from infection and starvation. The enzyme block may be generalised to many tissues, for example phenylketonuria and galactosaemia, or may be restricted to specific tissues as in urea cycle and glycogen storage disorders which primarily involve the liver. These localised deficiencies are still likely to have profound systemic effects because of the secondary impact of hypoglycaemia, acid–base imbalance and the circulation of toxic metabolites.

The abnormal accumulation of metabolites can usually be detected readily by chromatography of plasma and urine.

Phenylketonuria

Phenylketonuria (PKU) results from a block in the hepatic conversion of phenylalanine to tyrosine and causes severe mental deficiency, microcephaly and seizures. Infants with classical PKU have less than 1% of normal phenylalanine hydroxylase activity; less severe variants have milder deficiency, 1–5%.

PKU is a relatively rare, autosomal recessive disorder, 1 case per 10 000 births, but the effectiveness of prompt therapy justifies routine neonatal screening of blood phenylalanine levels. This is conveniently performed on capillary blood using the Guthrie bacterial inhibition technique in which a specific strain of *Bacillus subtilis* can multiply only in the presence of phenylalanine. To be valid the infant has to be established on milk, and the test is conventionally performed on samples collected at the end of the first week of life.

Dietary phenylalanine restriction must be established promptly and has to be carefully monitored to meet the dual aims of brain protection from toxic metabolites while allowing the supply of sufficient quantities of essential amino acids. The overall results of prompt diagnosis and careful treatment in early childhood are good with the prospect of normal schooling although with an increased incidence of behavioural and learning problems. Debate surrounds the issues of when and how to withdraw dietary restriction. Beyond the age of 6–8 years the nervous system is less vulnerable to elevated phenylalanine levels, and compliance certainly falls.

Guthrie test

Heel prick for a sample
of capillary blood

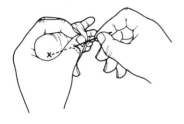

SCREENING BLOOD TEST (including PKU)	Baby's Surname (BLOCK CAPITALS)		
FOR LABORATORY USE	Baby's First Names		
	Mother's First Names		
	Hospital		Ward/Dept.
	Consultant/GP		
	Home Address		
	Baby's date of birth / /		Sex
	Date of first milk feeding / /		
	Date of Specimen / /		
No. 464391	Local Health Authority		
PAPER 'B'	Address to which reports of positive tests should be sent		
PLEASE PLACE ONE LARGE DROP OF BLOOD IN CENTRE OF EACH CIRCLE			

Maternal phenylketonuria is now increasing as a problem, and has devastating effects on the fetus, causing microcephaly, severe handicap and structural anomalies. This emphasises the long-term responsibilities of the health-care team who must retain patient contact, advise on planned conception and then reintroduce dietary restriction.

Organic acidurias

These are collectively more common than PKU, but individually each is rare. They have very varied presentation from fulminating neonatal illness to more slowly progressive neurodegenerative disease. Suggestive features should trigger analysis on blood, urine and possibly tissue samples. Defects of branched amino acid (leucine, valine and isoleucine) metabolism are a major cause of organic acidurias. Others are associated with defects of mitochondrial fatty acid oxidation.

Urea cycle defects

These result in toxic hyperammonaemia and deficiency of essential products of the urea cycle. The five enzyme steps of the cycle are present only in the liver and hence its key role in urea and amino-group nitrogen excretion. Hyperammonaemia may arise from inherited enzyme deficiency or from a range of other genetic or acquired liver disorders. The clinical presentation is relatively non-specific and the diagnosis has to be considered in infants and children presenting with unexplained collapse, liver failure or encephalopathy.

Ornithine transcarbamylase deficiency

Ornithine transcarbamylase (OTC) deficiency is X-linked and presents as a usually fatal neonatal illness in hemizygous males. 'Milder' illness presents with vomiting, fits, coma or retardation and occurs in females and some males. Biochemical markers are the very elevated ammonia, low urea, increased liver transaminases and increased urinary orotic acid. Enzymatic confirmation requires liver biopsy and there are gene probes for antenatal diagnosis. Milder cases are amenable to treatment with protein restriction, benzoate to promote alternative amino-nitrogen excretion via hippuric acid, and supplementary arginine.

Glycogen storage diseases

Enzyme deficiencies have been recognised for each of the steps in the pathways of glycogen synthesis and degradation. They enter into the differential diagnosis of recurrent hypoglycaemia, hepatomegaly, muscle weakness and congestive cardiac failure.

Type I: glucose-6-phosphatase deficiency is a serious disorder, usually presenting in infancy with hepatomegaly, hypoglycaemia and a metabolic acidosis. The enzyme deficiency prevents the normal glycaemic response to glucagon and can be confirmed by liver biopsy. Patients are unable to tolerate fasts beyond 2–3 hours, and overnight glucose polymer feeds are helpful in treatment.

Type III: debranching enzyme deficiency and type VI: liver phosphorylase deficiency present in a similar although milder fashion and can be diagnosed by measurement of leucocyte enzyme levels.

Galactosaemia

Galactosaemia is a rare, recessively inherited disorder and its importance lies in the disastrous consequences of being overlooked. It results from deficiency of the enzyme, galactose-1-phosphate uridyl transferase, which is essential for galactose metabolism. Affected infants are normal at birth but shortly after commencing milk feeds, the majority of infants develop jaundice, vomiting, diarrhoea or may collapse suggesting septicaemia. If the disorder remains unrecognised liver disease, cataracts and mental retardation will result. The urine contains galactose and is characteristically Clinitest positive but Clinistix negative, the latter being specific for glucose. Specific enzymatic techniques confirm the diagnosis and establish the necessity for a lactose-free diet.

Hereditary fructose intolerance

This is another rare enzyme deficiency in which prompt recognition can prevent the onset of life-threatening complications. The low activity of aldolase B not only results in the accumulation of fructose-1-phosphate but also causes a secondary inhibition of hepatic pathways responsible for maintaining normoglycaemia. In susceptible children, fructose-containing foods provoke abdominal pain, nausea, vomiting and symptoms of hypoglycaemia. In the longer term hepatomegaly, growth failure and liver failure occur. A detailed dietary history reveals normal health until the introduction of sucrose into the diet, and suspicion may be substantiated by a fructose tolerance test or by liver enzyme analysis. Therapy involves the elimination of all fructose containing items from the diet.

ENERGY PATHWAY BLOCKS WITH SECONDARY GENERALISED OR SPECIFIC TISSUE FAILURE

Energy pathway blocks with secondary generalised or specific tissue failure

Enzyme deficiencies in gluconeogenesis
  pyruvate carboxylase deficiency,
  pyruvate dehydrogenase deficiency

Fatty acid oxidation defects
  medium-chain acyl CoA
  dehydrogenase deficiency

Respiratory chain defects

These disorders arise mainly from enzymatic or transport deficiencies in the mitochondrial pathways which metabolise energy substrates to generate ATP. The resultant clinical picture varies depending on whether the block is distributed in all tissues causing life-threatening collapse or failure to thrive, or is limited to one or more of the more susceptible tissues, notably liver, myocardium, skeletal muscle and brain, resulting in varied patterns of hypotonia, cardiomyopathy, seizures and developmental regression. There may also be superimposed toxic accumulation of metabolites with systemic effects including hypoglycaemia and lactic acidosis.

Medium-chain acyl CoA dehydrogenase deficiency

This is the commonest variety of fatty acid oxidation defect. The mitochondrial defect interferes with hepatic metabolism of acetyl-CoA and $NADH_2$ which are essential to gluconeogenesis and ATP synthesis. There is also a block in ketone production which aggravates energy depletion to key tissues such as brain and cardiac muscle. Affected children may be entirely asymptomatic and without hepatomegaly until they are stressed by illness which within hours precipitates collapse or encephalopathy associated with hypoglycaemia and deranged liver function. It is suspected that undiagnosed medium-chain acyl CoA dehydrogenase deficiency (MCAD) is relatively common, 5–10 per 100 000, and that it contributes to unexplained infant mortality. Diagnosis has been simplified by the application of gene probe methodology and can be applied to dried blood on filter cards opening up the option for population screening.

MACROMOLECULAR CATABOLISM BLOCKS WITH ABNORMAL STORAGE

These are predominantly disorders of lysosomal function which result in progressive structural and functional disruption of tissues. Although a wide range of organs may be involved, the main target is the nervous system with profound disability and death. There are non-neuropathic exceptions in which the storage is focused in the reticuloendothelial system with hepatosplenomegaly and skeletal manifestations. The storage may be apparent in fetal life but most evolve during infancy or childhood; the rate of progression is not influenced by diet. Lysosomal disorders are inherited as autosomal recessive and are individually rare. However gene frequency rates for GM_2-gangliosidosis (Tay–Sachs disease) and Gaucher disease are high in certain ethnic groups, notably Ashkenazi Jews.

Macromolecular catabolism blocks with abnormal storage

Lipidoses
  GM_1-gangliosidosis, GM_2-gangliosidosis, Tay–Sachs disease, Gaucher disease, Niemann–Pick disease, metachromatic leukodystrophy

Mucopolysaccharidoses
  Hurler, Hunter, Sanfilippo, Morquio diseases

Glycoproteinoses
  sialodosis, mannosidosis, fucosidosis

Mucolipidoses

Others
  glycogen storage disease type II (Pompe disease), cystinosis

The biochemical basis of Tay–Sachs disease

Disorder	Storage material	Deficient enzyme

Ganglioside, GM_2
Tay-Sachs — ceramide — glucose — galactose — N-acetylgalactosamine / N-acetylneuraminic acid — hexosaminidase

Cerebroside
Gaucher — ceramide — glucose — glucocerebrosidase

Sphingomyelin
Niemann-Pick — ceramide — phosphoryl choline — sphingomyelinase

Suggestive clinical features include progressive neurological deterioration, hepatosplenomegaly, bone deformity, eye signs such as cloudy cornea and retinal changes, and a coarsening facies. A blood film may reveal vacuolated lymphocytes. The clinical pattern is used to select specific laboratory tests which include urinary chromatography, enzyme assays, gene analysis and tissue biopsy with electron microscopy. Treatment options are limited but a specific diagnosis is important for family counselling and for antenatal diagnosis.

GM_2-gangliosidosis (Tay–Sachs disease)

This results from deficiency of the lysosomal hexosaminidase complex leading to abnormal ganglioside accumulation in grey matter. Although rare in the general population it is relatively common in Ashkenazi Jews and has been a stimulus to successful voluntary heterozygote detection programmes in this population. The developmental regression with delayed motor milestones is usually obvious by age 6–9 months. An exaggerated startle response to sound, hyperacusis, is an early sign. Ophthalmoscopy reveals optic atrophy and cherry red spots on the maculae. Visual inattention and social unresponsiveness are part of the deteriorating course which includes convulsions and swallowing difficulty, and ends in death by 3–5 years.

Metachromatic leukodystrophy

This is the most commonly recognised storage disorder primarily involving brain white matter and usually becomes obvious in the second year. Sulphatides accumulate in the central and peripheral nervous system due to deficiency of the enzyme, aryl sulphatase, and resultant demyelination causes progressive motor deterioration and spasticity. The disease evolves with intellectual loss, blindness and convulsions. There are three main subgroups with the commonest arising in infancy. The diagnosis is made by demonstrating metachromatic material in urinary sediment or tissue biopsy, and establishing deficient aryl sulphatase activity in white cells or cultured fibroblasts.

Gaucher disease

This is the commonest lysosomal storage disease in which over 30 different mutations result in deficiency of glucocerebrosidase. The outcome is classified into the commoner type I or non-neuronopathic forms, and type II or neuropathic forms.

Type I Gaucher disease presents in childhood or early adult life with hepatosplenomegaly, hypersplenism and bone involvement, for example pathological fractures. Striated Gaucher cells can be identified in marrow or liver biopsy, and the diagnosis is confirmed by leucocyte enzyme analysis. The disease is compatible with a reasonable life span but the clinical course may be improved by regular infusions of glucocerebrosidase. Clinical trials are also being conducted into the use of retroviral vectors to transfer the glycocerebrosidase gene into haematopoietic stem cells of patients.

Type II presents in infancy with feeding problems, stridor and spasticity. There is prominent hepatosplenomegaly and death occurs within months. The blood–brain barrier reduces the prospect of successful enzyme or gene transfer therapy.

Niemann–Pick disease

This also causes abnormal storage in the reticulo-endothelial system and two of the four recognised varieties are neuronopathic. It may resemble Tay–Sachs disease and have a cherry red macular spot. It can also present in the differential diagnosis of neonatal hepatitis. Typical foam cells can be found in marrow and liver biopsy.

Mucopolysaccharidoses

These disorders result from abnormal accumulation of glycosaminoglycans, sulphated polysaccharides, in fibroblasts and chondrocytes resulting in coarsened skin, corneal clouding, skeletal dysplasia, progressive neurodegenerative disease and hepatosplenomegaly. The manifestations vary and not all have brain involvement. There are currently seven or eight subgroups which can be distinguished by inheritance, clinical picture, enzyme defect, and major storage substance.

Hurler syndrome

grossly retarded development

coarse facies
hazy corneas
enlarged tongue

cardiac abnormalities

hepatosplenomegaly
umbilical hernia
claw hand
joint deformities

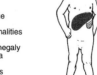

Hurler syndrome, an autosomal recessive disease, results from deficiency of L-iduronidase and manifests the entire spectrum listed above.

Hunter syndrome differs by having X-linked inheritance, no corneal clouding and a milder pattern of brain involvement. The enzyme iduronate-2-sulphatase is deficient.

Morquio disease causes severe skeletal deformity without brain or systemic involvement.

Glycogen storage disease Type II

Alpha-glucosidase deficiency (Pompe disease) results in excessive glycogen deposition in both liver and muscle, with cardiac muscle especially involved. The majority of affected infants present soon after birth with poor feeding, weakness, tachypnoea and cardiac failure. Muscle or leucocyte enzyme analysis confirms the diagnosis but treatment is supportive only.

MIXED MACROMOLECULAR ANABOLISM AND CATABOLISM BLOCKS

Peroxisomes share properties with mitochondria and the endoplasmic reticulum, for example a key role in beta-oxidation of fatty acids and their derivatives. They also synthesise a number of complex molecules including plasmalogens, components of myelin, and bile salts. Generalised peroxisomal failure has a profound impact on fetal organogenesis and brain differentiation such that effected infants appear dysmorphic and may have skeletal dysplasia, Zellweger syndrome. Partial failure resulting in more limited biochemical disruption may present later in life, for example X-linked adrenoleucodystrophy with adrenal insufficiency and progressive neurological disease.

MANAGEMENT OF METABOLIC DISEASE

The examples discussed above give some indication of the spectrum of potential treatments available but the main emphasis has to be on prompt recognition and specialist referral. A precise understanding of the biochemical basis of each disorder is essential to the introduction of more rational therapy. A small but important group of conditions which were until recently regarded as inevitably progressive and fatal can now be controlled by innovative drugs which manipulate enzyme pathways. Clinical trials of gene transfer are underway and obviously have enormous potential in these disorders.

Enzyme block	Metabolic disease: possible therapy	
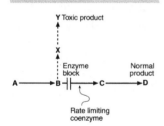	**Reduce supply of A, substrate** phenylketonuria, galactosaemia **Enhance enzyme activity to overcome block** cofactor responsive varieties of organic aciduria **Replace physiological requirements of C or D, essential products** thyroxine in inherited block of thyroxine synthesis **Block production of X or Y, toxic products** NTBC inhibition of tyrosine degradation in tyrosinaemia	**Remove toxic product by alternative pathway** benzoate linkage with glycine in urea cycle defects, penicillamine binding of copper in Wilson disease **Tissue or organ replacement** bone marrow transplant in certain mucopolysaccharidoses, liver transplant in alpha-1 antitrypsin deficiency **Enzyme replacement** glucocerebrosidase infusions in Gaucher disease **Gene transfer** adenoviral vector mediated transfer in cystic fibrosis

BIBLIOGRAPHY

Clayton B E, Round J M (eds) 1994 Clinical biochemistry and the sick child, 2nd edn. Blackwell Scientific Publications, Oxford
Nyhan W L, Oznand P 1997 Atlas of metabolic diseases. Chapman & Hall, London

17 Skin

RASHES OF EARLY INFANCY
ATOPIC ECZEMA
INFECTIONS AND INFESTATIONS
CONGENITAL SKIN LESIONS
OTHER COMMON SKIN
    DISORDERS

Man consists mainly of water and it is his skin which stops him from drying out. In addition, the skin protects the body from physical, chemical, microbial and ultraviolet light insult. The superficial layer of the epidermis, stratum corneum, with its compact horny cells provides an effective barrier to the passage of substances in either direction. The dermis, with its high collagen content, gives skin its ability to stretch and mould. Its numerous blood vessels and sweat glands are important in the control of body temperature.

The epidermis develops in the third week of fetal life, and is initially composed of two layers, an outer periderm and an inner basal layer. The periderm is equipped with absorptive microvilli and actively transfers substances between amniotic fluid and fetal tissues. It is normally shed long before term. The basal or germinative layer gives rise to the definitive multilayered epidermis, and this differentiation is largely complete when keratinisation establishes the stratum corneum in the sixth month of fetal life. An extremely premature infant has thin, poorly keratinised epidermis, and is therefore vulnerable to excessive skin water losses after birth. The sebaceous glands are active from mid gestation, and their secretion, together with the residue of the periderm, accounts for the vernix caseosa. The vernix provides a greasy coating to the newborn skin and may have bactericidal properties. Term infants are able to sweat within 2–5 days after birth, but there may be a delay of 2–3 weeks in the premature. Sebum and sweat retention are common in the newborn.

Lesions

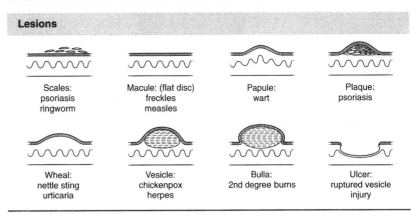

| Scales: psoriasis ringworm | Macule: (flat disc) freckles measles | Papule: wart | Plaque: psoriasis |
| Wheal: nettle sting urticaria | Vesicle: chickenpox herpes | Bulla: 2nd degree burns | Ulcer: ruptured vesicle injury |

RASHES OF EARLY INFANCY

Erythema toxicum. This is possibly the most frequent skin eruption in the first weeks of life. It arises as crops of asymptomatic papulo-vesicles on erythematous patches over the face, trunk and napkin area. It generally resolves spontaneously within 2–3 days.

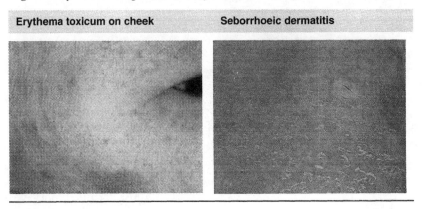

| Erythema toxicum on cheek | Seborrhoeic dermatitis |

Seborrhoeic dermatitis of infancy is a well demarcated erythematous and scaly eruption. Pityrosporum yeasts may play a causative role. It usually starts during the second or third month of life as excessive greasy scaling in the scalp (cradle cap) or as a glazed, red eruption in the napkin and axillary areas which may spread to the rest of the body. Unlike atopic eczema, the child is never ill and is not distressed by itching. It is distinguished from atopic eczema by the lack of rubbing/excoriations, distribution in the seborrhoeic areas (scalp, eyebrows, axillae and inguinal areas) and tendency for spontaneous disappearance after 6–12 weeks. If very extensive, very mild corticosteroid and antiseptic combinations such as 1% hydrocortisone with 3% clioquinol will usually hasten resolution.

Rashes in the napkin area are very common and not always indicative of poor mothering. The main causes are napkin dermatitis, candidiasis, seborrhoeic dermatitis of infancy and atopic eczema.

Napkin dermatitis is a form of irritant contact dermatitis caused by prolonged contact with wet napkins. Bacterial conversion of the urine to ammonia creates an alkaline irritant. Simple measures are usually effective; frequent napkin changes, careful washing at each change and the application of a protective cream such as zinc and castor oil ointment or white soft paraffin/liquid paraffin in a 50/50 mixture. Disposable napkins probably protect against this disorder providing they are changed regularly.

Candidiasis is commonly superimposed on a napkin rash and is characterised by small satellite erosions or superficial pustules on a background of erythema. It can be treated with nystatin cream or a short course of oral nystatin if very extensive.

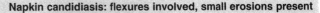

| Ammoniacal napkin rash: sparing flexures | Napkin candidiasis: flexures involved, small erosions present |

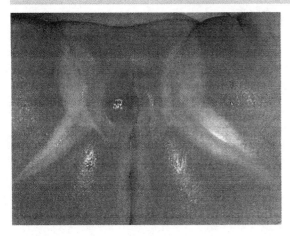 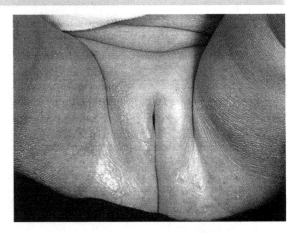

ATOPIC ECZEMA

Atopic eczema now affects 15% of children in Europe and usually has its onset between 2 and 18 months of age. There is often a family history of other atopic disorders such as hay fever or asthma. Itching is very prominent and scratching frequently results in secondary infection by *Staphylococcus aureus*. It has a fluctuating course with approximately 70% resolving by 11 years. Although skin prick tests for specific allergens are often positive, they provide little guide to clinical management as multiple factors are usually involved. The evidence that prolonged and excessive breastfeeding protects against the development of atopic eczema is conflicting.

Atopic eczema

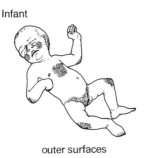

Infant

outer surfaces

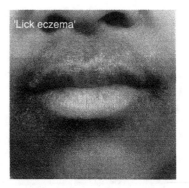

'Lick eczema'

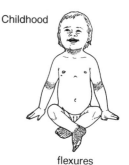

Childhood

flexures

Management. Atopic eczema is a very taxing illness for child and family. Disturbed nights, irritability and the often alarming appearance add to the burden. The parents have an active role in management and need lots of information and support as well as demonstration of application of creams and bandages. The skin is often dry; the avoidance of soap and the use of aqueous cream in its place helps to correct this. Emollients such as white soft paraffin/liquid paraffin in a 50/50 mixture should be used at least twice daily. Corticosteroid ointments applied once or twice daily benefit the affected areas but should be used sparingly and the potency kept to the minimum necessary to control the disease. One per cent hydrocortisone ointment, or betamethasone cream 1 in 10 ointment, are usually adequate for most cases. Occasionally, more potent preparations may be needed, especially for the stubborn discoid pattern of atopic eczema. These should be used in bursts of 5–10 days followed by rest periods using emollients only in order to avoid skin thinning. Widespread secondary infection is usually caused by *S. aureus* and a systemic antibiotic such as flucloxacillin or erythromycin should be given. Occasionally combined staphylococcal and streptococcal infection is seen. Control of scratching and the provision of undisturbed nights are important management objectives for child and family. Sedative antihistamines such as trimeprazine tartrate or promethazine may be helpful as a short course during an exacerbation. Other useful measures include using cotton underclothes rather than wool, keeping the bedroom cool at night and light bandaging of the limbs to protect against scratching. The hands must never be tied to prevent scratching. There is no contraindication to immunisation against diphtheria, whooping cough, tetanus and poliomyelitis. Primary infection with herpes simplex virus may give rise to a very severe eruption known as Kaposi varicelliform eruption. Such children usually require admission for parental acyclovir if there is systemic upset. Reduction of house dust mite around the home may reduce the severity and possibly the prognosis of childhood eczema. Dietary manipulation should ideally be carried out under the supervision of a paediatric dietitian.

INFECTIONS AND INFESTATIONS

Bacterial

Impetigo. This is a contagious superficial skin infection usually caused by staphylococci (but occasionally streptococci). It passes rapidly through a vesicular phase and usually presents with typical golden brown crusts on a red base. Topical treatment with fucidin or mupirocin cream is adequate for limited infection. More extensive lesions require a systemic antibiotic such as flucloxacillin or erythromycin, or an antistreptococcal agent if streptococci are grown from a swab. Refractory or atypical cases raise the possibility of an underlying cause such as scabies, scalp pediculosis or an immune deficiency.

| Impetigo: face | Bullous impetigo: abdomen | Erysipelas: leg |

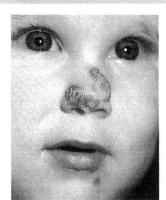 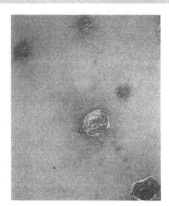 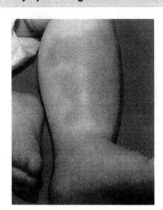

Staphylococcal scalded skin syndrome (SSSS or Ritter's disease). SSSS results from epidermal cleavage due to toxins of staphylococci (usually phage type 71). Typically, young infants and children develop acute inflammation and soreness which evolves into a generalised exfoliation, the scalded skin syndrome. Even ordinary handling can result in skin loss. As in burn victims, extreme care is necessary in nursing these children. Antistaphylococcal antibiotics may be needed as well as meticulous attention to fluid balance.

Viral

Primary Herpes simplex infection is usually asymptomatic but it can produce a gingivostomatitis in young children. It presents with fever, irritability and difficulty in swallowing. The latter is caused by extensive shallow ulcers of the buccal, gingival and pharyngeal mucosa. Occasionally there may be vulvovaginitis or a keratoconjunctivitis. Herpetic encephalitis is a rare but serious complication. Gingivostomatitis requires careful nursing to ensure an adequate fluid intake. Oral acyclovir can be used to treat extensive infections.

Herpes zoster. This is not uncommon in children and usually settles without post-herpetic neuralgia.

Viral warts affect most children at some time during childhood. They are harmless and self limiting, and treatment is only indicated if there is discomfort. This is most likely on the pressure bearing areas of the soles. The application of a salicylic acid based wart gel for 4–6 months or cryotherapy is usually all that is required.

Molluscum contagiosum. This is more likely to affect covered areas of the body. The individual lesions typically resolve spontaneously in 6–12 months. Sudden enlargement and redness of individual lesions usually indicate spontaneous resolution and not secondary bacterial infection. If treatment is required for very persistent individual lesions, these can be cleared by pricking the centre or cryotherapy.

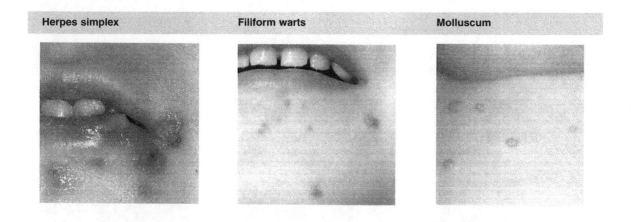

Herpes simplex · **Filiform warts** · **Molluscum**

Fungal skin infection

Tinea pedis is uncommon in children and needs to be distinguished from juvenile plantar dermatosis, a glazed, red scaly eruption of both forefeet, by skin scrapings taken for fungal microscopy and culture. Ringworm (tinea capitis and/or corporis) can occur in outbreaks and may be due to animal fungi like *Microsporum canis* which fluoresces under Wood's light or human such as *Microsporum audounii* or *Trichophyton tonsurans*. Treatment of skin fungal infection is with topical imadazoles but treatment of scalp infection *always* requires oral treatment with griseofulvin for 6–10 weeks.

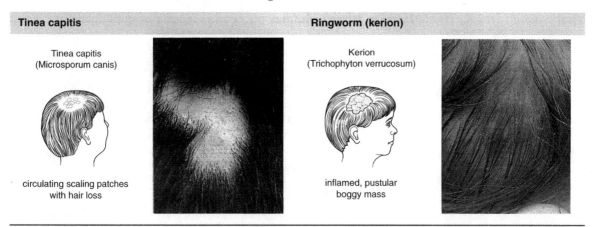

Tinea capitis · **Ringworm (kerion)**

Tinea capitis
(Microsporum canis)

circulating scaling patches
with hair loss

Kerion
(Trichophyton verrucosum)

inflamed, pustular
boggy mass

Infestations

Scabies is due to a mite which is spread by close physical contact and invades the horny layer of the skin where it lays its eggs. The 2–4 cm serpiginous grey/white burrows are generally over hands (especially finger webs), wrists, elbows, axillae, feet (especially ankles and soles) and genitalia but can occur on the face of babies. Infestations provoke an intense itch and a secondary erythematous papular rash. The mite may be identified using a low power lens and a needle. The whole family should be treated by a single application of permethrin to all the skin surfaces below the neck.

Pediculosis capitis or head lice infestation is common in our schools. It may present as a persistent itch with secondary dermatitis or be found on routine hair examination. The oval nits are easily seen firmly adhering to the hair shaft. The mature lice are less often visible. The application of 0.5% malathion solution or permethrin is effective against the lice and nits.

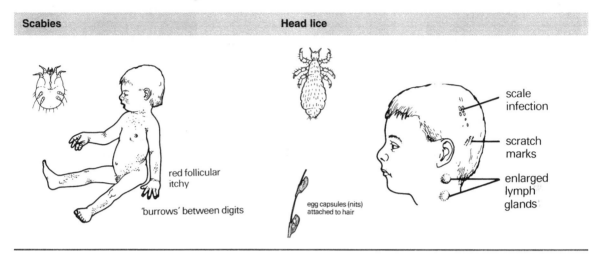

Scabies	Head lice

red follicular itchy

'burrows' between digits

egg capsules (nits) attached to hair

scale infection

scratch marks

enlarged lymph glands

CONGENITAL SKIN LESIONS

Birth marks

Strawberry naevus (immature capillary haemangioma). A third of these elevated lesions occur on the face and become conspicuous and grow rapidly in the first month of life. In spite of parental pressure, management of uncomplicated lesions is usually conservative with the reassuring knowledge that spontaneous disappearance occurs by the age of 5 or 6 years in most children.

Capillary naevus (port wine stain). This permanent vascular malformation of dermal blood vessels can occur anywhere but is commonest on the upper half of the body. There is no tendency to fade or spread. Usually it is an isolated cosmetic problem, but occasionally there may be meningeal involvement as well, for example in the Sturge–Weber syndrome. These lesions may be treated by pulsed tunable dye lasers with very good cosmetic benefit.

Pigmented naevi. Some naevi are evident at birth (congenital melanocytic naevi) but most start to appear throughout childhood. In childhood, melanocytic naevi are usually flat or only slightly elevated. Malignant melanoma is extremely rare in childhood and most occur as a complication of giant bathing trunk naevi at this age. A particular type of melanocytic lesion (Spitz naevus) may occur in childhood and is characterised by a reddish brown papule and benign nature. Extensive macular pale brown 'café au lait' spots are a feature of neurofibromatosis.

| Strawberry naevus | 'Salmon patch' | Sturge–Weber syndrome |

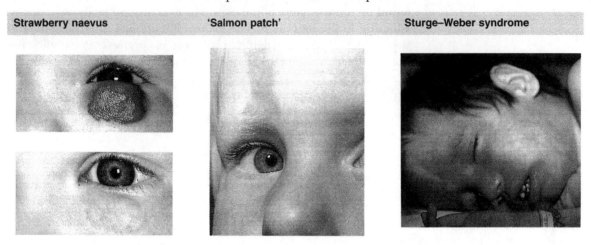

Ichthyosis. The most frequent form is an autosomal dominant condition (ichthyosis vulgaris) characterised by dry finely scaling skin which spares the flexures. It may coincide with and complicate atopic dermatitis. Restoration of skin moisture with an emollient such as white soft paraffin/liquid paraffin mixture or a urea-containing compound is the basis of treatment.

Congenital anhidrotic ectodermal dysplasia. This is a rare, sex-linked, recessive condition producing loss of sweat glands, dental hypoplasia, and sparse hair, eyebrows and eyelashes. Because they are unable to sweat, these children are intolerant of heat.

Epidermolysis bullosa. This condition is a pathological susceptibility to blistering and there are a number of genetic varieties. The severity ranges from blistering with unusual trauma to serious life-threatening scarring and deformity of digits, limbs and mucosal surfaces.

Incontinentia pigmenti. This rare X-linked dominant condition is almost exclusively restricted to females and is usually obvious at birth. Groups of vesicles evolve through warty papules to bizarre patterns of pigmentation. There is associated eosinophilia, dental and eye abnormalities.

Xeroderma pigmentosum. This autosomal recessive condition is manifest by marked photosensitivity and liability to skin freckling, keratoses and eventually malignant skin tumours such as squamous cell carcinoma and melanoma.

Acrodermatitis enteropathica. This produces progressive mucocutaneous ulceration and a dry eczematous eruption on extensor aspects of the limbs and around the mouth. It is usually associated with bowel pathology leading to poor absorption of zinc and responds to zinc supplementation.

'Café au lait' spots	Epidermolysis bullosa	Incontinentia pigmenti

 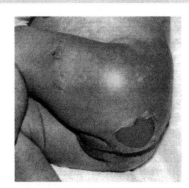 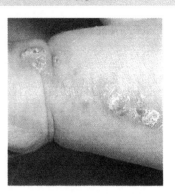

OTHER COMMON SKIN DISORDERS

Psoriasis

This commonly presents as an acute guttate (showers of lesions) rash following a streptococcal sore throat. An eruption of small (2 cm) discrete red scaling lesions may develop rapidly and cover much of the body. Resolution usually occurs after 2 months or so, but the existence of the psoriatic tendency has been indicated and the more typical plaques on elbows, knees and scalp may develop at any time. Treatment, if required, can be with a coaltar/hydrocortisone mixture. Sometimes ultraviolet light is added to clear an extensive and persistent eruption.

Pityriasis rosea

This is an acute self limiting eruption giving rise to erythematous scaling macules with a central distribution. It is thought to be a reaction to an as yet unidentified infectious agent. It may superficially resemble guttate psoriasis but is distinguished by a herald patch, which appears 3 or 4 days before the main eruption, and by the frequent presence of itching and fine scaling. A mild corticosteroid ointment may help resolution.

Guttate psoriasis	Pityriasis rosea (insert 'herald patch')	Granuloma annulare

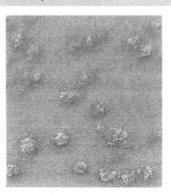 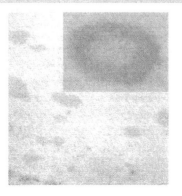 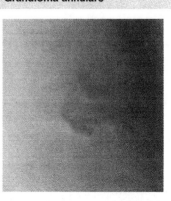

Granuloma annulare

These skin lesions consist of asymptomatic dermal nodules which evolve into irregular annular lesions with raised borders usually on the elbows, backs of the fingers or toes or dorsa of the feet. It is a harmless condition but resolution may take 1–2 years. Diabetes is a rare association for extensive granuloma annulare.

Alopecia areata

These areas of localised hair loss on the scalp have a smooth non-scaly appearance, often studded on the margin with occasional exclamation mark hairs. The alopecia usually re-grows in 6–9 months. Rare cases progress to alopecia totalis. It should be distinguished from habitual hair pulling, trichotillomania, and ringworm of the scalp in which there is an obvious inflammatory element.

Acne

Acne occasionally occurs in a child less than 18 months old and reflects physiological adjustments in the responsiveness of sebaceous glands to post-natal hormone changes. Its occurrence later in childhood, but before the onset of puberty, requires further investigation in case of underlying adrenal pathology. Acne is almost universal in adolescence and should be taken seriously as it may cause much psychological distress. It is linked with increased sebaceous gland sensitivity to normal levels of circulating testosterone, inflammation caused by *Proprionibacterium acnes* and blockage of pilosebaceous units. This results in comedones (blackheads), inflammation (red papules) and pustules (yellowheads). Treatment is directed at removing the keratin plugs, for example with 5% benzolyl peroxide or topical retinoids, and suppression of lipolytic bacteria. Topical antibiotics may be added and occasionally long-term oral antibiotics are required, although tetracyclines should be avoided in children because of the risk of staining the teeth.

Erythema nodosum

These tender erythematous nodules occur most frequently over the pretibial region. They appear in crops and may be associated with fever and arthralgia. An underlying problem may be streptococcal infection, tuberculosis, *Mycoplasma pneumoniae*, food or drug sensitivity. In the majority no underlying condition will be found.

Erythema multiforme

This is a local vascular reaction which may be triggered by viral infections like Herpes simplex and mycoplasma or drugs. The characteristic lesion is like a target or iris in shape, the rash is symmetrical and affects the limbs more than the trunk. When the reaction involves the mucous membranes, the Stevens–Johnson syndrome, the systemic reaction is more severe and there is a significant morbidity and mortality. Oral steroids probably do not affect the outcome.

| Erythema nodosum | Erythema multiforme | Stevens–Johnson syndrome |

BIBLIOGRAPHY

Cohen B A 1994 Atlas of pediatric dermatology. Wolfe, London
Higgins E, du Vivier A 1996 Skin disease in childhood and adolescence. Blackwell
    Science, Oxford

18 Bone and joint

ARTHRITIS
OSTEOMYELITIS
NORMAL POSTURAL VARIATIONS
SCOLIOSIS
HIP DISORDERS
KNEE DISORDERS
TALIPES (CLUBFOOT)
GENETIC AND BONE DISORDERS
BONE TUMOURS AND ALLIED
  DISORDERS

The immature joint

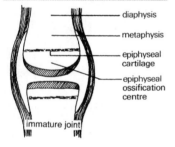

- diaphysis
- metaphysis
- epiphyseal cartilage
- epiphyseal ossification centre

immature joint

Bone tissue can be detected in the 8-week fetus. It arises from precursor mesenchymal cells which either evolve into osteoblasts and osteocytes capable of primary ossification, or into chondroblasts and chondrocytes which give rise to an initial cartilagenous model. Tissue oxygen concentration, mechanical stress and hormonal agents are some of the factors known to dictate the type of bone development. In the limbs there are also complex interactions between skeletal formation and the ectodermal covering. Mineralisation which is essential to bone structure depends on the transplacental passage of calcium, phosphate and vitamin D or its metabolites. This mineral transfer is maximal in later gestation and the calcium content of the fetus is doubled in the last month. The calcium deficit created by premature delivery increases the requirement for vitamin D in the postnatal period. Following delivery, the skeleton continues its growth, both in length and density. It also undergoes considerable remodelling, particularly in the first 2 years when the rate is 10 times that which occurs in adult life. Maturation is accompanied by progressive endochondral ossification with the appearance of epiphyseal centres and the disappearance of the growth cartilages. This maturation is subject to genetic and environmental controls and may be quantified to provide the bone age, a valuable parameter in assessing growth and its disorders.

Joint swelling in childhood	
Infection	Bacterial: pyogenic, tuberculosis Viral: rubella, mumps, parvovirus Arthropod borne: Lyme disease
Post-infectious	Post-streptococcal arthritis and rheumatic fever
Allergic	Henoch–Schönlein purpura
Collagen vascular disease	Juvenile chronic arthritis, systemic lupus erythematosis, Kawasaki disease
Haematological disease	Leukaemia, haemophilia, sickle cell disease
Gastrointestinal disease	Ulcerative colitis, Crohn disease
Trauma and synovitis	

ARTHRITIS

A swollen painful joint requires prompt evaluation as it may be the first sign of severe systemic illness. Young children present with fever, limp or reluctance to use their limbs rather than specific joint symptoms. When many joints are involved it is a polyarthritis. A monoarthritis is when a single joint is involved in which case a pyogenic infection must be excluded.

Pyogenic arthritis. In pyogenic arthritis the joint is usually hot, swollen and acutely tender and more than one joint may be involved. Movement of the affected joints is restricted and very painful. The joint must be aspirated and the fluid examined by microscopy and culture, and also blood samples taken for culture at the same time. Osteomyelitis adjacent to a joint may produce a sympathetic effusion but the tenderness will be on the bony metaphysis rather than over the joint. The commonest infecting organism is *Staphylococcus pyogenes*, and flucloxacillin given intravenously is the treatment of choice. Surgical drainage is frequently required if the diagnosis is delayed beyond 48–72 hours from the onset of symptoms. During the acute phase of the illness the joint is splinted, but later physiotherapy and mobilisation is essential to prevent joint flexion from developing into a permanent deformity.

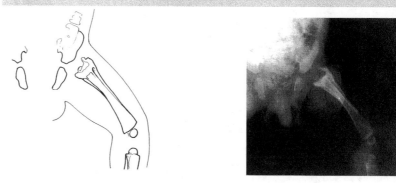

Septic arthritis and osteomyelitis in infants develop and destroy rapidly

Rheumatic fever. See Chapter 9.

Tuberculous arthritis is now very rare in Europe but occasionally presents in the spine and the larger synovial joints.

Viral arthritis may be confused with juvenile chronic arthritis or rheumatic fever.

Henoch–Schönlein purpura is a diffuse, self-limiting allergic vasculitis. It is common in young children but the precipitating factors have not been fully identified. The clinical picture is readily recognisable; the majority resolving quickly and requiring only analgesics. A minority have more severe gastrointestinal manifestation and may warrant a brief course of corticosteroid therapy. For renal lesion see Chapter 11.

Allergic polyarthritis. A transient allergic reaction consisting of an urticarial rash and synovitis is not uncommon. It may follow mild upper respiratory tract infections, drug or dietary allergen exposure.

Juvenile chronic arthritis

Chronic arthritis in children comprises a collection of disorders of unknown aetiology although there is growing evidence of genetic susceptibility with links to HLA tissue types. The diagnosis of juvenile chronic arthritis (JCA) must be based on clinical features and other disorders manifesting arthritis have to be excluded. There are three main forms of presentation: the systemic variety is the rarest, then more frequent a polyarthritis and the commonest form a pauciarticular onset in which joint involvement is limited to less than five joints. All these diseases are rheumatoid factor test negative. Some teenage girls present with an aggressive disease—juvenile rheumatoid arthritis which is seropositive and has features similar to the adult disease.

Systemic juvenile chronic arthritis (Still's disease) may not have any joint symptoms at onset. The diagnosis is made on clinical grounds with no single laboratory marker. It should be considered in an ill child with any of the following features—a remitting fever, variable rash, hepatosplenomegaly, anaemia, weight loss or abdominal pain. Acute leukaemia, metastatic neuroblastoma or septicaemia can produce similar features so a marrow examination and full septic screen may be necessary.

Clinical features of JCA

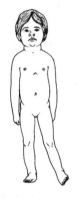

Lymphadenitis
transient pink maculopapular
   rash (prominent with fever)
pleurisy
pericarditis
hepatosplenomegaly
abdominal pain
variable symmetrical
   polyarthritis

Investigations:
   moderate normochromic
   normocytic anaemia
   ESR raised
   rheumatoid factor negative
   platelet count raised

Example of the fever and response to an antipyretic

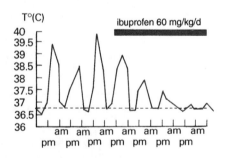

Polyarticular juvenile chronic arthritis presents with painful swelling and restricted movement in both large and small joints. It has a symmetrical distribution and characteristically involves the temporomandibular joints, the cervical spine, flexor tendons of the hands as well as limb joints. Systemic features are minimal with occasional weight loss and mild anaemia.

Pauciarticular onset juvenile chronic arthritis is a heterogeneous group of disorders with two main groups. In addition the arthropathy of psoriasis or inflammatory bowel inflammation (Crohn disease and ulcerative colitis) can present like this before becoming a polyarthritis.

Young girls frequently present with a swollen knee or ankle. They may have a positive anti-nuclear factor test and they are at high risk of developing chronic iridocyclitis. The latter should be screened for, as it can be asymptomatic until blindness occurs. This group generally has a good outcome but some progress to develop asymmetric polyarthritis.

Older boys may present with a swollen knee, tenosynovitis and a family history of HLA B27 related disease which may progress to a disease pattern of juvenile ankylosing spondylitis.

Management. The priorities in therapy are to reduce joint inflammation, maintain function and to prevent deformity. Non-steroidal anti-inflammatory drugs are used such as naproxen or ibuprofen. The latter in high dosage is useful for the control of fever in the systemic disease. Intra-articular steroids can suppress activity in single joints. Topical corticosteroids are used for iridocyclitis and oral or intravenous steroids are used to control features such as pericarditis in severe systemic illness. Oral and parenteral methotrexate is increasingly used early for uncontrolled systemic features and joint destruction.

Physical therapy is as important as the drug treatment. Daily exercises, hydrotherapy, day and night splints are all part of a personalised programme which is essential to maximize long-term joint mobility. With this most children can enter adulthood with an independent life even if their disease remains active.

Prognosis differs in the various subgroups but overall 75–80% should have no or only minor disability after 15 years.

OSTEOMYELITIS

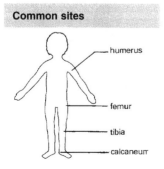

Common sites

- humerus
- femur
- tibia
- calcaneum

Osteomyelitis affects the metaphyses of long bones and is usually haematogenous in origin. The principal exception is at the proximal femur, as the metaphysis is intracapsular, the infection may spread to the bone by direct inoculation from a primary pyoarthrosis of the hip joint. The growth plate normally acts as a barrier to extension of infection from a primary metaphyseal focus to the associated epiphysis. *Staphylococcus pyogenes* accounts for 90%; *Streptococcus pyogenes* is a less common isolate. Children with sickle cell disease are susceptible to salmonella infections and the site is frequently atypical.

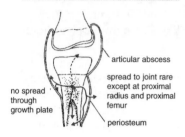

The anatomy of osteomyelitis

articular abscess

spread to joint rare
except at proximal
radius and proximal
femur

no spread
through
growth plate

periosteum

Clinical features. The infected limb is painful and held immobile. Swelling and occasionally redness may be seen if diagnosis is delayed. Examination of all inexplicably febrile children must include careful palpation of the limbs looking for areas of local swelling and tenderness. The adjacent joint may contain a sterile, sympathetic effusion. Repeated blood culture is the most satisfactory method of determining the responsible organism and therefore establishing its antibiotic sensitivity. X-rays are not of diagnostic help in the first 10–14 days. The first radiological signs are subperiosteal new bone formation and spotty rarefaction. Radionuclide bone scan will almost always demonstrate a zone of high emission at a much earlier stage and has proved to be a most useful tool to confirm diagnosis and localise the pathology.

Management. Prompt, effective parenteral antibiotic therapy is essential for a successful outcome. Neglected cases are liable to develop irreversible bone necrosis, draining sinuses and limb deformity. Appropriate antibiotic regimens include high dosage, intravenous flucloxacillin or fusidic acid (to cover staphylococcal infection) with ampicillin (to cover gram-negative organisms) until there is an unequivocal clinical response. This is followed by effective oral therapy for up to 6 weeks until all the clinical, radiological and haematological parameters indicate healing of the disease. Lack of response in the first 48 hours of therapy is an indication for surgical exploration and drainage.

NORMAL POSTURAL VARIATIONS

These are common problems which arouse much parental anxiety. Reassurance is usually more appropriate than expensive shoe modifications or unnecessary physiotherapy.

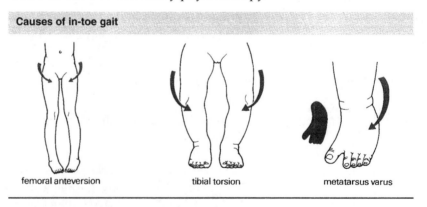

Causes of in-toe gait

femoral anteversion   tibial torsion   metatarsus varus

In-toe gait

This may originate in the foot (metatarsus varus), in the tibia (tibial torsion) or in the femora (persistent anteversion of the femoral neck).

These conditions are symmetrical, pain free and are accompanied by normal mobility. They generally resolve in 3–4 years.

Out-toe gait is also common in the first 2 years of life and may be unilateral. It always corrects spontaneously.

Genu varum (bow legs). Outward curving of the tibia is usually associated with internal tibial torsion, is not uncommon and always corrects with growth. Severe examples should raise the suspicion of rickets (nutritional in susceptible groups, or the congenital hypophosphataemic form).

Genu valgum (knock-knees). This is frequent in the 2–4-year age group and is usually innocent if symmetrical and independent of any other abnormality. Severe and progressive cases raise the possibility of rickets which is most frequently seen among Asian immigrant children. Rickets may be confirmed by the X-ray appearance of the typical frayed metaphyseal changes and by an elevated serum alkaline phosphatase.

Flat feet. The medial arch of the foot develops within 2–3 years of walking. It is largely obliterated by a fat pad in younger children. Persistent flat feet may be familial or reflect joint laxity. It is insignificant if the foot is pain free, mobile and develops an arch when standing on tiptoe. Neurological problems and pathological joint laxity are occasional underlying causes. Severe convex flat foot is occasionally due to congenital vertical talus, in which condition early surgical treatment can avoid crippling deformity in later life.

Genu valgum

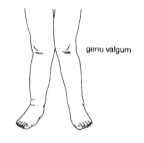

genu valgum

Pes planus

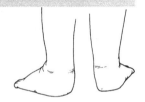

SCOLIOSIS

The anatomy of scoliosis

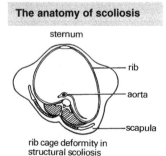

sternum

rib

aorta

scapula

rib cage deformity in
structural scoliosis

Scoliosis, refers to a spinal curve in the coronal plane. Scoliosis may be postural or structural. Structural curves are fixed and associated with vertebral rotation which produces, in the thoracic region, rib asymmetry detectable most easily when the child bends forwards. A postural curve will correct with adjustment of posture and is not accompanied by rotation. Such a curve will not evolve to a structural scoliosis.

Structural scoliosis. This may be idiopathic, either infantile ('early onset') or adolescent ('late onset'), congenital (with hemivertebrae or unsegmented lateral bony tethers) or secondary to other disease, such as osteogenesis imperfecta, Marfan syndrome or neurofibromatosis. Neuromuscular imbalance, as in cerebral palsy, or muscular dystrophy, can also result in a severe scoliosis.

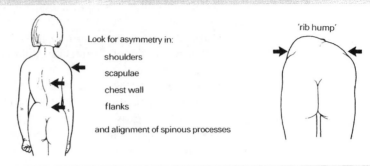

Structural scoliosis: clinical detection

Look for asymmetry in:

shoulders

scapulae

chest wall

flanks

and alignment of spinous processes

'rib hump'

Idiopathic adolescent scoliosis. Between 80 and 85% of all structural scoliosis falls into this group, affecting mainly girls in the age range 10–14 years. Great efforts have been made in the last decade to detect such cases early by programmes of school screening and this has resulted in many early curves being treated successfully by bracing; it is not, however, established that this has reduced the need for surgery. Thus, the value of screening programmes is uncertain and as the late onset curve, even allowed to progress unchecked, is unlikely to produce life-threatening cardiorespiratory compromise from thoracic deformity, the problem is primarily a cosmetic one, albeit severe. WHO has suggested that screening for cosmetic problems is not a justifiable resource allocation.

Physiotherapy has no place in the treatment of structural scoliosis. Curves of up to 40 or 50 degrees, depending on age of onset, are usually treated by a thoraco-lumbo-sacral orthosis (TLSO) which controls progression in about 70% of cases.

HIP DISORDERS

Congenital dislocation of the hip

Congenital dislocation of the hip (CDH) is now sometimes referred to as DDH—developmental dysplasia of the hip. Early detection of the lax hip at birth is important as it permits a relatively simple and safe treatment protocol with a high expectancy of a normal hip as the outcome. Delay in diagnosis leads to progressively severe dysplasia of both the femoral head and the acetabulum resulting in the need for more complex management, including the possibility of a long surgical programme. The precise aetiology is unknown. There is a high incidence of both shallow acetabulum and of congenital joint laxity in the first order relatives of CDH patients. There is wide variation in the geographical incidence of the condition. Established, irreducible CDH, in the absence of a neonatal screening and treatment programme, is found in about 1.5 per 1000 live births in most European groups. The Lapps and the North American Indians, who swaddle their infants with the hips extended and the legs together, have a much higher incidence; the Island Lake Manitoba Indian community, who still use the cradleboard, have a 4% incidence of CDH. It is a rare condition among ethnic groups who carry the infant with his legs astride the mother's pelvis, as in black Africans and the Chinese. It is against this background that it is believed that posturing the hips in subtotal abduction-in-flexion (the 'human' position as opposed to the 'frog' position) is believed to prevent the evolution of the lax neonatal hip into a fully established, irreducible dislocation. Screening for neonatal hip laxity and treatment by splintage is reducing the incidence of late diagnosis CDH.

Neonatal screening. These techniques must be learnt by practical instruction from an experienced clinician. The infant should be well fed, warm, relaxed and lain on a firm surface. The hips and knees are flexed to 90 degrees with one examining hand to each leg. The thumb should be on the inner side of the baby's knee and the ring and little fingers behind the greater trochanter. Gentle but firm pressure is applied in the line of the femur, so that a lax hip would be dislocated posteriorly. The thighs are then abducted fully with a gentle motion, at the same time lifting the greater trochanter forwards; this motion is less like opening a book and more like opening a surgical 'peel pack'. It is the movement which has to be learned. If a hip is lax, the reduction which occurs as the legs are abducted will be felt as a clunk or jumping sensation. Many normal hips 'crack' or click (like pulled finger joints!) and only experience can teach the distinction between clunks and clicks.

Ortolani test for congenital dislocation of hip

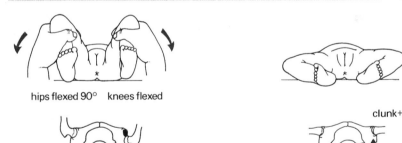

hips flexed 90°   knees flexed

clunk+

A variant of this test is to steady the pelvis with one hand with the thumb over the public symphysis and the fingers of the same hand behind the buttocks, and then with the other hand holding the examined leg as before, attempt to rock the head of the femur backwards and forwards in and out of the socket. This test must be applied in different degrees of abduction until the 'lax arc' is found. Any doubt about a hip should lead to referral to an orthopaedic surgeon with paediatric experience. Any child whose hip has been suspect should be followed up with ultrasound and at 5 months of age an X-ray. Infants statistically at risk are relatives of other lax hip children, first-born females, babies born by breech delivery (or by lower segment caesarean section after a breech intrauterine position) and those with foot deformities or sternomastoid 'tumour'. Babies at high risk of hip instability can have ultrasound examination to detect or monitor problems.

Congenital dislocation of hip: radiology and management

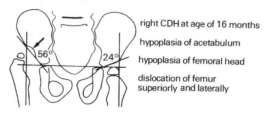

right CDH at age of 16 months

hypoplasia of acetabulum

hypoplasia of femoral head

dislocation of femur superiorly and laterally

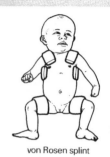

von Rosen splint

Congenital dislocation of hips (bilateral)

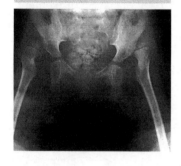

Management. The infant whose hips remain suspect should be splinted, such as with a Pavlik Harness. This needs careful application and adjustment. Three months of use is often all that is required. Ultrasound and X-rays must be used to confirm normal hip joint development until independent walking. X-rays are of little use under 5 months of age. The finding of limited abduction in flexion at the hip is a feature of the established dislocation and is, therefore, not a sign which develops until about 3–4 months of age. Conversely, the clunk will disappear at about 3 weeks of age when the hip first becomes irreducible.

It is unfortunately true that dislocated hips are still missed in spite of the widespread introduction of screening procedures. Suspicion is raised by a child with a shortened leg, or with a gait in which the affected foot is placed flat on the ground while the opposite knee is flexed. It does not generally delay the onset of walking but may well cause frequent falls. Bilateral cases have a symmetrical gait and tend to present even later if missed in the neonatal period. Attempted reduction of the hip involves initial traction followed by more prolonged splintage or in the event of failure, operative intervention. The latter may involve open reduction, femoral osteotomy and acetabular reconstruction.

Transient synovitis

This is the most common cause of limp, with hip and/or knee pain, in young children. It is a unilateral, self-limiting condition of ill defined aetiology although many follow a mild upper respiratory tract infection. Boys in the age group 2–12 years (average 6 years) are most susceptible. It usually has a sudden onset with limp, and pain of variable severity. Abduction, full extension and internal rotation are restricted and there may be tenderness over the anterior aspect of the hip. There is usually no leucocytosis, and the ESR is normal or only mildly elevated. X-rays are normal. The diagnosis can only be made after exclusion of an infective process at or adjacent to the hip joint, Perthes disease, slipped upper femoral epiphysis or even a primary neoplasm, benign or malignant.

Transient synovitis seldom lasts for more than a few days or weeks and treatment consists of simple analgesics and bed rest. Approximately 6% of cases considered to have transient synovitis subsequently develop features of Perthes disease.

Perthes disease

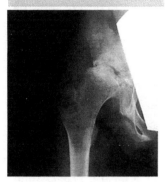

Necrosis of femoral head

This results from episodes of segmental avascular necrosis of the femoral head. The necrotic bone is gradually replaced by new bone, but recovery can be complicated by residual deformity of the femoral head. It is most common in the 4–8-year age group and the ratio of boys to girls is 5 : 1. The underlying cause has not been established but it is suspected that the femoral head disorder is part of a more generalised growth disturbance in which skeletal development is retarded.

Limp, with or without pain in the hip, knee or thigh, is the presenting complaint. Hip mobility, especially abduction and internal rotation, is limited. The hip X-ray reflects the natural history of the bone necrosis; initial increase in density followed by fragmentation and reossification. The identification of the femoral head at risk of deformity is central to management; the head at risk is usually treated by 'containment' in the acetabulum by femoral osteotomy. The healing phase during which the head requires protection lasts 2–4 years.

Slipped upper femoral

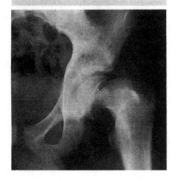

A slipped epiphysis

This condition, occurring during the adolescent growth spurt (10–14 years in girls; 12–16 years in boys), is a posterior slipping of the epiphysis of the femoral head in relation to its metaphysis, a shearing failure of the growth plate resulting. The slip may be acute after minimal trauma (massive trauma is required to displace a normal proximal femoral epiphysis) or gradual. Atypically early presentation should lead to the search for an underlying endocrine disease, the commonest being hypothyroidism. The condition is bilateral, but not necessarily synchronous, in about 25% of cases. Obese children with delayed secondary sexual development or tall thin boys appear to be especially susceptible. Pain in the hip, the thigh or the knee associated with limp in this age group demands urgent referral for investigation. Slipped upper femoral epiphysis is a true emergency, as massive further slipping may supervene without warning at any time. Traction and analgesics help pain.

CT or MRI scanning is useful in planning treatment. Mild slips need pin fixation while major slips need open reduction and fixation possibly combined with femoral osteotomy. The other side is usually pinned at surgery. Manipulation should never be attempted: it either fails to improve the position or, if it produces a reduction, avascular necrosis of the femoral head is then highly likely.

KNEE DISORDERS

The knee is a common source of complaint among adolescents. In assessing the cause of knee pain, the hip must also be examined as hip pain is often referred to the knee.

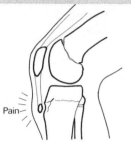

Tender tubercle

Pain

Osgood–Schlatter syndrome is a painful, tender swelling of the tibial tubercle due to repeated minor avulsion trauma at the site of insertion of the patellar tendon—a traction apophysitis. It is an example of an overuse syndrome and is caused by excess physical exertion before skeletal maturity. Some patients respond to anti-inflammatory drugs and limitation on sport, while others are managed with avoidance of sport and in some cases immobilisation for 6–8 weeks in a plaster cylinder.

Chondromalacia patellae indicates softening of the articular cartilage of the patellae usually as the result of indirect trauma, for example unaccustomed games activity. The retropatellar pain is worse on rising from prolonged sitting or on stairs, and is accompanied by crepitus. Avoidance of repetitive knee bending and minimising high impact sport is usually adequate advice. Occasional cases have patellar misalignment worthy of surgery.

TALIPES (CLUBFOOT)

Incidence of talipes		
Year	Numbers (England)	Rate per 10 000 births
1986	1823	29.2
1991	856	13.0
1995	659	10.7
1996	545	8.9

Talipes equinovarus. The fixed clubfoot is one of the most challenging deformities facing orthopaedic surgeons as it represents disruption of complicated interrelationships between bone, ligament and muscle. The incidence is 1.2 per 1000 live births, rising by 20-fold where there is an affected first degree relative. Males are more at risk by a ratio of 3:1, and 50% of cases are bilateral. All cases must be examined carefully to exclude an underlying neurological problem.

Treatment depends on the rigidity of the deformity. In the early stages gradual manipulative correction is combined with strapping. Tendo-achilles lengthening and further surgery is sometimes needed with plastering. The whole course of treatment may continue until at least 5 years of age. Failure to achieve early true correction may result in the need for corrective bone surgery later in childhood.

Talipes calcaneovalgus. In this deformity the foot is dorsiflexed and everted but the underlying structural abnormality is less profound and the foot is more amenable to simple manipulation.

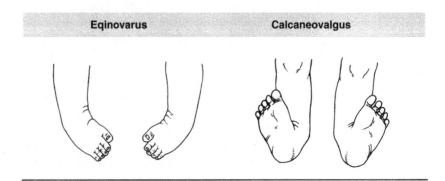

| Eqinovarus | Calcaneovalgus |

GENETIC BONE AND JOINT DISORDERS

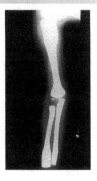

Radiodense bones of osteopetrosis

Marfan disease (autosomal dominant) consists of arachnodactyly, hypermobile joints, ocular abnormalities and a high arched palate. There are commonly associated deformities of the spine and chest. The prognosis is determined by associated cardiovascular problems such as dilated aortic root, dissecting aortic aneurysm and billowing mitral valve incompetence.

Osteogenesis imperfecta (autosomal dominant, occasionally recessive). In this condition there is an underlying failure in collagen metabolism resulting in multiple fractures of fragile bones, lax joints and thin skin. Blue sclerae, scoliosis, hypoplastic teeth and progressive deafness are also features. The congenital form may be so severe that the fetus dies in utero or shortly after birth.

Osteopetrosis or marble bone disease (autosomal recessive or autosoma dominant). The recessive form is more severe causing bone marrow failure and early death. The dominant or less severe form presents in childhood as facial paralysis, bone fractures and osteomyelitis. Bone marrow transplantation has had limited success in reintroducing normal osteoblast and osteoclast function.

BONE TUMOURS AND ALLIED DISORDERS

Features suggestive of a bone tumour include pain, swelling or a limp. Fortunately the majority of underlying lesions are benign; atypical osteomyelitis, incomplete fracture of normal bone, a simple cyst or an osteoid osteoma. Ewing tumour and osteosarcoma are described in Chapter 13.

Simple bone cysts

These are most frequently seen in the metaphyseal regions of long bones and are discovered usually only when they fracture and cause pain. The X-ray features are characteristic. They fill in spontaneously and disappear shortly after skeletal maturity. The fractures heal readily but the cyst often remains. Treatment is usually by washout of the cyst using two wide-bore needles inserted under anaesthetic and X-ray control, followed by the instillation of triamcinolone acetate.

Osteoid osteoma

Osteoid osteoma may present with intermittent and often nocturnal pain. X-rays show extensive periosteal thickening with a focus of dense new bone surrounding a centrally placed radiolucent nidus. The majority are so painful that surgical removal of the nidus is required. These lesions concentrate bone-seeking radionuclides such as technetium-99 m compounds and this can be exploited to locate them at surgery by the use of sterilisible miniature gamma ray detectors. Recurrence is virtually unknown after successful removal of the nidus tissue.

BIBLIOGRAPHY

Cassidy J T, Petty R E 1995 Textbook of paediatric rheumatology, 2nd edn. W B
    Saunders, London
Lloyd-Roberts G C, Fixsen J 1990 Orthopaedics in infancy and childhood. Butterworth-
    Heinemann, Oxford

19

Brain, cord, nerve, muscle

CEREBRAL PALSY
HEADACHE
EPILEPSY AND CONVULSIONS
ATAXIA
INTRACRANIAL INFECTION
NEUROMUSCULAR DISORDERS

Brain growth

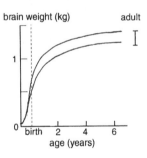

All who are concerned with the safe passage of children from conception to adulthood have as a prime goal the preservation of normal brain development. Potential hazards have effects which are largely determined by the degree of differentiation of the nervous system. In the first trimester genetic and environmental influences may disrupt embryogenesis and produce anomalies which either lead to abortion or reach term as malformations, for example anencephaly or lissencephaly. In later fetal life and during infancy insults are more likely to produce focal, irreversible pathology in differentiated tissue, lesions which may well be the basis of cerebral palsy.

In addition to interference with structural differentiation, the brain is also susceptible to problems during its various growth spurts. In the human fetus maximal neuronal proliferation occurs in the middle trimester and is relatively protected from maternal malnutrition and placental dysfunction, but it is vulnerable to viral infection, radiation, drugs and excessive alcohol. Glial multiplication and myelination occurs over a more extended period from the third trimester through the first 2 years of life and is therefore exposed to the effects of intra- and extra-uterine malnutrition, perinatal asphyxia and inborn errors of metabolism. We are only on the threshold of understanding how these hazards may influence the subtler components of growth, dendritic proliferation and synaptic connectivity.

CEREBRAL PALSY

Cerebral palsy is the leading cause of crippling handicap in children, with a prevalence of 2 per 1000. The label cerebral palsy implies that the underlying cerebral pathology is permanent and non-progressive. However in a developing child the resulting clinical picture will not be static. The disorder can be caused at any time during pregnancy, delivery or up to 5 years of age and, because it arises in early life, it interferes with normal motor development. The main handicap is one of disordered movement and posture, but it is often complicated by other neurological and mental problems. Cerebral palsy is due to brain

Causes of cerebral palsy

Cerebral malformation
Trauma
  birth
  postnatal
Hypoxia
Kernicterus
Hypoglycaemia
Infection
Cerebrovascular accident
Poisoning
Toxins

Classification

malformation or damage affecting those areas involved in motor functions. Congenital malformations of the brain include congenital cysts, fusion defects, failure of normal migration of grey matter and aplasias. Brain damage may occur during fetal life from infection or hypoxia-ischaemia. Birth related cerebral trauma or hypoxia-ischaemia is now considered an uncommon cause of cerebral palsy, perhaps 10%. Post-natal causes include severe neonatal illness, non-accidental injury, road traffic accidents, meningitis, encephalitis, near drowning and cardiopulmonary arrest.

Spastic cerebral palsy, which accounts for 70% of cerebral palsy cases, involves damage to the cerebral motor cortex or its connections, producing clasp-knife hypertonia, abnormally brisk tendon jerks, ankle clonus and extensor plantar responses. Hemiparesis affects just one side of the body and the arm is usually involved more than the leg. Quadriparesis affects both sides of the body, the arms being affected as much or more than the legs. In spastic diplegia both legs are spastic and the arms are less affected or not affected at all.

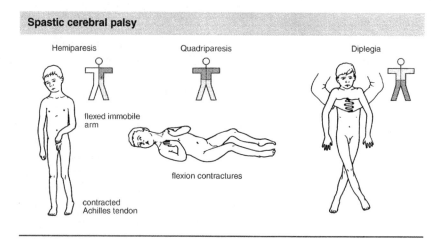

Spastic cerebral palsy

Hemiparesis — flexed immobile arm — contracted Achilles tendon

Quadriparesis — flexion contractures

Diplegia

Dystonic (athetoid) cerebral palsy. Ten per cent of cases are characterised by irregular and involuntary movements of some or all muscle groups. These may be continuous or occur only on voluntary active movement. Athetosis is the commonest form with slow purposeless muscle movements and extensor spasms.

Ataxic cerebral palsy. This is associated with hypotonia, weakness, uncoordinated movements and intentional tremor and accounts for 10% of cerebral palsy.

Mixed cerebral palsy. These form the remaining 10% of cases.

Clinical features

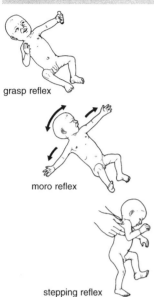

grasp reflex

moro reflex

stepping reflex

Management

Infants who show poor sucking ability, increased or decreased muscle tone, abnormal reflexes, irritability, convulsions or drowsiness in the newborn period are at risk of having cerebral palsy. However, many such infants do develop normally and great care must be exercised in anticipating future development. Usually cerebral palsy is not diagnosed until several months have passed, and when it becomes obvious that motor development is abnormal or delayed. For example, the infant may be brought to the doctor because he is not showing real head control at 3 months of age or he is not yet sitting alone at 10 months of age. His mother may say that he seems stiff on handling. An infant with a spastic hemiplegia will be noted to have developed hand preference before 1 year which is much earlier than normal. The persistence of primitive reflexes, such as the asymmetric tonic neck reflex, beyond the time they usually disappear is suspicious.

The characteristic involuntary movements of dystonic cerebral palsy are not usually obvious until near the end of the first year of life or even later. Affected children are usually very floppy and show delayed motor development in infancy. Children with ataxic cerebral palsy are also hypotonic and delayed in motor development but subsequently show an intention tremor.

The child with cerebral palsy requires a multidisciplinary assessment initially to define his strengths and weaknesses, and then to develop a structured treatment programme. Physiotherapy aims to encourage normal motor development, to inhibit abnormal motor development and to prevent contractures. The parents are taught to perform the exercises at home.

Some degree of learning disorder is seen in about 60% of children with cerebral palsy. However, it should not be forgotten that children with severe cerebral palsy may have normal intelligence; this applies particularly to the dystonic group. Epilepsy occurs in approximately 30% and is symptomatic rather than idiopathic. Visual impairment due to errors of refraction, disuse amblyopia, optic atrophy or visual cortical damage occurs in 20%. Squint due to external ocular muscle imbalance or paralysis is present in 30%. Twenty per cent have a degree of hearing loss which is often of the sensorineural type. Children with dystonic cerebral palsy are particularly liable to have associated deafness. Speech disorders are common and have a variety of causes, including hearing loss, perceptual defects, learning disorders and incoordination of tongue, palate and lip muscles.

Children with cerebral palsy often do less well in school than would be expected by their estimated abilities. One reason for this is the high frequency of perceptual defects. Behaviour disorders may be due to the frustrations of being handicapped, to strained family life brought about by the presence of a handicapped child, and to the hyperactivity which may be associated with brain damage.

Even with adequate physiotherapy, long-standing muscle weakness or spasticity may produce orthopaedic deformities. These are more

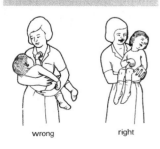

wrong   right

How to hold a spastic child

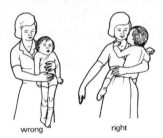

wrong   right

common in spastic cerebral palsy where the involved muscles develop dynamic contractures initially but eventually these may become fibrotic and fixed. Spasticity in the adductors of the thigh may lead to dislocation of the hips and operation may be necessary to correct this. Spasticity and contracture in the calf muscles may produce a fixed equinus deformity of the ankle which requires a tendo-achilles lengthening operation to allow the heel to be used for walking and weight bearing. Neglect of these deformities may lead to painful osteoarthritis.

Drugs have a limited role in the management of cerebral palsy, apart from the treatment of epilepsy. Schools for the physically handicapped provide physiotherapy and speech therapy, and have specially trained staff and equipment. There is, however, a deficiency of opportunity for the handicapped school leaver. The overlap between cerebral palsy and learning disorder is such that some children in schools for children with severe learning disorders also have cerebral palsy.

If a child with a physical handicap comes under your care enquire about his 'activities of living' from the child and the carers

What is their usual daily schedule?
What can they say?
How do they indicate—Yes, No, Want, Drink, Sleep, Toilet, Pain, Cuddly, Mummy, Daddy, etc?
How do they get about? Do they use a special chair or supports?
At meal times do they use special spoons and cups?
Do they wear glasses?
Do they wear hearing aids and when?

HEADACHE

Headache is a relatively common complaint in childhood. A self-limiting headache is a frequent accompaniment of many febrile illnesses. Severe headache of acute or subacute onset should always raise the possibility of intracranial inflammation, subarachnoid haemorrhage or brain tumour (see Chapter 13). Chronic intermittent headaches are usually either tension or migraine headaches but other causes such as dental caries, sinusitis, brain tumour, raised intracranial pressure, hypertension and ocular refractive error may need to be considered.

Migraine

Migraine affects about 5% of all children at some time. A family history and the characteristic symptoms of throbbing headache, visual disturbance, photophobia and nausea make the diagnosis relatively straightforward in the older child. There may be problems in the recognition of migraine in the handicapped or preschool child and it may be manifest by acute periods of distress, pallor and nausea. Attacks resulting in ophthalmoplegia or hemiparesis may occur. An underlying vascular malformation is a rare association. Treatment is initially with simple analgesics such as paracetamol given at the onset of symptoms with encouragement to lie down in a dark quiet room until the headache has passed. More severe cases may benefit from a regular migraine prophylactic drug such as pizotifen given for a period of a few months. Recently there has been renewed interest in the relationship between food allergy and migraine. Some children benefit from the exclusion of cheese, chocolate or citrus fruits from their diets. More severe exclusion diets (oligo-allergenic diets) have been tried with success in some children with difficult migraine.

Symptoms of migraine

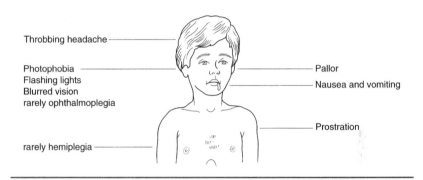

Throbbing headache

Photophobia
Flashing lights
Blurred vision
rarely ophthalmoplegia

rarely hemiplegia

Pallor

Nausea and vomiting

Prostration

Ocular headaches

Ocular headaches can result from constant muscular activity attempting to correct a latent squint or refractive error (usually long sightedness or astigmatism).

Benign intracranial hypertension

This term is used for an illness with raised intracranial pressure of unknown cause. It usually presents with vomiting, headache and papilloedema. CT scan shows small or normal sized ventricles and no space occupying lesion. It may be a complication of otitis media or occur after a non-specific viral illness; rarely it develops from too rapid reduction in corticosteroid therapy. Treatment is directed towards reducing the intracranial pressure in order to avoid secondary optic atrophy. A course of acetazolamide is usually successful but sometimes corticosteroid therapy is required. Rarely a theco-peritoneal shunt has to be inserted to reduce the raised intracranial pressure.

EPILEPSY AND CONVULSIONS

The diagnosis of epilepsy has major medical and social implications. Unfortunately diagnosis is sometimes mistaken and antiepileptic drug therapy commenced in error. The prevalence of epilepsy amongst schoolchildren is in the order of 8 per 1000. Epilepsy implies a disorder of the brain producing recurrent paroxysmal discharges which result in epileptic attacks. Because epilepsy is defined as a recurrent disorder, it can only be diagnosed if there has been more than one attack. A child who has only had one attack cannot be said to have epilepsy because he may never have another. A convulsion is a non-specific term and refers to all generalised tonic-clonic seizures both epileptic and non-epileptic.

Types of epileptic seizures

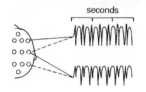

Typical absence seizure

seconds

3-second spike-and-wave
discharges

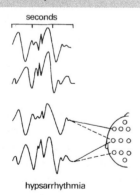

Infantile spasm

seconds

hypsarrhythmia

Simple absence seizures. The attacks consist of impaired consciousness without falling or involuntary movements. The child stops whatever he is doing and looks vacant for 5–20 seconds and then continues with what he was doing as though nothing had happened. Attacks can be brought on by having the child overbreathe for a minute or two. The EEG characteristically shows bursts of generalised 3 per second spike and wave discharges. This form of epilepsy is invariably idiopathic and usually carries a good prognosis.

Atypical absence seizures. These tend to be rather a mixed bag. Unlike simple absence seizures the episodes of impaired consciousness may last longer and be associated with involuntary movements such as chewing, myoclonic jerks, loss of postural tone, semipurposeful movements or peculiar sensations. Attacks may be difficult to differentiate from partial complex seizures on clinical grounds. The EEG will be helpful in this differential diagnosis as it will show generalised bursts of irregular fast or slow spike and wave activity. The prognosis is not as good as with simple absences.

Myoclonic seizures. Myoclonic seizures take the form of sudden shock-like jerks affecting one part or the whole of the body, the latter are usually bilateral and symmetrical. They may be predominantly flexor or extensor. Mild attacks take the form of sudden head drops but more severe attacks may cause a child to be thrown suddenly forwards or backwards, perhaps injuring his face or back of his head. They may be idiopathic and occur in children without evidence of any other neurological disorder, but more commonly they represent a type of symptomatic epilepsy and are associated with mental handicap or abnormal neurological findings. Myoclonic seizures are common in some rare cerebral degenerative disorders.

Infantile spasms are a kind of myoclonic epilepsy but are usually considered separately because of their particularly bad prognosis for future development. This is a relatively rare but serious type of epilepsy seen only in young children and usually commencing between 3 and 8 months of age. The majority of infants show typical flexion ('jacknife' or 'salaam') spasms which may occur several hundred times a day at their most frequent. The spasm involves sudden flexion of the neck and limbs and lasts 1–3 seconds only but they usually occur in clusters lasting 15–30 minutes.

Approximately half the children who develop infantile spasms will be found to have evidence of some underlying neurological disorder by history, examination or investigation. The prognosis for future development in such a child is almost always poor. The other infants have what are called idiopathic infantile spasms and have usually shown quite normal development until the spasms commence at which time they appear to regress developmentally. Sometimes the diagnosis is delayed because the spasms are thought to represent infantile colic or just fretfulness. Infantile spasms are an age-related type of epilepsy and usually cease spontaneously at 2–3 years of age though they may be replaced by tonic-clonic or other types of epileptic attacks. Idiopathic infantile spasms also have a poor prognosis but, after treatment, a minority (about 20%) subsequently make satisfactory developmental progress and turn out to be mentally normal.

Tonic-clonic seizures. The attacks start with sudden loss of consciousness, falling and often an initial tonic phase in which the limbs are extended and the back arched. This soon gives way to the clonic phase associated with generalised jerking during which micturition and salivation (foaming at the mouth) may occur. Respiration ceases during the tonic phase but recommences in an irregular fashion during the clonic phase. Commonly the clonic phase settles after a few minutes but if it continues beyond 30 minutes the term status epilepticus is used. When the clonic phase ceases the child gradually regains consciousness but usually remains sleepy for an hour or so afterwards.

Simple partial seizures. Simple partial seizures usually consist of twitching or jerking of one side of the face, one arm or one leg. Consciousness is usually retained or only slightly impaired and the child does not usually fall. Sometimes the jerking can be seen to start in one corner of the mouth and spread across one side of the face or start in one hand and spread up the arm; this is called a 'Jacksonian march'. A simple partial seizure may proceed to a generalised tonic-clonic seizure with loss of consciousness, falling and generalised convulsive movements. Temporary weakness of the affected side of the body is common after a simple partial seizure and is known as a Todd's palsy.

The so-called adversive attack is a rare kind of simple partial seizure which takes the form of turning of the head and eyes to one side and is usually associated with a discharging cortical focus in the opposite frontal cortex. Rarely simple partial seizures with sensory symptoms can occur in which the child complains of tingling or numbness starting in one hand or side of the face and spreading to affect the whole of that side of the body.

Complex partial seizure

seconds

Right mid-temporal spike focus

Complex partial seizures. Attacks consist of altered or impaired consciousness, usually without falling and associated with strange sensations or complex semipurposeful movements. The strange sensations may be visual (objects may look too big, too small or distorted, or there may be visual hallucinations), auditory (sounds or voices may appear too loud or too quiet, sensations of vertigo may be experienced or there may be auditory hallucinations), gustatory or olfactory (peculiar tastes or smell) or emotional (sensations of loss of reality, fear, sadness or excessive familiarity). The child may talk during the attack though what he says may not make sense. Commonly there are chewing, sucking or swallowing movements and these movements may accompany hallucinations of taste. The child may perform complicated manoeuvres such as getting up and walking about. If a sensation of fear accompanies an attack the child may rush to the nearest person and clutch him looking wide eyed and terrified. The attacks commonly last a few minutes and the child on coming round has little recollection of what has happened. A diagnosis of complex partial seizures is very dependent on a careful description of the attacks but the EEG may be helpful if it shows clear discharges arising from one temporal lobe.

Partial seizures with secondary generalisation. Any seizure discharge which starts from a cortical focus may be transmitted down to the deep subcortical grey matter, from which spread can then occur to both hemispheres simultaneously producing a generalised tonic-clonic seizure. Sometimes it is clear that the tonic-clonic seizure is preceded by a partial seizure (sometimes referred to as an aura), but at other times the initial partial seizure is so brief as to pass unnoticed. The EEG is helpful in distinguishing between tonic-clonic seizures which are primary and those which are secondary. In primary generalised tonic-clonic seizures the EEG shows generalised bursts of regular or irregular spike or polyspike and wave activity whereas in secondary generalised tonic-clonic seizures the EEG shows evidence of a cortical focus.

Assessment

All children with suspected epilepsy should be fully assessed. A careful and detailed history from someone who has witnessed the attacks is of the utmost importance. General examination with special emphasis on developmental and neurological aspects is also required. Fasting blood sugar and calcium estimations are sometimes indicated.

An EEG may help to decide if doubtful attacks are epileptic or not, and may give some help in deciding the kind of epilepsy present. Caution is necessary as a normal interictal EEG may be seen in a number of children with epilepsy, and conversely abnormal discharges may occasionally be seen in EEGs from children who have never had an epileptic seizure. A child with infantile spasms usually has a very severe EEG abnormality termed hypsarrhythmia. Some children have photosensitive epilepsy induced for example by television viewing. This may be confirmed by finding EEG discharges brought on by flicker from a strobe light. Partial seizures are associated with cortical spike foci. Bilateral symmetrical discharges of spike and waves are seen in the EEGs of children with primary generalised seizures.

A CT or MRI head scan may be required if there are clinical grounds to suspect a structural lesion of the brain or if the EEG shows a persistent slow wave focus.

Management

Children with epilepsy usually require regular drug therapy in an attempt to prevent further seizures. Experience has shown that certain categories of epilepsy respond best to particular groups of anti-epileptic drugs. Optimal drug dosage and susceptibility to side effects vary from individual to individual, and serum anti-epileptic drug levels may sometimes be helpful in assessing therapy. The regimen should be kept as simple as possible and it is seldom necessary to use more than two drugs.

Mode of action of the commonly used antiepileptic drugs. Some have more than one site of action

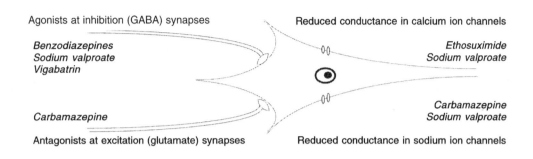

Agonists at inhibition (GABA) synapses

Benzodiazepines
Sodium valproate
Vigabatrin

Carbamazepine

Antagonists at excitation (glutamate) synapses

Reduced conductance in calcium ion channels

Ethosuximide
Sodium valproate

Carbamazepine
Sodium valproate

Reduced conductance in sodium ion channels

A diagnosis of epilepsy raises considerable fears not only in the family but among school teachers and social contacts. Children with epilepsy do not require much limitation of their activities. For obvious reasons they are advised not to cycle in traffic but they may swim provided there is a responsible adult in attendance. Learning difficulties and behaviour problems are more common than in other children but the majority of children with epilepsy attend ordinary schools and are average scholars.

Drug therapy in epilepsy

Type of epilepsy	Drug of first choice	Other drugs
Simple absences	ethosuximide	valproate
Atypical absences	valproate	clonazepam
Myoclonic	clonazepam	valproate
Infantile spasms	vigabatrin	ACTH
Primary generalised tonic-clonic	valproate	carbamazepine
Simple partial	carbamazepine	valproate
Secondary generalised tonic-clonic	carbamazepine	valproate
Status epilepticus	IV or rectal diazepam	rectal paraldehyde

More than 60% of children diagnosed as having epilepsy seem to 'grow out' of their seizure tendency during childhood and antiepileptic drug therapy can be discontinued if they have been free of attacks for 2–3 years. A very small minority of children continue to have frequent epileptic attacks despite anti-epileptic drug therapy. Nevertheless the overall prognosis for childhood epilepsy is good with modern management.

Treatment of status epilepticus. Parents of children who are known to be at risk of prolonged seizures should be taught how to manage them at home. The child should first be placed in the recovery position to protect the airway. If the fit has lasted 10 minutes by the clock, parents give a rectal tube of diazepam 0.5 mg/kg from a supply they keep at home. If their child is still fitting after a further 10 minutes they should phone for an ambulance to take them to the nearest accident and emergency department. If the child is still fitting on arrival, diazepam may be repeated but given intravenously in a lower dose of 0.25 mg/kg. Diazepam carries a slight risk of causing apnoea by this route so that it should not be used in the absence of facilities for resuscitation. Alternatively rectal paraldehyde 0.3 ml/kg mixed with an equal volume of arachis oil can be given.

Anti-epileptic drug dosage and side effects

Drug and dose	Infrequent side effects	Rare side effects
Carbamazepine 10–20 mg/kg/day	rash, fatigue*, dizziness*	bone marrow depression, hepatic toxicity
Sodium valproate 20–40 mg/kg/day	drowsiness*, nausea*, weight gain	thrombocytopenia (high dosage), hair loss†, hepatic toxicity, pancreatitis
Ethosuximide 20–40 mg/kg/day	nausea†, rashes	bone marrow depression
Clonazepam 0.05–0.2 mg/kg/day	drowsiness†, salivation†	
Vigabatrin 40–100 mg/kg/day	drowsiness*, ataxia†	behavioural change visual field defect

*Usually transient if drug continued　†Usually settles with slight dose reduction

Febrile convulsions

Age at time of first febrile convulsion

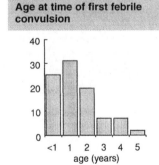

age (years)

Febrile convulsions are very common and affect some 4% of children, most often in the second year of life. They are strongly age related and hardly ever occur before 6 months or after 6 years of age.

The usual history is that the child is noticed to be unwell and hot and then has a major seizure lasting a few minutes. There is often a family history of febrile convulsions. On examination the child has a high temperature, and may have evidence of upper respiratory tract infection. More serious conditions such as meningitis or urinary tract infections must always be excluded. The attacks are considered to be benign if they last less than 10 minutes and there are no persisting neurological signs. The ultimate prognosis for children with febrile convulsions is good, though recurrences are common. The risk of recurrence may be minimised by advising the parents to take some of the child's clothes off and give an antipyretic whenever the child becomes febrile. Regular prophylaxis with sodium valproate 20–40 mg/kg/day will also reduce the risk of recurrence but is rarely prescribed for what is usually a very benign condition. The risk of developing epilepsy after one or more febrile convulsion of any kind is only 2%, but this risk is increased to 4% if any of the febrile convulsions are prolonged or atypical, and to 6% if there is pre-existing neurological abnormality.

Other causes of transient episodes

Breath-holding attacks. These are common in toddlers and are usually precipitated by 'not getting his own way'. The child cries, holds his breath and goes blue. The attack usually stops at this point but loss of consciousness sometimes occurs. Drug treatment is not necessary and the attacks cease spontaneously.

Reflex anoxic seizures. These occur in infants who have very sensitive vagal cardiac reflexes. Attacks are usually brought on by pain, especially unexpected bangs to the head. This causes reflex cardiac asystole with immediate loss of posture, deathly pallor and floppiness. The heart recommences beating itself and the child then recovers.

Syncope or fainting. This is not uncommon among older children. Careful history reveals likely predisposing factors such as prolonged standing, a hot environment or emotional upset.

Benign paroxysmal vertigo. This may present as sudden attacks of unsteadiness, swaying or dizziness but consciousness is not lost. Nystagmus may be noted by the parents. No treatment is indicated as these attacks are brief and disappear spontaneously.

Migraine, day dreams, night terrors and hysterical pseudoseizures. These also enter the differential diagnosis.

Tics or habit spasms. These are irregular contractions of muscle groups, for example blinking and jerking or facial grimacing. They can be controlled voluntarily for a while but feelings of tension increase until the movement has to be repeated. They are often a reflection of underlying emotional disturbance and should not be confused with focal epilepsy.

Fictitious seizures. Refractory seizures witnessed by only one carer may be a manifestation of Münchausen syndrome-by proxy. It is also possible for recurrent collapses in infants to be induced by partial asphyxia.

ATAXIA

Ataxia refers to a disorder of movement manifest by incoordination, clumsiness and poor balance. In the young child, hypotonia and delayed motor development may be the only obvious signs.

Ataxic cerebral palsy is caused by malformation or damage of the cerebellum or its connections. The commonest cause is cerebellar hypoplasia which may be inherited as an autosomal recessive. Dandy–Walker syndrome refers to congenital absence of the foramina of Majendie and Luschka with resulting cystic dilatation of the IVth ventricle. Affected children have a characteristic prominence of the occipital region and are often ataxic.

Acute ataxia in older children may be due to intoxication with drugs, for example solvent abuse, phenytoin or alcohol. If the history does not reveal a cause, the rapid recovery certainly suggests it. Cerebellar ataxia may also be a manifestation of viral encephalitis, especially that caused by varicella. The differential diagnosis includes an acute presentation of a cerebellar tumour such as medulloblastoma, but CT or MRI scanning rapidly resolves this concern.

Friedreich ataxia is the most common of the hereditary ataxias, and is an autosomal recessive condition initially characterised by pes cavus and a progressively clumsy gait. Examination reveals ataxia, loss of position and vibration sensation, and impaired leg tendon reflexes. There may, in addition, be optic atrophy and cardiomyopathy. The patients become increasingly handicapped and may be wheelchair users by early adult life.

Ataxia telangiectasia is inherited as an autosomal recessive disorder. In addition to slowly increasing cerebellar ataxia often commencing in infancy, there are characteristic groups of dilated capillaries (telangiectasia) which become obvious in the skin of the face and in the whites of the eyes. There is an associated impairment of cellular immunity which increases susceptibility to infection and predisposes to neoplasia, especially leukaemia and lymphoma.

There are rare metabolic disorders which result in ataxia; Hartnup disease in which there is a derangement of tryptophan metabolism, and Refsum disease in which phytanic acid accumulates.

INTRACRANIAL INFECTION

Acute infection of the meninges may be bacterial (acute purulent meningitis) or viral (aseptic meningitis) in origin. Meningitis may also be due to tuberculosis and rarer pathogens such as fungi and protozoa. Leukaemic cell infiltration can cause a sterile meningitis.

Acute purulent meningitis   Purulent meningitis is relatively common in childhood especially in preschool years, 35% of childhood cases occurring in the first year of life and 80% in the first 5 years of life. In the United Kingdom 1 in 500 children suffer from purulent meningitis between the age of 1 month and 10 years. It is essential to make an early diagnosis as delay increases the risk of death or neurological complications.

After the neonatal period meningococcus and pneumococcus are the commonest causes of purulent meningitis. *Haemophilus influenzae* used to be an important causal pathogen but is now rare following widespread infant immunisation with Hib vaccine.

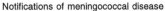
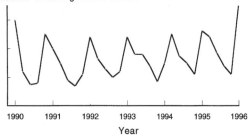

Meningococcal disease is commoner in the winter months and in children under 5 years of age (data from Communicable Disease Report 7 – 1977)

Notifications of meningococcal disease

1990   1991   1992   1993   1994   1995   1996
Year

Tests for neck stiffness— gently

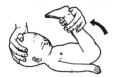

Tests for neck stiffness - gently

Clinical presentation. The characteristic features of meningeal irritation, neck stiffness and Kernig sign, are often absent in children under 18 months of age. Such young infants are more likely to present with a fever, poor feeding, vomiting and drowsiness. Some in this age group have a convulsion as the first sign of illness. An infant who has a fever with convulsion almost invariably warrants a lumbar puncture because of the difficulty of excluding meningitis on clinical grounds in this age group.

Children with meningococcal infections often have a widespread purpuric rash and are liable to develop septicaemic shock. Purpura in a febrile child suggests meningococcal septicaemia and must always be regarded seriously, because treatment should be commenced as soon as possible.

Diagnostic traps abound. The development of a complicating meningitis may be the reason why a child with an otitis media or other upper respiratory tract infection fails to respond to an antibiotic and becomes increasingly drowsy. On the other hand, children with an upper respiratory tract infection, cervical lymphadenitis or pneumonia may show meningismus, that is they have the signs of meningeal irritation in the absence of meningitis. Lumbar puncture is not always without risk in the child with meningitis, indeed in certain rare instances it is considered too dangerous and treatment is started after blood cultures have been taken.

Lumbar puncture

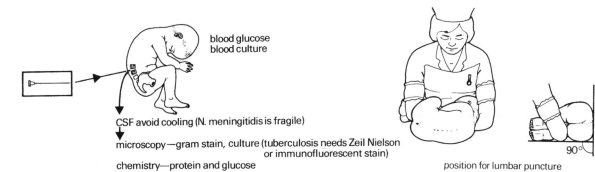

blood glucose
blood culture

CSF avoid cooling (N. meningitidis is fragile)

microscopy—gram stain, culture (tuberculosis needs Zeil Nielson or immunofluorescent stain)

chemistry—protein and glucose

position for lumbar puncture

90°

Treatment. For children older than 3 months intravenous treatment with a third generation cephalosporin such as cefotaxime 200 mg/kg/day is appropriate until the microorganism and its antibiotic sensitivities have been identified. *Haemophilus influenzae* is normally sensitive to cefotaxime but requires this dosage to be maintained for at least 10 days. *Neisseria meningitidis* and *Diplococcus pneumoniae* are usually very sensitive to parenteral benzylpenicillin, which is given in a dose of 300 mg/kg/day for 10 days. Prophylactic treatment with rifampicin to eradicate nasopharyngeal carriage and minimise the risk of contact cases is required for the index case and household contacts of all cases of meningococcal meningitis and those cases of *H. influenzae* meningitis where there is a child under 3 years of age in the household.

Cerebrospinal fluid findings in meningitis

	Normal*	Acute purulent meningitis	Aseptic (viral) meningitis	Tuberculous meningitis
Appearance	clear	cloudy	usually clear	opalescent
Cells/mm³	0–5 lymphocytes	10–100 000 polymorphs	15–2000 lymphocytes	250–500 lymphocytes
Glucose (mmol/l)	2.8–4.4 (CSF > 60% blood)	low (CSF < 60% blood)	normal (CSF > 60% blood)	very low (CSF < 60% blood)
Protein (g/l)	0.15–0.35	0.5–5.0	0.2–1.25	0.45–5.00

*In the postnatal period normal CSF contains a higher cell and protein content

Complications. Meningitis may be complicated by convulsions which require treatment with anti-epileptic drugs. Inappropriate anti-diuretic hormone release often accompanies intracranial problems and can lead to hyponatraemia which may be prevented by careful restriction of intravenous and oral fluids. Subdural effusions are probably frequent but the majority are small and insignificant. Occasionally, an enlarging head circumference and bulging fontanelle suggest a larger accumulation. This may be visualised by ultrasound, CT or MRI scanning, and confirmed by performing a subdural tap when a fluid containing a high protein content can be aspirated. A rapidly increasing head circumference may also be a consequence of hydrocephalus due to inflammatory obstruction of the CSF pathways. About 10% of all children surviving meningitis have long-term neurological abnormality; convulsions, deafness, spasticity, mental handicap or other learning difficulties. Recurrent meningitis raises the possibility of a congenital midline sinus, or a post-traumatic dural defect providing communication with an air sinus. An immune deficiency should also be considered.

Neonatal meningitis

This affects 1 in every 4000 babies. It is a very serious illness and is usually due to *E. coli* or group B haemolytic streptococci. It has a high mortality and a majority of survivors have some neurological sequelae. Therapy must be directed towards the ventriculitis which is usually associated. Systemic treatment must be with drugs like chloramphenicol or cefotaxime which are known to produce good concentrations in ventricular CSF.

Viral meningitis

Viral meningitis is commoner than realised, as mild asymptomatic meningeal inflammation may be part of many systemic viral infections. It can be accompanied by a macular rash or preceded by upper respiratory tract or gastrointestinal complaints. The symptoms of viral meningitis (headache and neck stiffness) are usually less abrupt and milder than those of acute purulent meningitis, and drowsiness is not usually a feature. CSF examination and culture are obviously essential to make the distinction. Serial viral titres, nasopharyngeal and rectal swabs may identify the virus.

Tuberculous meningitis

Tuberculous meningitis must be considered in every case of aseptic meningitis or encephalitis. It follows the rupture of a tubercle (Rich focus) into the CSF and evolves as the resulting inflammatory reaction and arteritis develops. The CSF examination is not always diagnostic in early cases. A tuberculin skin test is positive in 75% and a chest X-ray shows a suggestive lesion in 80%. Treatment is dealt with in the section dealing with tuberculosis and may have to be started when the diagnosis is just suspected, as any delay can be critical.

Brain abscess

This is a relatively rare condition, and there is usually a predisposing cause. Although it is essential to consider lumbar puncture in every child at risk of having intracranial infection, this procedure should be deferred if there are features of a space-occupying lesion and a CT or MR scan obtained in the first instance.

Encephalitis

Encephalitis produces fever, disturbed consciousness, convulsions and focal neurological signs. The majority of cases are viral and there may also be features of meningitis (meningoencephalitis) or spinal cord involvement (encephalomyelitis). Direct viral invasion of the brain results in inflammation and destruction of grey matter mainly. Systemic virus infections which do not invade the brain may nevertheless provoke an immunologically mediated demyelination of cerebral white matter (post-infectious encephalomyelitis).

An encephalitis-like illness without fever or cells in the CSF raises the possibility of a 'toxic' or metabolic encephalopathy. Lead poisoning and drug ingestion must always be considered.

Brain abscess

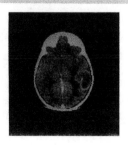

Herpes simplex encephalitis. This is the most common sporadic severe encephalitis. Only 10–15% have associated herpetic gingivostomatitis or skin lesions. Focal seizures and neurological signs are frequent and may suggest a temporal lobe space-occupying lesion.

The untreated mortality rate is 70% and neurological sequelae are frequent in the survivors. The CSF contains a variably elevated lymphocyte count and may be blood stained. Electroencephalography and CT or MR scanning help to distinguish this encephalitis from a cerebral abscess or tumour. The development of successful anti-herpes virus therapy, acyclovir, has emphasised the need for prompt treatment whenever the disease is suspected. Diagnosis can be made by polymerase chain reaction (PCR) for herpes virus DNA in the acute stage or later by showing increasing antibody titres to herpes simplex in blood and CSF.

The more common varieties of post-infectious encephalitis are measles 1 in 1000 cases, varicella 1 in 1000 cases, rubella 1 in 5000 cases, and (in the past) vaccinia 1 in 100 000 immunisations.

Measles encephalitis. This commences with irritability, drowsiness and multiple seizures 2–4 days after the appearance of the rash. The EEG shows a severe diffuse abnormality. The course varies from complete recovery in a few days to death in status epilepticus or grossly impaired recovery. There is no specific treatment.

Subacute sclerosing panencephalitis (SSPE) is a prototype of human slow virus infection and is now recognised as a late complication of measles. The disease may progress over a period of years or death can occur as soon as 6 weeks after onset. The persistence of virus in the brain may be due to a defective immune response when measles is acquired at an early age. It enters the differential diagnosis of degenerative brain disorders.

Varicella. This causes a relatively benign encephalitis, often an acute self-limiting cerebellar ataxia, although occasionally it can be more serious.

Reye syndrome. This refers to the association of acute encephalopathy with brain swelling and diffuse fatty infiltration of the liver. Viral infections, particularly influenza B and varicella, have been linked in some cases. Aspirin has also been causally implicated so that this drug is now no longer given to children for intercurrent febrile illnesses. Vomiting or symptoms of an upper respiratory tract infection often precede the onset of lethargy and seizures and hyperventilation frequently accompanies the increasing coma. A CT or MR scan shows cerebral oedema. CSF cells and protein are normal though lumbar puncture is best avoided if Reye syndrome is suspected because of the risk of coning. Clinical jaundice does not occur but a prolonged prothrombin time and elevated aminotransferases and ammonia in the blood give evidence of liver involvement. Blood and CSF glucose levels are sometimes reduced. The treatment of Reye syndrome is aimed at reducing the raised intracranial pressure by hyperventilation, hypothermia and osmotherapy. Mortality is 40% but the majority of survivors are neurologically intact.

NEUROMUSCULAR DISORDERS

Lower motor neurone and muscle disorders present as floppiness, delayed motor milestones, abnormal gait or progressive muscle weakness.

Muscle disorders

The muscular dystrophies are characterised by progressive degeneration of certain groups of skeletal muscles and are hereditary. A number of different forms have been distinguished on clinical and genetic grounds. Muscular dystrophy is the commonest cause of muscle disease in childhood.

Duchenne muscular dystrophy. This is the commonest and most serious type of muscular dystrophy with 1 in 3000 boys affected. A gene deletion at site 21 on the short arm of the X chromosome (Xp21) can be demonstrated with molecular genetic techniques in about 60% of boys with Duchenne dystrophy. This site is known as the dystrophin gene as it codes for the protein dystrophin which is present in all normal muscle cells. Dystrophin is absent in the muscle cells of boys with Duchenne dystrophy. Inheritance is as an X-linked recessive but new mutations are frequent and said to be responsible for 30% of isolated cases. The female carriers are usually asymptomatic.

Symptoms appear in the first 5 years of life and consist of delayed walking, frequent falls, a lordotic waddling gait and difficulty climbing stairs. Prominence of the calf muscles is an early feature and is called 'pseudo-hypertrophy' because the muscles though enlarged are weak. Due to weakness of the gluteal muscles, boys with this condition climb up their legs when they rise from the lying position (Gower sign).

The diagnosis of Duchenne dystrophy is made by finding a serum creatine kinase 10–200 times higher than normal, myopathic changes on electromyography and characteristic muscle biopsy features including absence of dystrophin staining. It is important to consider

Gower sign

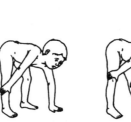
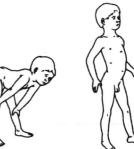

Duchenne dystrophy in any boy with unexplained generalised developmental delay or delayed walking past 18 months. The serum creatine kinase is always very elevated before muscular weakness becomes clinically evident and is a useful screening test in such cases.

Most of these boys are unable to walk by the age of 8–11 years and then become wheelchair dependent. They often develop scoliosis and an equinus deformity of the feet due to muscular weakness and imbalance. The pseudohypertrophy is replaced by muscle wasting. Respiratory infections precipitate death by age 15–25 years. Intellectual development is usually normal but there is a slightly increased frequency of learning difficulties.

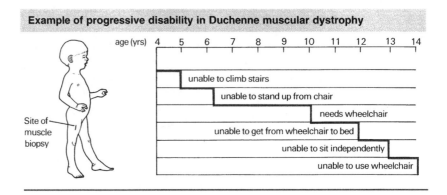

Example of progressive disability in Duchenne muscular dystrophy

Genetic counselling is important in Duchenne dystrophy, and female carriers may be detected by finding a moderately raised serum creatine kinase. When a woman is thought to be a carrier, prenatal diagnosis is usually possible by amniocentesis or chorionic villus biopsy. This is particularly true if the index case shows an Xp21 deletion.

Becker muscular dystrophy. This is a milder form of sex-linked recessive muscular dystrophy with a later onset of clinical muscle weakness. Becker dystrophy is now known to be allelic with the gene for Duchenne dystrophy. Muscle dystrophin is present in Becker dystrophy but reduced in amount.

Facioscapulohumeral muscular dystrophy. This has an autosomal dominant pattern of inheritance and presents in late childhood or early adolescence. There may be a marked variation in the severity of the disease within affected families. Shoulder girdle weakness is an early feature followed by facial involvement and inability to close the eyes tightly. Winging of the scapulae is another feature. This condition has a very slow progression and may be compatible with a normal life span.

Limb girdle dystrophy. This type of progressive muscular dystrophy is inherited as an autosomal recessive so that girls are affected as well as boys. The pelvic girdle muscles are more affected than the shoulder girdle muscles. It may mimic Duchenne dystrophy in a boy but muscle dystrophin is normal.

Myotonic dystrophy. This was previously considered to be a disease of adult life but it is now realised that onset in childhood may occur. It differs from the other muscular dystrophies, not only in the presence of myotonia, but also because of the involvement of other systems. Both males and females are affected and the inheritance is autosomal dominant. Recently it has been shown to be due to an abnormally large triple repeat (CTG) on chromosome 19.

The muscle weakness characteristically involves the facial and neck muscles producing a myopathic facies, ptosis, an open mouth and a sagging jaw. Myotonia is seen as delayed opening of the eyes after closure or difficulty in relaxing the grasp. Distal limb weakness may also be present. Other features which may occur include cardiac involvement, cataracts, testicular atrophy and diabetes mellitus.

In the congenital form infants are very floppy and have feeding and respiratory difficulties. Some die in the newborn period, Those who survive show considerable recovery in muscle tone and strength, although the majority have significant learning difficulties. It is of interest that in almost every congenital case the mother is the affected parent.

Congenital myopathies. These are a complex group of disorders which can only be characterised after detailed examination of muscle obtained at biopsy, for example central core disease and nemaline myopathy.

Metabolic myopathies. There are a number of rare metabolic disorders affecting muscle, for example type II glycogen storage disease due to acid maltase deficiency is an autosomal recessive condition in which muscle weakness is a major feature. In the infantile form (Pompe disease) infants present with cardiomyopathy, and gross hypotonia. The majority die before 18 months.

Acquired muscle disease

Dermatomyositis. This inflammatory disorder of muscle is rare in childhood. It is characterised by generalised proximal muscle weakness and a violaceous discolouration of the skin, especially over the butterfly area of the face, eyelids, elbows, knees and knuckles. The child is usually miserable and may be febrile. Blood creatine kinase is elevated and the ESR is sometimes raised. EMG shows myopathic changes and an inflammatory cell infiltrate is seen in muscle obtained at biopsy. Treatment with corticosteroids often produces a permanent remission.

Neuromuscular junction

Myasthenia gravis. This is now recognised as being an autoimmune disorder and is associated with circulating antibodies to acetylcholine receptors. It is more common in girls. The onset is usually gradual with ptosis, strabismus, difficulty in chewing, loss of facial expression and arm weakness. The weakness may be very variable and is characteristically induced by fatigue. The diagnosis is confirmed by showing prompt improvement after intravenous edrophonium. The treatment of myasthenia involves the use of long-acting anticholinesterase drugs such as neostigmine or pyridostigmine. Thymectomy may have a place. Infants born to mothers with myasthenia gravis are susceptible to a transient form of the illness due to transplacental antibody transfer.

Nerve fibre disorders

Infectious polyneuritis (Guillain–Barré syndrome). This presents as a rapidly evolving symmetrical flaccid paralysis of the legs, but trunk and arms usually become involved. Respiratory and facial muscles may be affected. The weakness is commonly preceded by symptoms suggestive of viral infection. The CSF typically shows a considerable elevation of protein but no cellular response. The weakness progresses over a matter of days and then remains stationary for some weeks before entering a slow recovery phase. Severe cases may be treated with intravenous gammaglobulin infusion which has been shown to improve the rate of recovery. A period of ventilation is required for respiratory paralysis in 10% of cases. Most children make a full recovery but this can take up to a year. It is essential to distinguish spinal cord disorders, which may need surgical treatment, from acute infectious polyneuritis.

Anterior horn cell disorders

Werdnig–Hoffman disease. This is the severe infantile type of spinal muscular atrophy (SMA) and has an incidence of 1 in 20 000 births. It is inherited as an autosomal recessive and recently has been found to be due to deletion of the SMN gene on chromosome 5. Mothers may notice poor fetal movements and the infants can be floppy and weak at birth. Symptoms are always present within the first few months of life. In spite of the extreme muscle weakness, the infants are alert and watchful. Muscle fasciculation, especially in the tongue, can be a feature. The diagnosis is made by electromyography and muscle biopsy. The condition is progressive and usually leads to death from respiratory failure before 18 months of age.

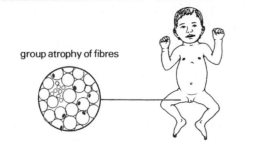

Werdnig–Hoffman disease: clinical features and muscle biopsy appearance

group atrophy of fibres

alert facial expression
fasciculation of tongue

deformed chest
see-saw respiration

frog position
absent reflexes

There are milder forms of spinal muscular atrophy with later onset, for example the Kugelberg–Welander syndrome (chronic spinal muscular atrophy).

Floppy infant syndrome

The term floppy infant describes babies who have marked hypotonia. A useful test is to hold the baby in ventral suspension. A floppy baby will drape over the hands like a rag doll whereas a normal baby will show postural tone appropriate to his age. Severe muscle weakness in addition to hypotonia suggests a neuromuscular disorder. Hypotonia in the absence of obvious muscle weakness suggests a non-paralytic cause for floppiness.

Hypotonia

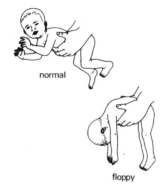

normal

floppy

Paralytic and non-paralytic causes of floppiness in infants	
Paralytic	Non-paralytic—examples
Neuromuscular disorders **Spinal cord lesions** birth trauma	**Brain disorders** cerebral palsy degenerative CNS disease Prader–Willi syndrome **Chromosomal disorders** Down syndrome **Systemic disorders** malnutrition congenital heart disease hypothyroidism **Connective tissue disorders** osteogenesis imperfecta **Benign hypotonia**

BIBLIOGRAPHY

Brett E 1997 Paediatric neurology, 3rd edn. Churchill Livingstone, Edinburgh
Dubowitz V 1995 Muscle disorders in childhood, 2nd edn. WB Saunders, Philadelphia
Levene M I, Bennet M J, Punt J (eds) 1995 Fetal and neonatal neurology and neurosurgery, 2nd edn. Churchill Livingstone, Edinburgh
O'Donohoe N V 1994 Epilepsies of childhood, 3rd edn. Butterworth-Heinemann, Oxford
Scrutton D (ed) 1984 Management of motor disorders of children with cerebral palsy. Spastics International Medical Publications, London

20 Seeing, hearing, speaking, and learning

SEEING

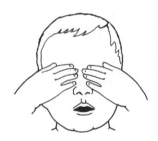

Vision is the most highly evolved of man's special senses. Binocular stereoscopic perception and interpretation requires not only an exact optic mechanism but also complex neural interconnections. The retina and eye are relatively mature at birth, and 75% of post-natal ocular growth occurs in the first 3 years of life. Myelination of the optic pathways is, however, still incomplete at term, and experimental work has recently confirmed the clinical impression that normal development of the optic radiation and visual cortex is dependent on undistorted light reception. It is therefore essential to act promptly when, for example, a severe ptosis or a cataract threatens the visual development of a newborn infant.

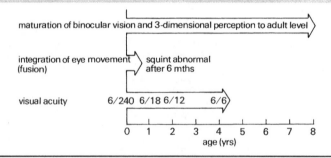

The development of vision

maturation of binocular vision and 3-dimensional perception to adult level

integration of eye movement (fusion) — squint abnormal after 6 mths

visual acuity — 6/240 6/18 6/12 6/6

0 1 2 3 4 5 6 7 8
age (yrs)

Assessment of vision

Before the age of 6 months, vision may be assessed by the response to a moving face, a slowly moving ball and by attention to hand–eye skills. By 6 weeks of age all babies should show clear evidence of visual fixation with some following provided they are not sleepy or upset. Vision must always be considered in the context of general development. Quantification of visual acuity is possible in infancy using a preferential looking test in which the baby is presented a striped and a uniformly grey target simultaneously. Targets with narrower stripes are presented until the baby no longer gives them preferential attention compared with the uniformly grey target. After 3 years single letter Stycar letter matching cards and after 5 years Stycar letter charts can be used. The Stycar letters have been specially selected as those which cause young children least confusion. Adult type Snellen charts can be used after 7 years.

The assessment of vision

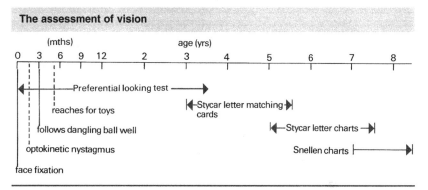

Squints

Testing for a squint

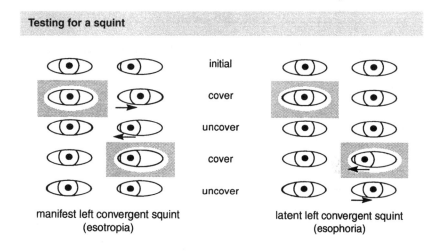

manifest left convergent squint
(esotropia)

latent left convergent squint
(esophoria)

Squints are common in early childhood. A fixed squint at any age and a variable squint which persists to age 6 months requires careful evaluation. Having detected a squint, expert assessment involves full examination of the eyes to exclude, for example corneal opacities, cataracts and refractive errors. The usual cause of infantile strabismus is an ill-understood failure to develop binocular fusion at the normal time. Other important causes include refractive errors, particularly hypermetropia and astigmatism, neurological disorders which interfere with the normal function of the extraocular muscles, and eye diseases such as cataracts or retinoblastoma. Whatever the cause, the image of the squinting eye is suppressed thereby avoiding diplopia, but if neglected, this may lead to an irreversible failure of development of the visual cortical neurones related to the squinting eye (amblyopia).

The blind child

For educational purposes a child is defined as blind if he requires education by methods which do not involve sight, for example Braille, and as partially sighted if he requires special educational consideration but can use methods which depend on sight, for example large print books. In practice, most blind children have some vision even if it is only recognition of light and dark, or perception of shapes.

In the United Kingdom about 500 children each year are newly registered blind or partially sighted, a prevalence of approximately 1 in 2500 children, but the true prevalence may be higher because of incomplete registration. As many as 50% of blind children have additional handicaps, for example physical disability, learning disorder, hearing and language difficulties. In their survey of visual handicap, Schappert-Kimmijser et al (1975) reported that the main causes of visual handicap in childhood were optic atrophy (18%), congenital cataracts (16%) and choroidoretinal degenerations (15%). Overall the conditions causing visual handicap were genetically determined in 45% of children and due to some perinatal disturbance in 33%. The incidence of retinopathy of prematurity dramatically decreased in the early 1960s, possibly due to greater care when giving oxygen therapy in the newborn period.

Causes of childhood visual handicap

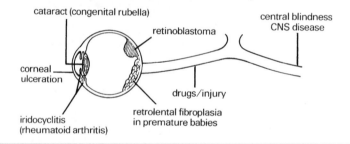

Blindness must be suspected when an infant shows pendular nystagmus or roving, purposeless eye movements. Normal children cease to show uncoordinated eye movements by 6 weeks of age. Some blind children poke their eyes in a characteristic fashion, probably to produce pleasurable visual hallucinations of retinal origin (phosphenes).

With the exception of cataracts, most causes of blindness in children are not amenable to medical treatment. Recent advances in cataract surgery allow early removal of a congenital cataract and the immediate provision of a lens implant or contact lens thereby avoiding stimulus deprivation amblyopia.

Parents of a blind child need expert, sympathetic advice from a very early stage. Peripatetic preschool teachers from the Royal National Institute for the Blind or local education authority fulfil this role in the United Kingdom. The parents must be taught to stimulate their infant using non-visual means, touch and speech. The home should be adapted so that the child can explore his environment safely. Residential school may sometimes be necessary for the blind child who needs to learn Braille. The child with partial sight is usually managed in an ordinary school with the support of a special teacher.

HEARING

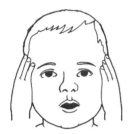

Hearing refers to the reception of sounds, their transduction to nerve impulses and transmission to the relevant areas of the cerebral cortex. Listening implies an attention to the sounds and their interpretation and is a prerequisite for language development. The fetus is sensitive to noise and from the moment of birth there is an important sound interplay between mother and infant. Hearing provides for emotional contact, language development, identity with the environment and assists in the awareness of posture and body orientation. All children should be screened for deafness by tests which are appropriate to their stage of development and it is usual for these tests to be performed at 6–9 months of age, and again at the preschool examination.

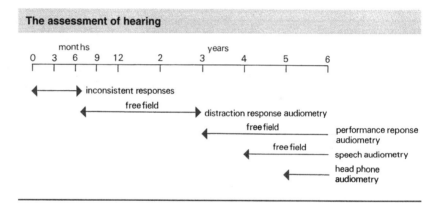

The assessment of hearing

Assessment of hearing

Babies up to about 7 months show inconsistent responses to noises and reliable testing can only be done with sophisticated apparatus such as brainstem evoked response audiometry. From 7 months infants will turn their head and eyes towards the source of a quiet sound (distraction responses). It is essential to have a contented child in a quiet room. The examiner stands 1–3 feet (0.30–0.90 m) to the side of the child and just outside his range of vision. The sound stimulus should be given at ear level. Sound makers employed are a high pitched rattle, spoon in cup, tissue paper, hand bell and selected speech sounds, for example 'oo' and 'ss'. A free field pure tone audiometer may be used to generate the sound stimuli. From 3 years, a child will play a game of putting a toy in a box whenever he hears the sound (performance responses). From 4 years, picture cards or toys can be used. The child is asked in a quiet voice to show the examiner a certain picture or toy from an array in front of him (speech audiometry). Most children of 5 years and over will tolerate wearing headphones and give reliable pure tone audiograms showing both air and bone conduction thresholds.

The final proof of adequate hearing is the imitation and comprehension of normal speech. Although pure tone audiometry has a place in defining the hearing of children, it cannot replace clinical speech tests.

Causes of childhood deafness

Conductive deafness (4% of school children)	Sensorineural deafness (0.3% of school children)	
Glue ear following otitis media (almost all cases)	Genetic—various types 50%	
	Intrauterine (8%)	congenital infection, e.g. rubella maternal drugs, e.g. streptomycin
	Perinatal (12%)	birth asphyxia severe hyperbilirubinaemia
	Postnatal (30%)	meningitis encephalitis head injury

Types of deafness

Whereas hearing loss of up to 20 dB normally has little effect on the child's development, a loss of over 40 dB creates problems in the development of ordinary speech. Testing over a range of frequencies may show a widespread loss or a loss purely in the high frequency zone. Deafness is classified into two categories, sensorineural and conductive. In sensorineural deafness there is damage to the cochlea or auditory nerve whereas in the conductive type there is middle ear dysfunction. Most severe deafness in children is sensorineural in type and is present from birth. The two types of deafness can be distinguished in older children by pure tone headphone audiometry. In the sensorineural type, there is equal impairment of bone and air conduction of sound; in the conductive type, there is an air–bone gap with bone conduction hearing better than air conduction.

Four per cent of all schoolchildren have mild deafness, usually a conductive middle ear deafness due to glue ear. Two in every 1000 children have moderate deafness sufficient to require them to use a hearing aid, and one child in every 1000 is severely deaf and requires special education.

Treatment of deafness

More careful management and follow up of children susceptible to otitis media may reduce the incidence of glue ear. In established cases of glue ear the deafness is usually reversed by aeration of the middle ear by means of a grommet inserted into the tympanic membrane, and removal of hypertrophied adenoids which may block the eustachian tubes

Audiograms: three patterns of hearing loss

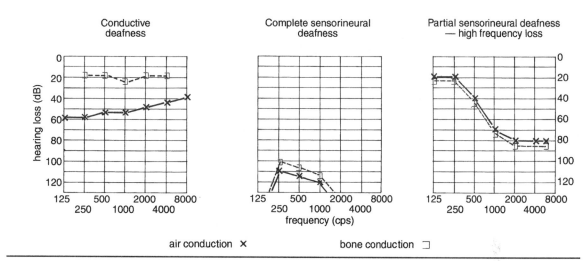

air conduction ✕   bone conduction ☐

There is no specific therapy for sensorineural deafness apart from cochlear implant surgery which is only suitable for a minority of such children. If there is some residual hearing, a hearing aid is useful. This is simply a device for amplifying sounds within the frequency range of the spoken voice. There are problems in that the receiver is not selective and is liable to cause distressing exaggeration of environmental and background noises, for example rustling clothes. Careful instruction in its use is required as well as attention to such items as the ear moulds. It must be emphasised that the provision of an aid is only part of a more general process of rehabilitation and education. Parents of the young deaf child need expert guidance on how to encourage him to talk and develop language. Such help is given by the peripatetic teacher of the deaf. Learning a sign language for the deaf is now considered valuable and is not thought to interfere with the development of oral speech. Many moderately deaf children can attend a normal school, but the more severely affected require specialist education, either at a school for the deaf or in a partial hearing unit attached to a normal school. As genetic causes are present in 50% of children with sensorineural deafness, genetic counselling is often indicated.

SPEAKING

Language is essential to our culture as it provides the symbolic code for communication and for our thought processes. The early development of vocalisation (exploratory sounds) and verbalisation (meaningful sounds) is closely linked to the development of hearing and listening. There is a wide age range among normal children for the development of vocabulary.

Some children with slow speech and language development may be excellent at non-verbal communication and clearly have a well

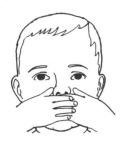

developed inner language. In others, there may be much more profound disturbance affecting all aspects of communication. Occasionally in a child with speech delay, the physiological mechanisms for speech development are considered to be intact but progress with speech and language is hindered by detrimental family relationships, social factors or psychiatric disturbances. It is recognised for example that children in institutional care may have delayed speech development and this is probably due the fact that relationships with carers cannot be expected to be as nurturing as those with natural parents.

Assessment of speech

Speech development must be considered in the context of the wide range of normal development. The parents of the 2-year-old boy with obviously normal development but a vocabulary of only 10–20 words may be comparing him with the little girl of similar age down the road with a vocabulary of 200 words. Both are within the normal range. Assessment must consider general development as well as environmental factors. Comprehension and free conversation during play are useful guides before embarking on more specific diagnostic exercises. An experienced speech therapist plays a valuable role in assessing and treating these children, and will be able to make a distinction between comprehension and expressive speech and language delay. It is essential to make sure hearing is normal in any child who is showing delayed speech development.

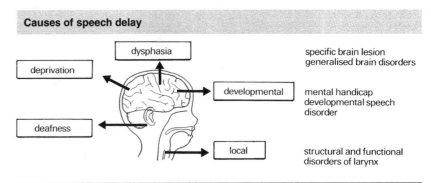

Causes of speech delay

The developmental speech and language disorder syndrome

About 6% of 3-to 4-year-old children show significant delay in speech and language development. In half of these children the cause is cerebral palsy, deafness or an underlying general learning disability. The remainder have a developmental speech and language disorder syndrome. It is more common in boys and there is often a family history. With the help of speech therapy the majority eventually catch up with speech and language development but some of these show later difficulties with reading and spelling (dyslexia). Only a minority, perhaps 1 in 1000 of all children, continue to have major problems with speech and language in later childhood, and the term developmental dysphasia is sometimes used for them. Such children require specialised teaching and may benefit from learning a non-verbal form of communication such as the Bliss or Paget–Gorman systems.

Dysrhythmia (stammering)   It is common for children between 3 and 4 years of age to have a so-called physiological stammer. This usually corrects itself spontaneously and must not be made a focus of attention. A more persistent stammering or stuttering has a familial predisposition. In younger children, therapy is largely directed towards diverting attention away from the speech difficulty with the expectation of spontaneous improvement. In older children, more formal exercises such as syllable timed speech may be necessary for the most disruptive cases.

LEARNING

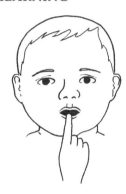

The level of medical care provided within a community may be assessed by the prevalence, identification and care of those who have a severe learning disorder. Better services result both in fewer people being affected, and in the early recognition of those who are affected due to the effects of deleterious genetic, environmental and social factors. The care offered must also be as supportive and humane as the community can afford.

The words used to describe learning disordered children have changed with the years for they quickly become terms of abuse (e.g. moron, idiot, cretin, mongol). Recently the terms 'mental retardation' and 'mental handicap' have been largely replaced by 'learning disability' or 'learning disorder'. Children with severe learning disability have difficulty in learning to walk, dress, feed and communicate. The more mildly affected have difficulty acquiring the skills required to look after themselves and earn a living when they reach adulthood.

Aspects of mental ability or intelligence can be measured by a variety of tests. They measure what an individual has achieved at the time of the assessment and, although they may be a guide to what he might achieve, they do not necessarily measure potential reliably. The results of the tests are expressed as a quotient, the child's 'mental' age over chronological age. The distribution of intelligence follows a Gaussian or normal distribution with a distortion in the lower range due to the effects of deleterious genetic, environmental and social factors. Fetal and early infant death counteracts some of this distortion.

It is helpful to divide children with learning disability into two groups, moderate and severe. The moderately handicapped have IQs between 50 and 70 which represents the lower end of the normal distribution range. Children with moderate learning disorder tend to come from families of lower ability and poorer social background. The severely handicapped with IQs below 50 more often have some underlying organic disorder, for example a recognised inherited metabolic disorder or a brain malformation syndrome, and there is little correlation with social class. Obviously there is some overlap in these respects between the moderate and severe groups.

Causes   The following list emphasises the extensive number of disorders which may contribute to learning disability; each chapter in this book contains problems which may produce this end result.

A classification of the recognised causes of learning disability

Causes of mental handicap	Examples
A Genetic	
• Chromosomal disorder	Trisomy, e.g. Down syndrome Deletion, e.g. cri du chat syndrome Sex chromosome anomaly, e.g. fragile X syndrome
• Metabolic disorder	Amino acid, e.g. phenylketonuria Carbohydrate, e.g. galactosaemia Organic acid, e.g. isovaleric acidaemia
• Cerebral degenerative disorder	Gangliosidoses Lipidoses Mucopolysaccharidoses Leucodystrophies
• Structural disorders	Tuberous sclerosis Familial hydrocephalus
B Intrauterine	
• Nutritional deficiency	Iodine deficiency
• Congenital infection	Cytomegalovirus Rubella Toxoplasmosis
• Drugs	Phenytoin, alcohol
• Cerebral malformations	Holoprosencephaly, lissencephaly
C Perinatal	
• Problems during pregnancy	Pre-eclamptic toxaemia Antepartum haemorrhage Premature onset of labour
• Problems during labour and delivery	Prolonged labour Fetal distress Trauma Asphyxia
• Neonatal problems	Intraventricular haemorrhage Hypoglycaemia Meningitis Severe hyperbilirubinaemia
D Postnatal	
• Trauma	Accidental or non-accidental injury
• Infection	Encephalitis, meningitis
• Anoxia	Asphyxia, status epilepticus, near drowning
• Metabolic and endocrine	Hypoglycaemia, hypernatraemia, hypothyroidism
• Poisoning	Lead, carbon monoxide
• Psychological	Infantile psychosis/autism

Identification

Routine developmental checks should be available for all infants, and for those where suspicion arises there must be ready access to specialist assessment. It is important that prompt, confident reassurance is given to the parents of children who demonstrate innocent variation of development, and that sensitive explanation is provided where abnormality is likely.

Following careful assessment, the cause of severe learning disorder will be found in roughly 80% of cases. The history, examination and investigations may all contribute to the diagnosis. Cerebral palsy although strictly not a cause of mental handicap is an associated finding in 25% of severely mentally handicapped children. A number of dysmorphic syndromes are associated with learning disorder. A single minor anomaly, for example a single palmar crease or low set ears, is relatively common and occurs in 14% of newborn infants, but the presence of three or four minor anomalies carries a 90% risk of an associated major defect including learning disorder. Particular attention should be paid to eyes, ears, palate, hair pattern, hands and feet. There are invaluable reference atlases which link such features with defined dysmorphic syndromes.

Congenital hypothyroidism and phenylketonuria should not cause learning disorder nowadays as they are diagnosed by routine neonatal screening tests and treated before they cause permanent damage. Progressive deterioration in performance emphasises the need to look for metabolic, storage or neurodegenerative disorders. Modern techniques and the identification of specific enzyme deficiencies have improved the yield of such investigations.

Management

Getting dressed

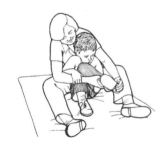

Domestic skills

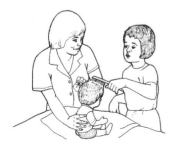

Children with learning disorders and their families require a multidisciplinary approach. In addition to general assessment, the child's social, motor, language, hearing and visual abilities must all be considered. A therapeutic programme must begin as early as possible with parents playing an active role together with physiotherapists, speech therapists, and play counsellors. Health visitors and social workers assist the parents in coming to terms with their problems and advise on financial and equipment help. Seizure disorders and behavioural problems may require specific drug therapy.

The Education Act of 1970 legislated for special schools to be available for all handicapped children. More recently the 1981 Education Act established the basis for a more enlightened framework, moving away from traditional categories of handicap and promoting more integration with normal schoolchildren in mainstream schools. Although special schools are classified as dealing with moderate learning disordered (MLD) children or severe learning disordered (SLD) children, the system has to be flexible to accommodate coexisting physical problems. Some children with IQs in the 50–70 range benefit from the high staff : pupil ratio available in MLD schools. On leaving school 80% of MLD children are capable of open occupation and the remainder may be provided with employment in sheltered workshops. SLD children rarely become independent and in adult life may need help with the routine activities of daily living such as dressing and feeding. Education at SLD schools is primarily aimed at training the children to become as socially competent as possible. As the children become older parents may find it increasingly difficult to look after them. Up to the age of 20 years only a minority of such young people are in residential care but after this age the proportion increases rapidly. Residential facilities vary considerably but there is a tendency towards smaller units which attempt to retain the family structure and links with the surrounding community. Those remaining at home usually attend a day centre run by the local social services department. Community based learning disability teams play a major role in the provision of services for adults with severe learning disorder and their carers.

Features on history, examination and investigations which may identify the cause of mental handicap

Historical items

Family history of affected males	fragile X syndrome
Maternal alcoholism	fetal alcohol syndrome
Light for dates	placental dysfunction, congenital infections
Pica	lead poisoning
Deterioration	cerebral degenerative disorder

Clinical findings

Floppy infant	Prader–Willi syndrome, congenital myotonic dystrophy, Down syndrome
Obesity	pseudohypoparathyroidism, Prader–Willi syndrome
Funny smell	organic acidurias, maple syrup urine disease
Cerebral palsy	perinatal asphyxia
Hepatosplenomegaly	Niemann–Pick disease, Gaucher disease, Hurler syndrome
Cardiac abnormalities	Down syndrome, congenital rubella, infantile hypercalcaemia
Coarse facies	hypothyroidism, mucopolysaccharidoses
Deafness	congenital rubella, mucopolysaccharidoses
Large head	Soto syndrome, hydrocephalus, neurofibromatosis, mucopolysaccharidoses
Microcephaly	Congenital infections, maternal phenylketonuria, fetal alcohol syndrome, Smith–Lemli–Opitz syndrome, perinatal asphyxia, genetic microcephaly
Large fontanelles	pseudohypoparathyroidism
Hypertelorism	agenesis of the corpus collosum, cri du chat syndrome
Hypotelorism	holoprosencephaly
Slanted palpebral fissures	Down syndrome
Synophrys (eyebrows meeting)	DeLange syndrome
Congenital ptosis	Smith–Lemli–Opitz syndrome
Cataracts	congenital rubella, galactosaemia
Corneal opacities	mucopolysaccharide disorder
Lens dislocation	homocystinuria
Retinal pigmentation	Laurence–Moon–Biedl syndrome, congenital rubella, Leber amaurosis
Hypopigmented macules	tuberous sclerosis
Café au lait patches	neurofibromatosis
Port wine stains on face	Sturge–Weber syndrome
Pigment whorls	incontinentia pigmenti
Hirsutism	DeLange syndrome, mucopolysaccharidoses
Polydactyly	Laurence–Moon–Biedl syndrome
Small hands and feet	Prader–Willi syndrome
Large hands and feet	Soto syndrome
Broad thumbs	Rubenstein–Taybi syndrome
Simian creases	Down syndrome, DeLange syndrome, Smith–Lemli–Opitz syndrome
Joint contractures	mucopolysaccharidoses, sex chromosome disorder
Cryptorchidism	Smith–Lemli–Opitz syndrome, Prader–Willi syndrome
Hypospadias	Smith–Lemli–Opitz syndrome

Investigations

Thyroid function tests	hypothyroidism
Serum and urine aminoacids	aminoacidurias
Blood lead level	lead poisoning
Blood calcium	pseudohypoparathyroidism
Blood acid–base balance	organic acidurias
Chomosome studies	chromosome abnormalities
Skull X-ray	intracranial calcification
CT or MRi scan	cerebral malformation, hydrocephalus, leucodystrophy
White blood cell enzymes	cerebral degenerative disorders

REFERENCE

Schappert-Kimmijser H, Hansen E, Haustrate-Gosser M M, Lindstedt E, Skydsgaard H, Warburg M 1975 Documenta Ophthalmologica 39: 213

BIBLIOGRAPHY

Birch H G, Richardson S A, Baird D, Illsley R 1970 Mental subnormality in the community. A clinical and epidemiological study. Williams and Wilkins, Baltimore
Clarke A M, Clarke A D B, Berg J M 1985 Mental deficiency: the changing outlook, 4th edn. Methuen, London
Craft M, Bicknell D J, Hollins S (eds) 1985 Mental handicap: a multidisciplinary approach. Ballièrie Tindall, London
Haggard M P, Evans E F 1987 Hearing. British Medical Bulletin 43: 775–1042
Heaton-Ward W A, Wiley Y 1984 Mental handicap. Wright, Bristol
Russell O 1985 Mental handicap. Churchill Livingstone, Edinburgh
Yule W, Rutter M 1987 Language development and disorders. Mac Keith Press and Blackwell Science, Oxford

21

Emotions and behaviour

BRAIN DISORDERS
SPECIFIC DEVELOPMENTAL DELAY
INTERACTION BETWEEN THE
   CHILD AND HIS WORLD
BEHAVIOURAL PROBLEMS
EMOTIONAL DISORDERS
MANAGEMENT
MALTREATMENT OF CHILDREN

Until recent years, doctors treating children tended to ignore unusual emotions or deviant behaviours, believing them to be the responsibility of the parents or, if the problem was particularly troublesome, the child psychiatrist, social worker, teacher or the welfare services. However, it is a mistake for a family or hospital doctor caring for children not to have studied the behavioural and emotional disturbances, for on the one hand many childhood illnesses are associated with some disturbance in behaviour, indeed some organic diseases may present with a behaviour problem, and on the other hand children in emotional conflict with themselves or their family or their surroundings may present with symptoms which mimic organic diseases.

Problems with childhood behaviour, or emotions that are severe or prolonged enough to interfere with everyday life are classified as psychiatric disorders. The sociocultural context, and the child's stage of development, must be taken into account when deciding whether or not a symptom is abnormal. In different parts of the world, epidemiological surveys using this definition have reported 1-year prevalence rates of about 1 in 10. Surveys of paediatric patients have shown that about 1 in 4 suffer from a significant psychiatric disorder.

Virtually all the symptoms of psychiatric disturbance in children are non-specific. For example temper tantrums may be a symptom of a mood disorder, such as anxiety or depression. They may also be a sign of disturbed relationships, developmental immaturity or a reaction to a recent stressful event. Of course temper tantrums can be quite normal in preschool children. In view of the non-specificity of symptoms when they are considered in isolation, it is important to look at the total picture. A child who is miserable and seems depressed, but has no other associated symptoms, is unlikely to suffer from a depressive disorder; but a child who is occasionally tearful and at the same time has disturbed sleep and appetite, tends to be irritable and expresses feelings of hopelessness and worthlessness, is very likely to be suffering from a significant depressive disorder. The context in which a symptom occurs is also important. Stealing, for example, may be quite normal if it occurs in the context of a family where antisocial behaviour is considered acceptable, and where the child may have actually been taught how to steal. On the other hand, a 4 year old who takes something valuable without asking can hardly be said to have stolen it, because their sense of moral value is still developing;

People and places

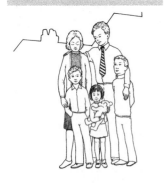

therefore, in the context of the child's developmental stage the stealing does not signify disturbed behaviour.

Child factors that make emotional and behavioural problems more likely to occur

Boys: more likely to develop behavioural problems when younger
Girls: more likely to develop emotional problems when older
Physical illness: especially temporal lobe epilepsy
Difficult temperament
Developmental delay and learning difficulties
Communication problems: deafness or language disorder
Poor self image: low self esteem, feeling of failure
School failure
Poor peer relationships

Family factors that make behavioural and emotional problems more likely to occur

Marital difficulties, separation and divorce
Death: close relative, friend or pet
Poor discipline: inconsistent, unclear or hostile
Rejecting attitudes
Abuse: emotional, physical or sexual
Poverty: poor housing, unemployment
Four or more children in family
Psychiatric illness in the mother
Criminal behaviour in the father

Social and cultural factors that make emotional and behavioural problems more likely to occur

Bullying
Antisocial influences from other children
Disorganisation within the school
Social/cultural expectations
Social policy

Protective factors that make emotional and behavioural problems less likely to occur

Consistent loving relationships
Age appropriate care
Above average ability
Regular adequate income
Stable family relationships
Support for mother outside the family
3 or more years between children

The different factors that work together to cause a child to develop a disturbance of behaviour or emotions usually interact with each other in such a way that the whole is more than the sum of the parts. For example, a child who is physically ill and has missed school may have no problems, but if academic failure results, then the resulting problems may interact with the child's feeling of ill health and produce a low self esteem and a feeling of hopelessness, ultimately leading to a depressive disorder. In this instance, the depression was not caused by the physical illness, or by missing some time from school; it was the way in which these two factors interacted with each other that caused the problem. In reality, these interactions are usually much more complicated, especially where family factors are involved. In order to understand what is happening to a child it is, therefore, important to consider not only the different factors that might be causing the child's disturbance, but also the way in which they interact. An awareness of this interactive process can be helpful in working out where to target treatment to have the maximum effect. So in the example given, additional teaching help for the child may be more effective than treatment of the depression.

BRAIN DISORDERS

Diseases affecting the brain It is important to avoid falling into the trap of considering physical and psychological problems as quite separate entities. Every physical illness has a psychological aspect and every emotional or behavioural disorder will have an associated physical component. There are three ways in which diseases of the brain can affect a child's psychological stage.

Specific effects. Direct damage to the brain can lead to loss of cognitive skills, for example difficulties with language and communication, or with mathematical calculation or problem solving. These problems may combine with short- or long-term memory loss to present a typical picture of dementia. Hallucinations, particularly if they are either visual or tactile, are characteristic of cerebral dysfunction. Unusual repetitive behaviour and perseveration of spoken language that is abnormal for the child's stage of development, are both commonly associated with abnormal brain function. Finally, clouding of consciousness and disorientation in time, place and person are perhaps the most obvious signs that there is abnormal brain function.

Non-specific effects. Brain dysfunction can result in both emotional and behavioural abnormalities that are not specific to a damaged brain and could occur as a result of a number of different causes. For example, disinhibited behaviour can be the result of brain damage, but it can also result from immaturity of social awareness, or inadequate social training. Similarly, emotional lability is commonly associated with an abnormally functioning brain, but is also typical of immature personality development. Likewise, bizarre behaviour may result from a number of different causes but it is also commonly associated with an abnormally functioning brain.

Secondary effects. Any disease process that interferes with brain function to a sufficient extent to cause cognitive difficulties is likely to lead to secondary emotional and behavioural problems that are secondary to these symptoms. For example, memory loss and difficulties with cognitive skills can lead to academic failure; clouding of consciousness and hallucinations may lead to secondary delusional ideas.

Epilepsy Epilepsy of whatever form is associated with an increased incidence of behaviour disturbance. This is probably caused mainly by brain dysfunction or by the drugs used to control the fits or by the social handicap that epilepsy brings to the child in his relationships. Temporal lobe epilepsy is particularly associated with psychiatric disorder with a prevalence rate of 70% compared with 25% in other epilepsies and 10% in the general child population.

Learning disability

Learning disability (mental handicap) whether due to obvious brain injury or to an uncertain mix of genetic and early environmental factors may present primarily with emotional or behaviour difficulties. These disturbances may be more of a burden to the child, his parents and his teachers, than his basic learning problem. Such difficult and challenging behaviour is often as much to do with the way the child is handled in early life as with the abnormal brain function.

There is no doubt that parents of a developmentally retarded child tend to have strong feelings of guilt and distress about the child. These strong feelings are often channelled towards either rejection or overprotection, and it is not unusual for parents to have many misconceptions about what their child can do. Parental expectations that are either too high or too low in relation to the child's natural ability can easily lead to tension in the parent–child relationship, and subsequent emotional behavioural problems.

The prevalence of psychiatric disorder increases as the level of ability decreases, and children with an IQ below 50 are five times more likely to have an emotional or behavioural disorder than a child whose ability falls within the average range. Unlike most other psychiatric disorders in children, boys and girls with severe learning disability are equally affected, suggesting that there is an aetiological factor that overrides the more usual childhood factors that make boys more vulnerable. Cerebral dysfunction is the most likely explanation for this. There is no type of psychiatric disorder that is specifically associated with severe learning disability, but psychosis, hyperactivity, self-injury and stereotypes occur more frequently than normal. When assessing a child with developmental delay, it is particularly important to keep in mind the developmental stage that the child has reached before deciding whether or not a psychiatric disorder is present. For example, it would be quite reasonable for a 12-year-old child who is developmentally at a 2-year-old stage to have temper tantrums of the type that would be normal in a toddler.

SPECIFIC DEVELOPMENTAL DELAY

Children with generalised delay in development will have reduced abilities in all areas, so-called global retardation. However the delay may be in one area only and, with time, the child may learn to overcome the difficulty or to bypass it. Thus the child may have a specific delay in motor control, language, reading, bladder and bowel control. All specific developmental delays occur three or four times more commonly in boys than in girls. They tend to occur in families and follow a normal developmental course, though more slowly than normal. The prognosis is therefore generally good, though it is likely that there will remain a disparity between the specific area of developmental delay and other fields. The relatively slow progress of the specifically delayed area of development can be speeded up using training techniques. So, for example, bladder training exercises will help enuresis and motor control exercises will help clumsy children. Specific delays in development can lead to emotional and behavioural problems if a sense of failure is allowed to develop as a result of the special area of difficulty the child has. On the whole, young children are remarkably resilient and quickly bounce back from failure, but as self concept develops, between the ages of 7 and 9 years, children become increasingly vulnerable to the experience of repeated failures which may then lead to the development of poor self image, and its associated psychological problems.

Clumsiness or dyspraxia

This is a good example of the type of problem that can be caused by a specific developmental delay. In its severe form developmental dyspraxia may result in a child being so uncoordinated that he has problems at home, at school and at play. Fine motor coordination problems result in untidy writing and children with gross motor incoordination are delayed in learning to dress themselves and have difficulty with sports, particularly ball game. They continually knock things over and frequently fall over themselves. The academic and social difficulties which follow can cause the child considerable unhappiness and lead to behavioural problems if they are not recognised and dealt with sympathetically. Specific training programmes to improve coordination may help.

Specific reading retardation

Reading is a complex activity which requires a great number of skills, and therefore reading difficulties might be due to a variety of factors. For example children with a general learning problem are slow to read, as are children who are understimulated or badly taught. But apart from those in whom a reading delay might be anticipated, there are many otherwise normal children who have specific reading retardation. Some experts consider that up to 8% of school children have such a problem. As with other specific delays in development, boys are more often affected than girls and there is often a family history. Some children may be a little slow to develop speech and characteristically they have even more difficulty with spelling than with reading so that, for them, dictation is a nightmare. They may also be delayed in developing handedness. There is an argument for screening all children at 7 years for specific reading retardation, not only so that their reading exercises can be approached with insight and sympathy but also to ensure that their general education is not hampered by their limited reading ability. Dyslexia, specific learning difficulty and 'word blindness' are the names given to the most overt form of this problem.

Specific speech and language problems

Hearing, intellectual or psychosocial impairment are more common factors leading to speech delay than a specific developmental disorder. Nevertheless, there is a small group of children, around 2%, of those with speech delay, who have normal intelligence and hearing and come from a happy, stimulating environment but who are unable to speak clearly. Speech difficulty, which is mostly due to motor coordination problems of the tongue and structural abnormalities of the mouth and palate, are distinguished from language difficulties. Children with specific language difficulties have the ability to pronounce words correctly, but they make the same mistakes of grammar and syntax that would be typical of a much younger child. It is possible to distinguish between receptive and expressive language disorders but they both present as delay in the acquisition of language. The most extreme form of specific language disorder is infantile autism where all aspects of communication are affected, but other skills are often preserved. It is therefore not surprising that milder forms of specific language delay such as Asperger syndrome are associated with autistic like symptoms, such as habits and mannerisms, social difficulties and difficulty coping with change. Sometimes children with specific language delay present later on in childhood with bizarre behaviour and abnormal social relationships with a history of being delayed in learning to talk. It is only when their language is carefully analysed that abnormalities of sentence construction, and limited use of words and abstract concepts can be identified. These children require an individualised education programme aimed at increasing language and social skills.

Nocturnal enuresis

Involuntary emptying of the bladder during sleep is a common and troublesome problem. Generally the majority of children are dry at night by 3 years of age, some 10% of children regularly wet the bed at 5 years of age, and somewhat less than 5% still do so at 10 years of age. One or two in every hundred will have an organic problem, either a congenital abnormality of the urinary tract, a urinary infection, polyuria or neurogenic bladder. A careful history, thorough examination and urine examination for glucose, infection and specific gravity should exclude these possibilities. Only rarely is a history of nocturnal enuresis alone sufficient to justify radiological investigation of the renal system. In another small percentage nocturnal enuresis will be the presenting symptom of an emotionally upset child. Gentle probing enquiry should bring this to light and point the interview in the appropriate direction. In the majority, clinical enquiry gives no indication of the aetiology. Often there is a family history and there will be relatively more children from poor and unhappy homes than might be expected. There is no evidence to support the parents' suggestion that their child's bladder capacity is too small or that they pass excess amounts of urine during the night, and sleep more deeply than other children. The most likely explanation is that enuresis is due to immature neuromuscular coordination of the bladder muscles and sphincters. Many children improve, some surprisingly quickly, with whatever method of management is used, whether it be habit training with star charts, a pad and bell or simple suggestion and encouragement. A distinction is sometimes made between primary and secondary enuresis where primary enuresis is lifelong, and secondary enuresis starts after a period of being dry. Unfortunately this distinction is not very helpful because both types of enuresis share the same characteristics and respond in the same way to treatment. The notion that enuresis is a sign of hidden emotional distress is usually inaccurate and treatments for emotional disturbance are remarkably ineffective with enuresis. There is some evidence that enuresis itself may cause emotional distress as children become older. In this situation the symptomatic treatment of enuresis results in remarkable improvement in the child's mental state. There is some evidence, however, that children who have experienced social adversity during the first 5 years of life are more likely to suffer from enuresis. The most likely explanation for this is that normal toilet training has been interrupted by the social disruption. Although the majority of children will eventually become dry, the spontaneous remission rate becomes progressively less as children grow older. At the same time, the secondary, emotional and social consequences of enuresis become more serious. Children who continue to wet over the age of 8 years old are at risk of developing a sense of failure and low self esteem. As long as they continue to wet themselves, they are likely to remain rather immature because it is difficult to feel grown up while at the same time wetting the bed, or the pants. The bell alarm which is placed in the child's bed so that the alarm rings when the child wets is said to help over two-thirds of those who use the system correctly. Medication may be useful for symptom relief in the short term, for example when staying overnight with a friend. Desmopressin has an 80% success rate, but the relapse rate is quite high.

Faecal soiling

Most children are clean by 2 years of age and soiling may be viewed as abnormal after 4 years of age and certainly by the time the child goes to school. Whatever the reason for soiling, as with enuresis, most forms of soiling are more common in boys, and can be seen as a specific developmental immaturity. Inadequate or disruptive training, or irregular bowel habit, are predisposing factors, as is constipation. One of the main problems with soiling is that it elicits strong negative reactions from those around the child, especially at school, and it does not take long for children who soil to become emotionally distressed, purely as a result of the soiling and its consequences. At the same time children who are emotionally stressed are more likely to have difficulties with bowel control, and it is easy to see how a vicious circle soon develops. The term 'encopresis' is used to describe the passage of formed faeces in unacceptable places. This may be in the pants, but it can also be behind the settee, in a drawer, or indeed anywhere except in the toilet. Occasionally this behaviour is directly linked to a stressful event, and it is clearly meant to be a provocative act. This type of severe encopresis may be difficult to resolve, and expert psychiatric advice is required. Children who are chronically constipated may develop overflow incontinence and they soil continuously without passing a formed stool. Dealing with the constipation always leads to resolution of the soiling. The secondary repercussions of soiling are so serious for a child that it is important to deal with the problem actively, rather than waiting and hoping that the child will eventually grow out of it. There are three aspects of treatment:

Toilet training. This involves regular toileting at intervals that are frequent enough to keep the child clean. On each occasion the child is expected to sit on the toilet for about 3 minutes. If a motion is passed, great pleasure and appreciation is shown to the child. It is helpful to keep a record of the child's progress, and it may also be helpful to use a star chart, or some other reward system, for success.

Diet and exercise. An appropriate diet with adequate amounts of high fibre foods and other foodstuffs that promote bowel action will help, as will appropriate levels of physical activity.

An empty bowel. The bowel should be kept as empty as possible. Most children who soil only partially evacuate the contents of the bowel. If regular toileting has not been effective, then regular laxatives, and in more severe cases micro-enemas, may be necessary. It is important to continue an active treatment regimen for 3–6 months after the child has become clean, otherwise a relapse is likely. If a child fails to respond to the above regimen, the most likely explanation is that it has not been carried out to the letter. However, in a minority of cases, the lack of response to treatment may be because the child is seriously emotionally disturbed, and the causes for this should be sought and dealt with. In the majority of children, once the soiling has stopped, they start to flourish and mature rapidly.

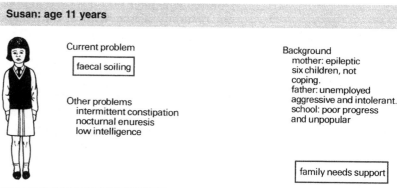

Susan: age 11 years

Current problem

| faecal soiling |

Other problems
intermittent constipation
nocturnal enuresis
low intelligence

Background
mother: epileptic
six children, not
coping.
father: unemployed
aggressive and intolerant.
school: poor progress
and unpopular

| family needs support |

Tics

Tics are sudden repetitive coordinated movements of no apparent purpose. They can effect any muscle groups but commonly take the form of blinking, facial grimacing, twisting the head or shrugging the shoulders. The usual age of onset is between the ages of 5 and 8 years and it has been reported that as many as 4% of children develop marked tics at some time and a much larger number develop mild tics. Tourette described a bizarre syndrome where vocal tics, often rude words, accompany gestures which might be equally embarrassing. In 25% of children with tics there is a family history. In some there is evidence of brain damage or other features of delayed maturation. Tics are more common in boys and are often associated with hyperactivity or obsessional symptoms. Usually the tics disappear spontaneously, sometimes in weeks or months, often in late adolescence. Only rarely do they persist into adult life. Tics are made worse by stress and they are also worse when a child is excited or relaxed. Anything that draws attention to the tics will make them worse.

Hyperkinetic syndrome and attention deficit disorder with or without hyperactivity (ADHD or ADD)

There has been some confusion around the different terms used to describe children who have a particular difficulty in developing self control. There is now general agreement that the three core problem areas are:

- overactivity
- short attention span
- poor impulse control.

Typically, the symptoms are present from an early age, and are associated with other developmental delays and often cause problems soon after starting school. Between 3 and 5% of children are said to suffer from this condition which, like other specific delays of development, is about four times more common in boys and tends to run in families. Overactive children who have never been taught to have self control can easily be misdiagnosed as having ADHD. Similarly, children who are emotionally stressed or abused may present with restlessness and poor concentration, but not suffer from ADHD. The diagnosis of ADHD is especially difficult when it occurs in children who have been exposed to poor parenting. Preschool children are naturally active with a short attention span and parents may mistake this normal stage of development for hyperactivity. School age children are quickly identified as disruptive and fidgety in the classroom. The typical child with ADHD is easily distracted, often interrupts, has difficulty delaying gratification and may engage in dangerous, thrill seeking activities. Most children with ADHD soon become unpopular at school and fall behind in academic achievement. In adolescence, though the hyperactivity is less, their learning difficulties with socially disruptive behaviour may lead to further problems and the link between hyperactivity and conduct disorder is a close one. As adults they are more likely to have trouble with the law or need psychiatric help.

Management starts with a careful evaluation of the child's problems and continues by full discussions with parents, teachers and anyone else concerned. Each programme is individual and involves teaching self control and having a regular routine to daily life. Brain stimulants, methylphenidate and other amphetamine related drugs may benefit some affected children, but should only be prescribed by appropriately trained clinicians in conjunction with a treatment programme involving the family and the school aimed at training the child to develop more self control. There is no evidence that hyperactivity is caused by certain foods; however, some parents claim that exclusion diets can improve behaviour. One explanation is that it is the parents' constant firm line that brings about the improvement rather than the exclusion diet itself which carries the risk of nutritional deficiencies. Fortunately, most children with ADHD grow out of it to an extent that they are able to function reasonably well as an adult in much the same way that children with dyslexia improve provided they receive appropriate individual training.

Autism and Asperger syndrome

Autism is rare: in a population of one million some 20–40 children might be identified. Boys are affected three or four times more frequently than girls. Characteristically, autistic children fail to develop social relationships, they are slow to speak and have little non-verbal communication. They also follow ritualistic behaviour patterns and endlessly perform repetitive movements. Parents seek advice because they wonder if the child is deaf and again later because of delay or absence of speech development. Often the infant's behaviour has been unusual from birth and only occasionally is the child's development for the first year or so apparently normal. There is a strong genetic component to autism, and the organic nature of the disorder is highlighted by the fact that some 40% of autistic children develop epilepsy during adolescence. It seems likely that autism is at the extreme end of a continuum of specific language disorders that include Asperger syndrome, semantic pragmatic disorder and developmental dysphasia. Most autistic children are mentally retarded. Those with a non-verbal IQ below 70 have the worst prognosis. Even those with average intelligence have great difficulty coping when they grow up. Only a few manage to be gainfully employed and they always find close relationships difficult to manage successfully. The essential abnormality in autism is a severe deficit in language ability that affects all aspects of communication and imagination. To be an autistic child is rather like living in a foreign country where not only is the language difficult to understand but gestures and sign language are incomprehensible as well. One of the most difficult problems autistic children have to face is that they look normal, and as they grow older they may achieve reasonable language competence, but they are rarely able to master abstract concepts and the subtleties of relationships. This makes them unusually vulnerable and frequently misunderstood.

Autistic children need detailed assessment by experts and to have access to ongoing treatment programmes for the wide range of associated behavioural problems. Management involves intensive training of communication skills, and providing as much routine and regularity in everyday life as possible. Specialist support for their families and teaching in special schools or units is the main focus of treatment, but because of the rarity of autism and similar communication difficulties it is often difficult to provide this for all children while maintaining strong home links. Drugs currently play only a small part in management, but may have a role during adolescence when it is not unusual for autistic children to have episodes of extremely disturbed behaviour.

Some children only develop autistic like symptoms after a period of several years apparent normality. This type of disorder is called disintegrative psychosis and is thought to be triggered by some form of organic brain disease. It is important to distinguish autism, Asperger syndrome and disintegrative psychosis from schizophrenia which is a totally different disorder. The typical onset of shizophrenia is later on in adolescence or early adulthood. The symptoms and the genetic loading are quite different from autism.

THE INTERACTION BETWEEN THE CHILD AND HIS WORLD

A child may develop symptoms of physical disorder or behaviour problems or educational difficulties due to conflicts and confusion within himself, or with his family, with his peers, with school or with society at large. If a schoolgirl gets stomachache because she hates her ballet lessons or dislikes her new stepfather, then eliciting that information may be just as important for that child as testing the urine in another suspected of having urinary infection. This section merely points to some of the more obvious factors which might lead to problems.

The child

Acute organic disease frightens children possibly more than adults, and they show it in different ways according to their maturity. It can be difficult to distinguish the symptoms and signs due to this reaction from those due to the underlying pathology. A terrified 2 year old with croup may improve dramatically in the arms of a friendly, confident, capable nurse or become even worse if placed on a strange bed surrounded by flashing lights and stainless steel.

Chronic organic disease makes extra demands on the child. The majority of children cope marvelously well but in others the continuing difficulties are just too much and secondary symptoms or behaviour problems add to their difficulties. The burden of the disease for some children can be very heavy; what, for example, can be said to an adolescent with muscular dystrophy or cystic fibrosis when he learns by one means or another of the prognosis of his condition? Sometimes it is the parents who cannot accept or have difficulty managing the child's condition. It is always sad when a child with asthma exaggerates his bronchospasm, or a child with diabetes deliberately breaks diet to precipitate hyperglycaemia, in order to gain admission to hospital where they feel more secure, and where the pressures of coping either with the family or the outside world are avoided.

Deformity and disability present at birth may lead to problems if one or both parents have difficulty accepting their own abnormal child; they feel ashamed about him when they should be showing him off. Later as the child grows up he may have trouble at school, for children go through a period of wanting to be the same and of mocking those who are different. Just being different can lead to problems. Fortunately, most children and their families cope remarkably well with disability and bullying in school is usually not directed at those who have a very obvious deformity.

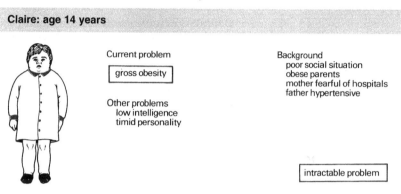

Claire: age 14 years

Current problem

gross obesity

Other problems
low intelligence
timid personality

Background
poor social situation
obese parents
mother fearful of hospitals
father hypertensive

intractable problem

Illness behaviour. Some children present with symptoms that suggest a physical illness, but lack the appropriate physical signs and pathological findings. In such cases it is important to avoid getting into a debate with parents as to whether the condition is physical or psychological because all illnesses are a mixture of both. The aim is to reach agreement with the child and parents that the condition is not life threatening or life long. All therapeutic effort should be directed at convalescence and gradual return to normal function by insisting that the child does a little more each day. This approach is effective for most cases of chronic fatigue and the post-viral syndrome. More resistant cases may benefit from detailed psychiatric assessment and a combined physical and psychological treatment programme.

Intelligence is determined by a mixture of genetic and environmental factors. Happily, in the main, parents have children of similar abilities but misfits occasionally occur, a slow child in an academic family, an awkward child in an athletic family, a gifted child in an average family, a swan among ducks. All may lead to conflict and result in bodily symptoms, behaviour disturbances and underachieving. In general, there is an inverse relationship between intelligence and psychiatric disorder. Children with severe learning difficulties have four to five times the risk of developing emotional or behavioural problems.

Temperament likewise appears to be genetically and environmentally determined. A child's temperament is not only a factor in the risk of disorders developing but may also determine the mode of expression.

An outgoing, extrovert child is more likely to develop behaviour problems, while a sensitive, timid child is more likely to internalise conflicts and have anxiety or disorders of bodily function. The success of any management programme depends on those concerned knowing the child for whom they are making plans. Children with a difficult temperament can be recognised at birth and the combination of strong negative moods, irregular functioning and poor adaptability is associated with an increased risk of behaviour disorder

The family

A great deal has been written recently about the qualities required of parents. A child needs not only food, warmth and physical protection but also to be loved, to feel important, to be stimulated and encouraged to make the most of his abilities, and to be controlled and guided in the ways of his society. It is the privilege and responsibility of parents to meet these needs and most parents delight in the task. Many factors, some beyond anyone's control, can interfere with the relationship between parents and child. Of course the child is constantly changing and developing and a special task for parents is to modify their management as the child matures.

Maternal bonding. The bond between the mother and her child starts as soon as she knows that she is pregnant. Important stages in the attachment process occur when she first feels the child move and then later at the moment of birth, and the first few weeks after that. The 'bonding' of a child to the mother is also a gradual process. Although a child is able to distinguish between some characteristics of his own mother and those of other mothers, clear evidence of bonding only becomes apparent when a child is around 5–8 months. It is at this stage that stranger anxiety and separation anxiety are first seen; they are part of normal development. The bonding of the child to the mother continues to strengthen over the next few years, and is generally secure by the age of 5 or 6 years. Children who are separated from their mother before the age of 5–8 months usually show no particular symptoms. Separation before the age of 2 or 3 years causes much less distress than later on, and very young children adapt remarkably well to alternative parenting.

Fathers also become attached to their children, but not only is this a more gradual process, it is also very variable and depends upon the

Some reactions a toddler might show on admission to hospital

protest   despair   denial

degree of involvement that the father has with the child. Young children who are separated from their main carer characteristically show three stages of reaction. These are:

- protest, screaming and extreme distress, followed by
- restless searching and frequent crying, and finally
- withdrawal and despair.

For most families brief periods of separation are not as harmful in the long term as was originally thought but they can be in the context of hostile and rejecting family relationships. If either the mother or her dependent infant needs hospital care, they should be admitted together if it is at all possible. One is often important in the other's recovery. The effect that the death of a parent has on a child varies with his maturity. It is not until 6–8 years old that children develop a reasonably clear concept of death. A disturbed child may be considerably helped by having the opportunity to talk frankly about it with a sympathetic but uninvolved adult.

Family breakdown. Unhappily for children in western societies divorce rates are increasing. At least 1 in 5 children will experience the separation of their parents before they reach 16 years of age. Couples seeking divorce are tending to be younger and the duration of their marriages is shorter. Illegitimacy rates are also increasing, and good alternatives for child care have not become available at the same rate as the increase in working mothers. Such situations add to the children's problems and may limit the care they receive. In the year following family breakdown about 80% of children show some significant disturbance and it continues to be higher than normal over the next few years. Boys are more likely to become disturbed than girls.

John: age 8 years

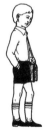

Current problem

| stole money from school and home to buy sweets |

Other problems
  high IQ
  reading retardation

Background
unmarried mother who despised and did not mention his father. Catholic school taught the sanctity of marriage

| he wanted to be told about his father |

Parental abilities and attitudes. If a parent is sick, what of the child? If a child has stomachache it is well to ask about the family symptoms. Children are quick to note how adults gain sympathy and avoid the unpleasant, and they assume that there is no reason why they should not use the same tactics. A parent with a chronic illness may add to the child's anxieties and responsibilities and push the child beyond his limit. A parent with a psychiatric disorder, for example, depression, may have a devastating effect on the child. The key factor that determines the effect on a child is the amount of involvement that the child has in the parent's illness. Thus a parent with obsessional cleanliness may have a profound effect, while a psychotic parent who is admitted to hospital when ill will often have much less of an adverse effect. Sometimes it is the child's behaviour which draws attention to the parent's need. Unclear limit setting and unpredictability are especially linked with an increased risk of disturbed behaviour. Even when both parents are well and able to provide a comfortable home, their attitudes and expectations of their children can still lead to difficulties. In the extremes they may overprotect them or overdiscipline them or ignore and reject them or they may wish to dominate them, even when they are capable of being independent. On the other hand, they may have unrealistic expectations of their abilities; for example, a mother who expected a 6-month-old infant to use a pot, a father who expected his children to move at the blow of a whistle, a professional woman who thought her 7 year old should realise when she wished to be left alone. Although the unhelpful attitudes may be obvious to everyone else, it often requires very lengthy and sensitive counselling to help parents to change.

Adoption and alternative families. The situation of a couple longing for children that they cannot have and adopting into their family an unwanted child has its own peculiar problems. Inevitably the child has those characteristics, appearance, abilities and personality determined by his genetic make-up from his parents but also he is influenced by the environment provided by his new home. Because adoptive parents are usually specially selected as being capable, adopted children usually do better than they would have done in their natural family. The rate of emotional-behavioural problems in adopted children differs very little from the general population. It has been said that bad parents are better than no parents. This is not true. However, in the absence of a larger family to embrace a child who loses both parents, the best efforts of the social services often fall well short of the child's needs. It is easy to be pessimistic about the long-term prognosis of such children. Nevertheless, many children build happy and successful lives out of appalling childhoods. One important factor to determine outcome is a continuing stable and caring relationship with an adult who specially values the child. This does not have to be the main carer but could be a teacher, a relative or any concerned adult.

Environment

Ineffectual parents tend to be poor and to live in bad housing in deprived sections of the towns or country. It is difficult to be sure of the extent that a child's problems are due to his make-up, the care and attitudes of his parents or to his physical surroundings. But there is no doubt that poverty, overcrowding and poor housing are associated not only with increased rates of illness and death in infancy and childhood but also behaviour problems and school failure. It is also difficult for children from such backgrounds to become good parents themselves.

The poor are at a threefold disadvantage; they are more likely to fall ill, they have less family reserves to meet new problems and they are less able to make use of the support the state provides. Even in the UK with a National Health Service, the deprived are still at a disadvantage in comparison with the middle classes and almost a million children are being brought up in poverty. Wealth is relative, and poverty as defined in western societies need not bring misery. It has been shown that the prevalence of health and social problems varies considerably from one community to another with apparently similar levels of wealth, housing, and services. In some communities there is stability and mutual responsibility, in others there is aggression, cruelty and conflict. Race, culture, religion, and poverty can all lead to a family being rejected by the neighbourhood. Families continually on the move may create problems of insecurity for their children.

School

School is where children go to work, where they make friends and enemies, where they test out their personality against others, where they find out how other families think and behave. So problems at school may be far more than difficulties with learning. A child who has difficulty with his school such that special education is considered necessary, should have a thorough and expert medical assessment so that the handicap due to a medical condition is reduced to a minimum. Schools vary quite significantly in the rate of behaviour problems shown by their pupils over and above that which can be explained by social factors. In other words, some schools have a positive effect on children, whereas others make it more likely that children will be disruptive and difficult. Schools with high staff morale, low teacher turnover, good organisation, clear methods of discipline, and a detailed knowledge of children as individuals, tend to have a low rate of antisocial behaviour.

BEHAVIOURAL PROBLEMS

From what has been said so far it can be appreciated that many factors may contribute to the genesis of any particular problem which brings a child to the doctor's attention. The physician is particularly concerned with symptoms which suggest physical disease but have their origins in a psychological disturbance, and with behavioural problems which are a consequence of a physical disorder, either as a direct effect of brain disturbance or indirectly due to the difficulty the child has coping

The preschool child

Feeding problems. Interaction between an uncertain or insecure parent with a healthy baby, or a happy parent with a determined or difficult baby may lead to the baby vomiting, refusing food or failing to gain weight satisfactorily. Sometimes the problem is resolved by patience and counselling either from the health visitor, relative or friendly neighbour but it is not uncommon for a child to have to be admitted to hospital to exclude an organic cause and to reassure both mother and her baby. Battles over food are always best avoided. Anxiety reduction for all concerned is the most effective approach, relying on the child's natural thirst and hunger drive to take enough food.

Sleep problems. Adults used to a regular biological rhythm differ in their tolerance of the baby's desire for a feed in the middle of the night. Occasionally infants appear to scream and cry through most of the night and this may be tolerated when the baby is young and weak but a playful demanding toddler in the middle of the night can stretch the patience of most parents. A regular pattern of sleep/waking is usually established by 6 months. But if not, the temptation for the parents is to take the child in their bed or for one or other parent to sleep with the child to comfort him but this is really no solution and can lead to further problems. Adults without sleep become irritable and perform poorly in their work and this adds to the strain. In this situation there is an argument for establishing a regular bedtime routine and not responding to a child's crying. This approach is usually rapidly effective, but can only be carried out if the child is obviously well and not in pain, and the parents are sure that their child is safe in the bedroom or in the cot. Night sedation is best avoided, it should only be used as a last resort.

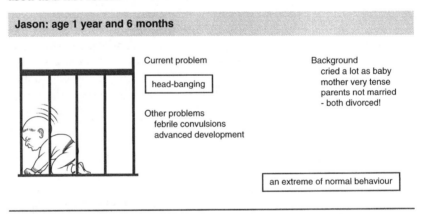

Jason: age 1 year and 6 months

Current problem

head-banging

Other problems
febrile convulsions
advanced development

Background
cried a lot as baby
mother very tense
parents not married
- both divorced!

an extreme of normal behaviour

Breath-holding attacks. Infants and toddlers quickly find that they can control their parents by refusing to do what they are asked. For example, they may refuse to eat or go to the toilet, but perhaps their most dramatic card to play is to refuse to breathe. Breath-holding attacks to the point of going unconscious, when they may or may not provoke a fit, are not uncommon. They certainly terrify the parents and may reduce them to quivering slaves. From the medical point of view it is important to distinguish the episodes from convulsions due to other causes and to reassure parents about the nature of the attacks. In the vast majority of cases the children come to no harm and parents should be encouraged to take no action during the episode. These determined, often stubborn youngsters need to be handled firmly and consistently.

Rhythmic behaviour and habits. Head rocking, head banging, thumb sucking, self stimulation, baby behaviour and many other variants may all occur during normal development. They are more likely to appear when the child is bored, anxious, excited or tired. In the very disturbed, autistic or retarded child they can become bad habits and strategies need to be devised to avoid or suppress them by diverting, disrupting or preventing the behaviour.

Delayed development and regression. Understimulation with or without undernutrition may limit a child's development and growth. It is not surprising perhaps that a child left alone for hours with no toys in a high rise flat is quite withdrawn, apathetic, and has little muscle tone or strength, and delayed motor, social and mental development. Physical illness or emotional stress frequently causes regression with the loss of the more recently acquired skills and a return to a more immature stage of development.

Bowel and bladder control. Again inappropriate training or anxiety and conflict will interfere with the development of bodily control and appropriate social habits. Nocturnal enuresis which in the main is probably due to a disorder in maturation and encopresis have been discussed in the first part of this chapter.

School age children

Recurrent abdominal pain. One of the common symptoms which bring children to clinic is recurrent pains usually in the abdomen or head, occasionally in the limbs. A few will have organic disease and so all require a careful clinical evaluation. In others it may be a cry for help, the child having a psychiatric disorder or a terrible domestic situation. But for the majority, the clinical investigations will be negative and there will be no major psychosocial problems. There may have been mild or moderate disturbances in the child's life, and the symptoms become a way of communicating distress. Finding words to express emotional problems is difficult for children and most parents respond more quickly to physical symptoms than to emotional reactions in their children. A thorough examination and reassurance with explanations will help many. However in those referred to

---

Jane: age 8 years

Current problem

recurrent abdominal pain

Other problems
none

Background
quiet, sensitive shy child
mother had migraine
father travelling salesman
away from home.
brother—big and extrovert

sibling rivalry

hospital, a good percentage continue to have recurrent pains into adolescence and adult life. Headaches rather than abdominal pains tend to persist, especially if there is a positive family history.

Periodic syndrome describes a condition where attacks of abdominal pain are associated with severe vomiting. The vomiting can sometimes result in dehydration to a degree that requires correction by intravenous therapy. In this situation it is difficult to believe that the child has not got an organic disease but so far no pathology has been identified. However in its milder form it merges with the clinical entity of 'recurrent abdominal pain'.

School refusal and truancy. Illness is the commonest reason for school absence, but occasionally children are kept away from school by their parents to help in the home. It is important to distinguish these two categories from those children who refuse to go to school because they are anxious, frightened or depressed, and from those children who play truant from school because they dislike the atmosphere in which they appear to fail and are subject to ridicule and, as they see it, to unfair discipline. The distinction between school refusal on the one hand, and truancy on the other, is characteristic of the contrast between neurotic disorders and conduct disorders. School refusal is a neurotic/emotional disorder and is associated with: school phobia, depression and separation anxiety. It has equal frequency in boys and girls and occurs in children from a stable family background and where there is good progress at school. The family is typically close, overinvolved and there may be high levels of emotional distress. By contrast, the families of children who truant are typically large and disorganised, with poor supervision, marital disharmony and open expression of aggression in the family. There may be social deprivation together with antisocial behaviour and poor achievement at school The main distinction between school refusal and truancy is that in the former, everyone knows where the child is, but in the latter the child disappears during school hours and may turn up at home after school as if it were just another ordinary school day. It can sometimes be helpful to distinguish between school phobia and separation anxiety. In separation anxiety there is characteristically a long history of separation problems, the problems of going to school are at their worst on leaving home. On the other hand, school phobia is often triggered by a distressing event at school and the symptoms become progressively worse as the child approaches the school.

Truancy is rare in primary school and if it does occur it usually has a very poor prognosis. However, truancy becomes increasingly frequent in secondary school and reaches a peak in the last year of schooling. The treatment for school refusal is to return the child to school in what ever way is possible. This will either work or will reveal the underlying cause which can then be dealt with. Truancy is best managed by increasing supervision and cooperation between home and school.

School refusal is a neurotic/emotional disorder and is associated with:	Truancy is a conduct/antisocial disorder and is associated with:
School phobia, depression and separation anxiety	Disruptive and aggressive behaviour
Equal frequency in boys and girls	Higher frequency in boys
Stable family background	Disrupted family background
Good progress at school	Academic failure
Close, overinvolved family	Lack of supervision at home
Emotional distress in the family	Social deprivation

Conduct disorders. Often parents are concerned because their young children are unacceptably aggressive, destructive, cruel or antisocial. Again individual tolerance will depend on the family and the community. In some lively teenagers, outbursts of aggressive, destructive, foolish or antisocial behaviour may be dismissed as high spirits but in others living in inner city areas with mixed cultures and limited outlets it results in delinquency.

It is now clear that as children grow older, persistent aggressive or antisocial behaviour has an increasingly poor prognosis. In fact the continuity of aggression after the age of 5 is almost as strong as it is for intelligence. Aggressive children are significantly more likely to grow up into adults who have a poor employment record, are convicted criminals and form unsatisfactory relationships. It is therefore unwise to expect persistently aggressive and antisocial children to grow out of it. How parents manage the temper tantrum phase between 18 months and 2 years is thought to be a critical determining factor in the future control of aggression. Inconsistent and excessively harsh discipline tends to cause childhood aggression, so also does a lax or tolerant attitude to antisocial behaviour. Children who have witnessed frequent aggression at home or on the TV are at risk for this type of behaviour. Children who are hyperactive or have difficult temperaments are similarly at risk, as are children who have low self esteem.

Peter: age 14 years

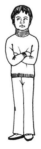

Current problem:

unprovoked outbursts of aggressive behaviour

Other problems
 severe epilepsy
 low intelligence
 nocturnal enuresis

Background
 low birth weight
 abandoned by teenage mother.
 fostered—
 then adopted

requires protective environment in special school

EMOTIONAL DISORDERS

Children, like adults, can get unduly anxious; they may suffer from unreasonable fears and they can have outbursts of 'hysterical' behaviour. By nature, children are usually optimistic and confident about the future, but occasionally even without obvious cause they can become severely depressed and may even attempt suicide. These children should have the counsel of a child psychiatrist.

Anxiety states

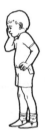

Children frequently experience worries and fears in much the same way that adults do, and there is a similar variation in the way that some are much more reactive and sensitive to fearful situations than others. Normal fears do not interfere with the child's everyday life, and usually fade away after a few weeks. On the other hand, pathological anxiety is disruptive to the child's life to the point where family functioning may also be affected. It is often appropriate to see anxiety as being 'infectious', in that it is very easy to pick it up from other people. It is therefore helpful to consider 'where does the anxiety come from, who does it belong to?'. The source of the problem has to be identified before the child's anxiety can be addressed.

Fears at different ages	
Strangers	0.5–3 years
Animals	2–4 years
Darkness, storms, imaginary monsters	4–6 years
Mysterious happenings	6–12 years
Social embarrassment, academic failure, death and wars	12–18 years

Anorexia nervosa

Anorexia nervosa is diagnosed when more than 20% of the expected body weight is lost and in girls past the menarche, the monthly period has stopped. Ninety per cent of cases are female and the incidence is between 0.1 and 1% of adolescents. No aetiological organic pathology or avoidable environmental factors are usually identified and any change is usually secondary to starvation. Young people either just before or during puberty deliberately avoid food so that they lose weight, and they often go on losing weight until they become tragically thin. They have a morbid fear of being fat and a preoccupation with reducing calorie intake and increasing exercise. It used to be thought that they have an irrational fear of growing up, of becoming sexually and physically mature, but there is little evidence that this is any more than in the normal teenager. Usually they are able youngsters, if somewhat obsessional and precise. Rarely are there major psychological problems which need attention.

The most effective approach is to find a way to feed the child up again by whatever means. It is often necessary to be very firm and determined, even to the point of feeding by nasogastric tube if necessary. Treatment of any underlying psychopathology is best left until the weight is no longer a matter of concern. Child psychiatric help is usually needed for the more complex cases.

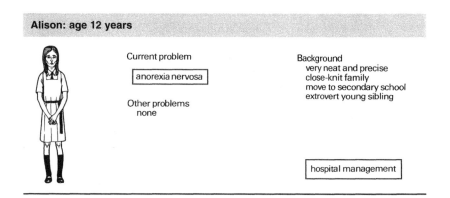

Alison: age 12 years

Current problem

anorexia nervosa

Other problems
none

Background
very neat and precise
close-knit family
move to secondary school
extrovert young sibling

hospital management

Depression

Babies cry a great deal, but this does not mean that they are depressed. Indeed, crying in very young children can have a wide range of meanings, including 'I am hungry', 'I am in pain', 'my nappy needs changing' and 'I am just bored and fed up'. The term 'depression' can be used as a general description for everyday distress and unhappiness. When it is used in the technical sense, there is in addition to feelings of misery, thoughts of hopelessness about the future and feelings of worthlessness about oneself. Thus, in order to be depressed, a child must have developed to the stage where there is a clear concept of time in order to understand hopelessness for the future, and a clear concept of the self in order to feel worthless. Both of these abilities become reasonably well established between the ages of 7 and 9, and it is not until this stage that children are developmentally able to experience a depressive disorder. Even then, it is rare and requires a high level of stress to trigger it. Additional symptoms of depression include poor concentration, deterioration of school work and some or all of the symptoms of emotional distress, such as alterations to appetite and sleep patterns, psychosomatic aches and pains and other symptoms of physiological disturbance.

The development of a depressive disorder during childhood has a very serious significance. This is partly because a child must have been subjected to high levels of stress for depression to occur in the first place, but also because relationships and progress at school are often adversely affected and the child becomes stuck in a vicious circle. Recent research indicates that the long-term prognosis for depressed children is very poor.

Phobias and obsessions

The link between phobias and obsessions is quite strong. For example, obsessional cleanliness could be described as dirt phobia, or dog phobia could be described as an obsessional avoidance of dogs. Both conditions are classified as neurotic disorders and occur with equal frequency in boys and girls.

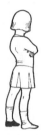

A phobia is an overwhelming but unrealistic fear which is accompanied by avoidance behaviour. Mild phobic reactions occur quite commonly in young children, reaching a peak between 5 and 7 years of age, and occur in approximately 1% of children. The prognosis for single phobias is good, but if they are multiple or complex, the phobic reactions tend to continue, with one being replaced by another.

An obsession is an irresistible urge to repeat a thought or action. The term 'compulsion' is used to describe an obsessional behaviour or ritual. Overall the condition is known as 'obsessional compulsive disorder' (OCD) and occurs significantly less frequently than phobias. Both conditions are classified as neurotic disorders and occur with equal frequency in boys and girls. Children between the ages of 5 and 7 commonly go through a phase of ritualistic behaviour, where they insist that something is done in exactly the same way on each occasion. This is often motivated by a fear that something bad will happen if the routine is not followed. Where obsessions or phobias are complex or severe, they have a tendency to persist, even into adult life. Treatment is focused on preventing or disrupting the obsessional process and getting the child to gradually face the feared situation.

MANAGEMENT

Management of emotional and behavioural disorders includes identifying the contributing factors and conferring with the other people concerned. The latter may include the family doctor and other members of the primary care team, the health visitor, the school teacher, school health services and school welfare officers, the educational psychologist and social service workers. When, after review, a programme of care has been agreed, it is essential that a person is identified to be responsible for counselling the child and parents, and ensuring that all concerned are properly informed. Being thorough at the outset can avoid many problems later. With the more intractable emotional and conduct disorders a child psychiatrist will be the key person, but the majority will fall within the responsibility of the health visitor or the family doctor or the paediatrician. Perhaps the most important factor in determining a successful outcome in the management of children with emotional-behavioural problems is to achieve an agreed understanding and approach to the problem. It is particularly important to gain cooperation and agreement between all adults who have direct care of a child. This will usually involve a considerable amount of time spent in delicate negotiations. However, agreement and understanding are not sufficient in themselves. One of the most common reasons for treatment plans being ineffective is that they are not carried through. The role of the key person should be to make frequent checks to ensure that the agreed treatment approach is in fact being carried out, and to arrange further discussion with those involved if no progress has been made. The detailed treatment programmes that are currently available are beyond the scope of this book, but there are some general guidelines which should be considered in each case.

Guidelines for management

—Child's emotional-behavioural problems may be the symptom of disturbance elsewhere, for example in the family or in the school, in which case treatment needs to be directed, not at the child, but at the source of the problem

—The younger the child the more likely it is that the source of the problem is outside the child. Treatment approaches for young children should therefore be directed at changing a child's family and environment

—As children approach adolescence it is increasingly important to consider individual treatment needs and the child's inner world

—Behaviour problems respond best to clear limit setting, high levels of supervision, and training in appropriate behaviour

—Developmental problems, such as soiling, wetting and specific language problems, require intensive training programmes aimed at increasing competence and confidence in the skill that is delayed

—Anxieties and phobias are best tackled by finding ways in which the child can be helped to face up to them. This can either be done very gradually, or by going in at the deep end. This latter approach is often rapidly effective, but it is important to have the agreement of all those concerned if this approach is going to be used

—Miserable and depressed children are unlikely to respond to treatment unless the cause has been identified and dealt with

—Medication has a very limited role to play in the treatment of childhood behaviour and emotional problems, and should only be prescribed by those who have specialised knowledge of this area

—Children easily become stuck in a vicious circle that maintains the psychiatric disorder. Treatment can be directed at any part of this circle and still be effective, even if it is not directed at the problem itself. For example, a child with academic failure, leading to school phobia, may be helped merely by treatment directed at boosting self image

—It is never acceptable to wait for a child to grow out of a problem, even though behavioural and emotional problems eventually often resolve spontaneously. Children easily become stuck in particular patterns of behaviour and develop characteristic emotional reactions. If these are maladaptive, a range of adverse consequences quickly follows, such as rejection, scapegoating and hostility, which will leave the child psychologically damaged, even though the problem may have been resolved

---

THE MALTREATMENT OF CHILDREN

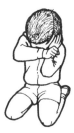

Deviant behaviour by adults may take the form of injuring their children. Child murder, child cruelty, child neglect, child abuse, child molesting and the use of children for pornography all fall into this category. The obvious examples are easily recognised, but defining the limits of child abuse or child neglect is difficult. It might be considered that it is the right of every child to be allowed to develop to his full potential. Child abuse could then be defined as any action or omission by an adult responsible for that child which either temporarily or permanently interferes with that development. In a real world we must settle for something less. What we are able to achieve is a good measure of our success as a society. In this section we will not be concerned with mental or social abuse or educational ineptitude, not because these are unimportant, but because they are not primarily medical problems.

Child physical abuse

Clinical features. Non-accidental injuries (NAI) and other forms of child abuse occur when parents, at their wits end, strike out at their helpless but demanding infant. It also happens when ignorant, inept, cruel, selfish, irresponsible or mentally sick parents do not exert reasonable self control. Gripping and shaking the baby may produce fingertip bruising on his chest and arms. Forcing his mouth open to give food may cause similar bruises on the cheeks. The frenulum may be torn or the palate scratched by objects pushed in the mouth.

Gripping injuries

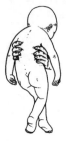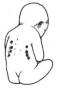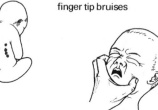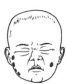

finger tip bruises

Slapping and hitting the infant may cause black eyes or characteristic strap marks. The skin of the attacked infant may also show scratches, bite marks, cigarette burns of scalds. Rough handling may fracture long bones, ribs or skull. Swinging the baby by the legs or arms can cause epiphyseal separation at the end of the long bones. Squeezing the limbs with rotation can separate the periosteum and cause periosteal haematomas. Repeated injuries of the same bone leads to large callus formation.

Other non-accidental injuries

cigarette burns

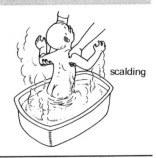

scalding

bite marks

Banging the head not only produces fractures of the skull but haemorrhages in the eyes and occasionally blindness. Shaking the head can tear superficial veins over the brain and cause subdural haematomas. The child may weather the initial injury, but the blood clot may then draw in fluid; the infant then develops the clinical features of a space-occupying lesion of slow onset. He may present with vomiting or fits or changes in the level of responsiveness and activity. The fontanelle is full and there may be papilloedema and retinal bleeds. This injury may kill the child; if it does not, it often leaves him mentally retarded, hemiplegic or blind.

Bony injuries

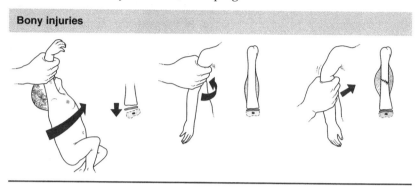

All the baby's injuries must be noted in detail and photographed if possible. A careful enquiry is essential. The parents often delay in bringing the child for medical attention. Their story does not accord with the injuries. Their explanation for the injuries may change if they are pressed. Their concern for the child may be inappropriate, they may show too much concern or anger or they may be off-hand and indifferent. Often they are relieved when hospital admission is advised. Sometimes they will talk at length about their own anxieties and problems and say how difficult and demanding the baby has been. It is very important to record precisely the history as it is given, with an evaluation of the parents' attitudes.

The injury that can kill or leave a child with brain damage

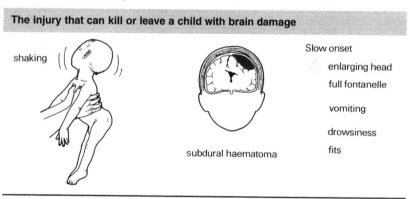

shaking

subdural haematoma

Slow onset
enlarging head
full fontanelle
vomiting
drowsiness
fits

Child abuse occurs in families from all walks of life but it is more common in the underprivileged and in families where actions speak louder than words. As Professor Kempe has suggested, the setting in which child abuse might occur includes a number of elements:

1. The parents have usually had troubled childhoods themselves; they may be from broken homes or have suffered deprivation or abuse themselves when children.
2. There are problems with the marriage; for example the marriage may be between two young people from disturbed homes who

married for the wrong reasons, perhaps because they wanted to leave home or were in need of affection. Some people mistakenly believe that a pregnancy will help to reverse a breaking relationship.

3. The child may be difficult to rear, he may have been premature or have a blemish or handicap. More often than not the child's problems are imaginary, the baby's first cry is seen as rejection, he fails to respond as his mother feels he should to her and this is felt to be his fault. An unloved child may be difficult, a difficult child may be unloved.

4. Against this background there may be added stresses, for example the father in trouble with the law or there may be financial or housing problems.

5. Finally, there are no life lines available, no close friends to whom the parents can turn for advice, support and relief.

Management. If a health visitor, social worker or casualty doctor suspects non-accidental injury the child must be admitted to a place of safety until a fuller enquiry has been made. This might be a police station, a social service institution or a hospital. If his parents are deliberately injuring him, society has a responsibility to protect him. If the parents are unwilling to release their child then he may have to be taken from them on the grounds laid down to obtain the necessary care order.

While providing temporary protection, the primary medical responsibility is to identify and treat the injuries, attend to the child's general wellbeing, and to exclude possible contributing factors and alternative diagnoses. It is equally important for others to evaluate the parents and the family situation and provide support and guidance if this is appropriate.

The distribution of the bruises is usually diagnostic. Babies when they begin to walk frequently fall and bruise their foreheads and shins, but do not bruise their upper arms and chests. Nevertheless bleeding diseases should be excluded. Brittle-bone disease is a rare condition where bruising as well as bone fractures occur with the slightest injury, but the fractures are in the shaft and not at the end of the long bones. Although some bony injuries are obvious, others are not, so a full skeletal survey by radiography is essential.

The social work team will usually take the lead in planning the strategy for management, but they depend on the full cooperation of medical and nursing personnel involved and the police. Initial policy is usually worked out at a case conference held as soon as possible after the diagnosis is firm. Subsequent management will depend on the background and on the attitudes of the parents. When investigations have been completed a full case conference with representatives from all agencies concerned in attendance is held to decide what legal action is required, what social work activity is to be attempted and what medical surveillance is desirable. Many children may be allowed home, initially under supervision, and though they may not live happily ever after they do appear to thrive and to be content.

Occasionally it is necessary to take the child away from his parents and put him into the care of others. The decisions are very difficult and even those with most knowledge and experience can get it wrong. Unhappy experiences in this area can harden the hearts of the wisest and kindest of men and produce vicious reaction in others.

Child neglect

A child may also be harmed by omission. This might be due to unavoidable circumstances, or ignorance or ineptness on the part of his guardians as well as deliberate attempts to hurt or punish him. The children are generally undernourished and undersized, the skin and hair are often in poor condition and they may be dirty and infested. Nasty rashes may be present in those places where the most dirt collects, the skin creases and nappy area.

Sexual misuse or abuse

Sexual abuse, that is a child being involved by an adult in sexual activities that he or she is not old enough to understand, or to give informed consent to, and which breaks the community taboos and expectations, appears to be on the increase. Although there is a notion that such activities happen at the hands of strangers, in fact it is three times more likely to occur within the family or within a circle of trusted friends. The first step is to recognise the problem for what it is, for both the adult and the child involved need expert counselling.

Emotional abuse

It is important to remember that emotional abuse may occur on its own in the form of open hostility, rejection or scapegoating, in which case it is obvious, or it may occur in less obvious ways, for example by not recognising the child's emotional need for affection, security and consistent care. All forms of child abuse and neglect involve emotional abuse. It is always necessary to attend to the emotional needs of abused children.

Deprivation

A child in a repressive atmosphere may appear to be well nourished and clean, but still fail to thrive, his hands and feet may be cold and small, and his growth suppressed. These more subtle forms of negligence or abuse are more difficult to recognise and define. The management as with most of the problems in this chapter includes a thorough clinical evaluation, a detailed enquiry about him, his family life and his neighbourhood, and a programme of care which is realistic and accepted by all concerned.

Münchausen syndrome by proxy

This is a bizarre form of child abuse in which one of those who cares for a child, usually the mother, persistently fabricates symptoms and signs such that the child becomes ill or is in danger of, or is subject to, unnecessary investigations and treatment. The diagnosis should be considered in any child whose illness is unexplained and prolonged or extraordinary in some way; when the child's signs and symptoms seem particularly inappropriate or incongruous, or only occur when the parent is present. It should also be suspected when treatments are surprisingly ineffective or not well tolerated. As in other instances of child abuse the parent may be inappropriately concerned, or alternatively not concerned about the severity of the child's supposed problems, or they may in some way benefit from the child's illness by way of support, attention or money.

Making a firm diagnosis can be difficult. There is no alternative to taking a clear history, particularly noting the time and place of the events described, and then making enquiries from others for supporting evidence. This means seeking information from other members of the family and other health professionals concerned with the child's care. If the diagnosis is suspected, it is important that the child and the parent be observed carefully. Perhaps the easiest way of making the diagnosis is to see if the signs and symptoms disappear when the parents are excluded.

Management can be difficult and it is vital for the child's sake for it to be firm and determined. This will involve case conferences and may mean keeping the child in a place of safety at least in the short term until the situation has been clarified.

BIBLIOGRAPHY

Garralda M E (ed) 1993 Managing children with psychiatric problems. BMJ Publishing Group, London
Goodman R, Scott S 1997 Child psychiatry. Blackwell Science, Oxford
Hoare P 1993 Essential child psychiatry. Churchill Livingstone, Edinburgh

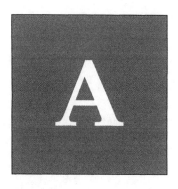

A Normal values

CLINICAL CHEMISTRY

These values are offered as a guide only. Local laboratories may differ. Check normal values with the laboratory you use. For less common tests check with your local laboratory.

Acid–base	pH 7.3–7.45 P_{CO_2} 4.5–6 kPA (32–45 mmHg) P_{O_2} 11–14 kPA (78–105 mmHg) Bicarbonate 18–25 mmol/l Base excess –4 to +3 mmol/l
Alanine amino-transferase (ALT)	Newborn–1 month up to 70 iu/l; infants and children 15–55 iu/l
Albumin	Preterm 25–45 g/l; newborn (term) 25–50 g/l; 1–3 months 30–42 g/l; 3–12 months 27–50 g/l; 1–15 years 32–50 g/l
Alkaline phosphatase	Newborn: 150–600 u/l; 6 months–9 years: 250–800 u/l
Ammonia	Newborn < 80 μmol/l; infants and children < 50 μmol/l
Amylase	70–300 iu/l
Aspartate amino-transferase (AST)	<45 iu/l
Base excess	See acid–base
Bicarbonate	See acid–base
Bilirubin	Full term day 1 < 65 μmol/l; day 2 < 115 μmol/l; 3–5 days < 155 μmol/l; > 1 month < 10 μmol/l
Calcium (ionised)	Adult value is 1.19–1.29 mmol/l
Calcium (total)	Preterm 1.5–2.5 mmol/l; infants 2.25–2.75 mmol/l; > 1 year 2.25–2.6 mmol/l; correction for protein binding—measure Ca^{2+} + (40 – albumin/40 g/l) mmol/l
Calcium (urine)	Children < 0.1 mmol/kg per 24 hours
Chloride	95–105 mmol/l
Creatine kinase	Newborn < 600 iu/l; 1 month < 400 iu/l; 1 year < 300 iu/l; children < 190 iu/l (male), < 130 iu/l (female)
Creatinine	0–2 years 20–50 μmol/l; 2–6 years 25–60 μmol/l; 6–12 years 30–80 μmol/l; > 12 years 65–120 μmol/l (male), 50–110 mmol/l (female)

Creatinine clearance	0–3 months 17–50 ml/min/m²; 3–12 months 26–75 ml/min/m²; 12–18 months 36–95 ml/min/m²; 2 years–adult 50–85 ml/min/m²
Creatinine (calculation of GFR from serum level)	GFR = 38 x ht (cm)/plasma creatinine (μmol/l)
C-reactive protein	< 20 mg/l
Gammaglutaryl transferase (GGT)	Neonate < 200 iu/l; 1 month–1 year < 150 iu/l; > 1 year < 30 iu/l
Glucose	Newborn–3 days 2–5 mmol/l; > 1 week 2.5–5 mmol/l
Glycosylated haemoglobin	4.5–7.5%
Lactate	0.7–1.8 mmol/l
Liver function	see Bilirubin, AST, GGT and Protein
Magnesium	Newborn 0.7–1.2 mmol/l; child 0.7–1.0 mmol/l
Osmolality	275–295 mmol/kg
Phosphate	Preterm first month 1.4–3.4 mmol/l; full term newborn 1.2–2.9 mmol/l; 1 year 1.2–2.2 mmol/l; 2–10 years 1.0–1.8 mmol/l; > 10 years 0.7–1.6 mmol/l
Potassium	0–2 weeks 3.7–6 mmol/l; 2 weeks–3 months 3.7–5.7 mmol/l; > 3 months 3.5–5 mmol/l
Protein (total)	1 month 50–70 g/l; 1 year 60–80 g/l; 1–9 years 60–81 g/l
Sodium	135–145 mmol/l
Urea	0–1 year 2.5–7.5 mmol/l; 1–7 years 3.3–6.5 mmol/l; 7–16 years 2.6–6.7 mmol/l (male), 2.5–6.0 mmol/l (female)

HAEMATOLOGY

Normal haematological indices for various ages

Age	Hb (g/dl) Mean (range)	MCV (fl) Mean (range)	WBC (× 10⁹/l) range	Reticulocyte (%) range
Birth	18.5 (14.5–21.5)	108 (95–116)	5–26	3–7
1 month	14.0 (10.0–16.5)	104 (85–108)	6–15	0–1
6 months	11.0 (8.5–13.5)	88 (80–96)	6–15	0–1
1 year	12.0 (10.5–13.5)	78 (70–86)	6–15	0–1
6 years	12.5 (11.5–14.0)	81 (75–88)	6–15	0–1
12 years	13.5 (11.5–14.5)	86 (77–94)	5–15	0–1

Note: an artefactual high neonatal WBC may be reported because automatic cell counters may wrongly include in the WBC the many normoblasts (red cell precursors) in the neonate

Blood pressure

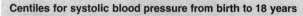

Centiles for systolic blood pressure from birth to 18 years

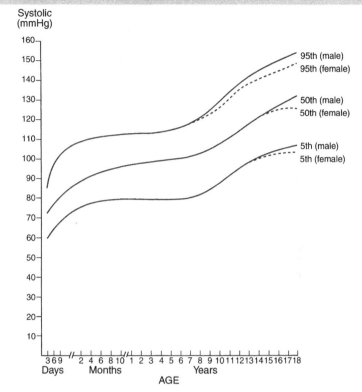

Centiles for diastolic blood pressure from birth to 18 years

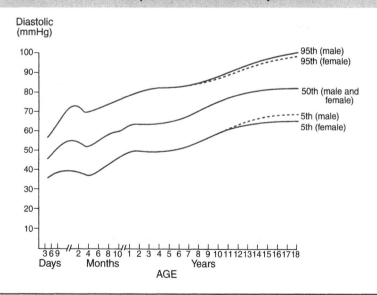

CALCULATING THE BODY SURFACE AREA FROM HEIGHT AND WEIGHT

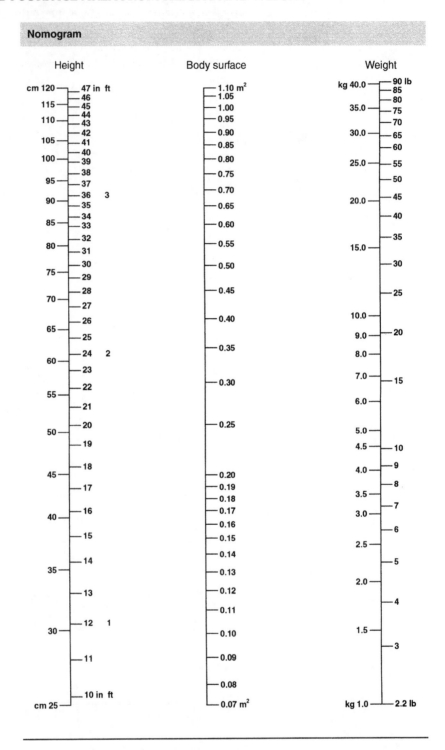

The nomogram may be used to calculate the body surface area from the weight and height of the patient. Note the patient's height on the left-hand scale and weight on the right-hand scale, and put a ruler between the two points; the point at which the line intersects the centre scale indicates the patient's body surface area.

Surface area and weight

	Weight (kg)	Surface area (m²)
Newborn	3	0.2
1 year	10	0.5
3 years	15	0.6
5 years	20	0.7
9 years	30	1.0
14 years	50	1.5
Adult	70	1.7

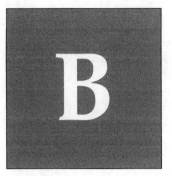

National immunisation schedule

Derived from Salisbury DM, Begg NT 1996 Immunisation against infectious disease. Department of Health, HMSO, London

---

INFANT

Birth	BCG for babies in Asian and other immigrant families with high TB rates and those in contact with active respiratory tuberculosis
2 months	Polio + diphtheria/tetanus/pertussis (DTP) + *Haemophilus influenzae* B (Hib)
3 months	Polio + DTP + Hib
4 months	Polio + DTP + Hib
12–15 months	Measles, mumps and rubella (MMR)

PRE-SCHOOL

3–5 years	Booster polio + diphtheria/tetanus (DT) + MMR 3 years after primary course

---

SECONDARY SCHOOL

10–14 years	BCG after tuberculin skin test

SCHOOL LEAVING

15–19 years	Polio + tetanus/diphtheria (Td) MMR if not received previously

---

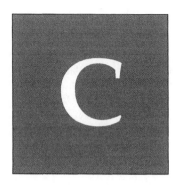

Child health promotion programme

The following is taken from *Health for All Children* edited by David Hall.

THE CORE PROGRAMME

The Child Health Promotion Programme consists of three main elements: immunisation (primary prevention of infectious disease), health education to minimise hazards and promote optimum physical and mental health and screening tests leading to early detection and intervention (secondary prevention). Emphasis has shifted to give greater prominence to the health education elements of the programme. Those providing the programme require knowledge of normal growth and development (physical, mental and emotional), understanding of how these may be influenced by social family and environmental attributes and communication and teaching skills. Recognition of child abuse and local child protection procedures are important parts of the training that is required. Recognition and referral of 'Children in need' (Children Act 1989), as well as recognition of physical and developmental problems, is an important part of child health surveillance.

The core programme of surveillance for all children incorporates those screening procedures which can be supported in the light of the available evidence. It consists of a series of checks and reviews which, it is hoped, will strike a balance between the risk of 'missing' children with problems on the one hand, while on the other avoiding an excessive number of examinations. In individual cases, parental concern or professional judgement may dictate that the child is seen on more or different occasions. In a minority of families, more intensive support and guidance may be needed, targeting health promotion information and support where it is most needed. No two primary care teams will function in exactly the same way and each will tailor the service to meet the particular needs of its population. Nevertheless, each of the key reviews has a different content and are delivered by GP, health visitor and practice nurse following a common protocol in which their complementary roles are identified. A District Child Health Promotion Co-ordinator, usually a consultant community paediatrician, is responsible for the District policy and its implementation. Clearly signposted referral pathways are required for problems that are identified through this programme.

The following is a summary of the recommended programme:

• incorporates details of the specified health checks and immunisations
• gives examples of topics for health education at each age
• stresses the importance of record systems that facilitate communication, clinical audit and epidemiological monitoring.

Consideration should always be given to social and psychological aspects of family life, whatever the nature of the examination or review. Housing and financial problems, parental depression and illness, and difficulties with siblings, are all relevant to the health and development of the individual child.

The commonest disabilities in childhood—behaviour, communication and continence problems—should be identified through a well run Child Health Surveillance (CHS) programme with the primary health-care team working in partnership with parents.

Neonatal examination

This would usually be the responsibility of suitably trained hospital staff, but should be the responsibility of the primary care team in the case of home deliveries, babies born in GP obstetric units and very early (<6 hours) discharges.

Content of review. Elicit and consider any concerns expressed by parents. Review of family history, pregnancy and birth. Full physical examination including weight and head circumference. Check for congenital dislocation of hips (CDH) and testicular descent. Inspect eyes, view red reflex of fundus with ophthalmoscope but do not attempt fundoscopy. If high risk category for hearing defect, the policy in many districts is for otoacoustic emissions (OAE) or brainstem evoked response (BSER) test of hearing. Phenylketonuria (PKU) and thyroid tests to be done at usual time. Haemoglobinopathy screen if specified in local policy.

Completion of record sheet, preferably in Parent Held Record.

Topics for health education could include: feeding and nutrition; baby care, sibling management; crying and sleep problems; transport in cars.

First 2 weeks

Many GPs consider it good practice to visit all new babies as soon as possible after discharge from hospital. This provides an opportunity to evaluate any concerns raised by the parents, and to cement the relationship with the family. In addition to the immediate benefits, this contact can be the prelude to an effective programme of surveillance and helps the members of the primary care team to estimate the level of support and assistance that each new parent is likely to require. Further physical examination should be undertaken if appropriate. Check hips again (this may be done by either a doctor or a nurse, provided that the person is adequately trained).

Topics for health education could include: nutrition; supine sleeping position and clothing; effects of passive smoking; accident prevention—bathing, scalding by feeds, fires, dangers of shaking baby; immunisation; reason for doing PKU and thyroid tests (and haemoglobinopathy if indicated); sibling management.

6–8 weeks

This check should be undertaken by the doctor responsible for the child's surveillance. The presence of the health visitor facilitates the sharing and follow up of any anxieties. The examination may be undertaken at the same visit as the first immunisation and/or the post-natal check for the mother; this is a matter for individual practices to decide.

Content of review. Check history and ask about parental concerns. Consider risk factors and relevant family history. Physical examination, weight, (+ length if indicated), and head circumference. These should be plotted on the centile charts on the personal child health record and explained to the parents. Check for CDH. Check heart and femoral pulses and testicular descent in boys. Boys with undescended testes should be referred at this examination. Enquire particularly about concerns regarding vision, squint and hearing. Inspect eyes, looking for abnormal appearance and movements and look for red reflex. Do not attempt hearing test (there is no simple clinical test of hearing suitable for primary care use in this age group). If a high risk hearing screening service is provided, check again whether baby is in high risk category for hearing loss and refer if necessary. Give parents checklist of advice for detection of hearing loss ('Hints for Parents'), or draw parents' attention to relevant information in Parent Held Record. Handling the baby during the examination will give an idea of tone and responsiveness. A thorough physical examination with the child completely undressed will ease concerns about the possibility of physical abuse or neglect in a small number of babies. Observation of parental handling and parent–child interaction is important.

Discuss immunisation. Signed consent is NOT essential, but should be obtained at this visit if thought desirable by individual practitioners. Record and explain results of neonatal biochemical screening tests.

Complete the record and ensure information is transferred to the agency responsible for monitoring the CHS programme (Health Authority/Health Board).

Topics for health education could include: immunisation; nutrition; dangers of fires, falls, overheating and scalds; recognition of illness in babies and what to do, sleeping position and passive smoking. Discussion of social security benefits and other sources of support should be provided for families on low income or other children in need. Specific enquiry may be required. Information from the home visit at 2 weeks may prompt such discussion.

2, 3 and 4 months

The baby should receive the primary course of immunisations at these ages. No specific checks are required, but the parent should have the opportunity to discuss any concerns with the appropriate member of the primary health care team. Weaning advice, promotion of social and language development, as well as praise and reassurance are important tasks especially for parents of first children and those who lack family support.

Weighing in the first 6 months. Regular weighing of normal healthy babies is of uncertain value. There is no doubt that parents value this procedure because of the reassurance it gives them that all is well, but health professionals should be aware of both the unnecessary anxiety and the false sense of security it can provide. Facilities for weighing should be available as part of a CHS service. The parent(s) should be encouraged to weigh the baby themselves, if they so wish.

6–9 months

This examination can be regarded as primarily the health visitor's responsibility, provided that the essential items of physical examination are undertaken (on an opportunistic basis if necessary); or it can be undertaken by the health visitor working together with the doctor.

Content of review. Enquire about parental concerns regarding health and development. Ask specifically about vision and hearing. Check weight if parents request or if indicated. Measure length if indicated. Look for evidence of CDH. Check for testicular descent. Observe visual behaviour and look for squint. Carry out distraction test of hearing. Note: TWO adequately trained staff, and suitable testing conditions, are essential for this test.

Complete the record and ensure information is transferred to the agency responsible for monitoring the CHS programme.

Topics for health education could include: accident prevention: choking, scalds and burns, falls, anticipate increasing mobility, i.e. safety gates, guards, etc. nutrition; dental prophylaxis; reinforce advice about safety in cars and passive smoking; developmental needs; sunburn.

18–24 months

This review is concerned primarily with parental guidance and education. It is often carried out at the family home and it is suggested that the health visitor is the most appropriate person to take responsibility for this examination. The doctor provides support and advice where necessary. In some families, however, opportunistic review by the doctor may be desirable, for example where the health visitor experiences difficulty in contacting the family at home. The amount of time devoted to this review in each case should be decided on the basis of the primary care team's overall knowledge of the child and family.

Content of review. Enquire about parental concerns, particularly regarding behaviour, vision and hearing. Confirm that the child is walking with a normal gait; and that speech production and comprehension are appropriate for age. Do not attempt formal tests of vision, hearing or language development. Arrange detailed assessment if in doubt. Remember the high prevalence of iron deficiency anaemia at this age. Carry out Hb estimation if local policy or if there are clinical concerns and plot on chart. Measure length or height IF child is sufficiently cooperative for accurate measurement.

Complete the record and ensure information is transferred to the agency responsible for monitoring the CHS programme.

Topics for health education could include: accident prevention: falls from heights including windows, drowning, poisoning, road safety; developmental needs: language and play; need to mix with other children—playgroup, etc. avoidance and management of behaviour problems. Diet remains an important topic for discussion. Parents frequently need guidance on toilet training.

Special educational needs of children and the Education Act 1996

The Education Act of 1996 requires the Health Authority to notify the Local Education Authority if it believes that a child has, or may have, Special Educational Needs, when the child reaches the age of 2 years (or sooner than this if the parents so wish). The primary care team should ensure that the specialist paediatric services are informed if there is ANY anxiety about a child's educational potential, so that the doctor with responsibility for liaison with the Education Authority can arrange further assessment and where necessary notification. This would usually involve discussion between the local educational psychologist, paediatrician, health visitor and other involved professionals, for example speech therapist or preschool parent–teacher counsellors. This provision of the Act was designed to ensure that children and parents benefit from the expertise of specialist teachers in the preschool years, and deserves the support of all professionals.

36–48 months

This can be regarded as a 'school readiness examination'. The aims are to ensure that the child is physically fit and that there are no medical disorders which may interfere with education; that the immunisations are up to date; and to determine whether there are problems with development, language or behaviour which may have educational implications. The review is usually carried out by the health visitor.

Content of review. Enquiry and discussion about vision, squint, hearing, behaviour, language acquisition and development. If any concerns, discuss with the parent whether the child is likely to have any special educational problems or needs and arrange further action as appropriate. Measure height and plot on chart. Check that testicular descent has been recorded and if not the child should be examined. If concerned about possible hearing impairment, perform hearing test IF adequately trained and equipped, otherwise refer.

Complete the record and ensure information is transferred to the agency responsible for monitoring the CHS programme.

Topics for health education could include: accidents: fires, roads, drowning; begin to teach road safety; preparation for school; nutrition and dental care.

5 years (school entry—range approximately 54–66 months)

The school entrant medical review is undertaken by the school nurse. Although child health surveillance now moves from the primary health care team to the school health service, effective communication must always be maintained. Some authorities believe that ALL school entrants should be offered not only a physical examination but also a full developmental evaluation. However, in most Districts and Boards, the universal 'cohort' examination of all school entrants has been discontinued, because the yield of new abnormalities is small. Only selected children are examined, on the basis of previously inadequate or poorly documented preschool surveillance, or concerns raised by parents or teachers. Whichever policy is adopted, it seems likely that a well conducted preschool surveillance programme, as outlined above, will progressively reduce the need for, and the yield of, detailed school entrant examinations. History is most important and may reveal concerns about general health, development and behaviour or identify 'a child in need'. For ALL children the following are recommended at school entry:

Enquire about parental and teacher concerns. Review preschool records, including immunisation status. Measure height and weight and plot on chart. Check vision using Snellen chart. Check hearing by 'sweep' test.

Complete the record and ensure information is transferred to the agency responsible for monitoring the CHS programme.

Health of school children

In many schools these checks are combined in a health interview in which the opportunity is taken to provide health education relevant to school health. Important topics include adjustment to school, accident prevention, medication needed in school, sunburn, and health services available within school.

The older child of school age will continue with a programme of child health promotion. The focus moves from screening procedures (with the exception of vision, colour vision and growth monitoring), towards health education ideally linked to national curriculum based teaching. The school nurse is well placed to provide individual advice on topics such as diet, exercise, smoking, substance misuse, relationships, stress management and sexual health. Self referral is encouraged. Review in school year 10 (age 14–15 years) has as one of its aims to provide career advice relevant to particular conditions and to liaise, where needed, with the careers service.

Index

A

Abdomen, examination, 6
Abdominal pain, 159–164
  acute, 159–163
    causes, 160
  key features, 159
  recurrent, 163–164
    psychological causes,
      343–344
  vomiting and, *see*
    Periodic syndrome
Abdominal wall defects,
  anterior, 66
ABO incompatibility,
  maternal–fetal, 63
Abortion, spontaneous,
  chromosomal
  abnormalities, 13
Abscess, brain, 307
Absence seizures
  atypical, 298
  simple, 298
Abuse, *see* Child abuse
Accessory skin tags, 45
Achondroplasia, 240
Acid maltase
  (α–glucosidase)
  deficiency, 267, 311
Acidosis, metabolic, 60–61
Acne, 278
Acrodermatitis
  enteropathica, 171,
  276–277
Acute organic disease,
  psychological impact,
  336
Addison's disease, 251
Adenitis
  cervical, 93
  mesenteric, 160
Adenoviruses in gene
  therapy, 29
Adolescent scoliosis,
  idiopathic, 286

Adoption, 340
Adrenal glands, 249–51
  carcinoma, 228
  congenital hyperplasia,
    250
  failure/insufficiency, 238
    primary adrenocortical,
      251
Adrenarche, premature,
  247–248
Aggressive behaviour, 345
AIDS, *see* HIV disease
Airways, 121–135, *see also*
  Respiratory disorders
Alcohol poisoning, 118
Alimentary tract disorders,
  see Gastrointestinal
  disorders
Allergens in asthma, in
  pathogenesis, 132
Allergic polyarthritis, 282
Allergy, food, *see* Food
  allergy
Alopecia areata, 278
Alpha–1–antitrypsin
  deficiency, 178
Alpha–fetoprotein (AFP), 33
Alpha–thalassaemia, 209
Alzheimer disease and
  Down syndrome, 15
Aminoacidopathies, 262
Aminoaciduria, 184
Anaemia, 202–212
  aplastic, 204
  haemolytic, *see*
    Haemolytic anaemia
  infantile causes, 202
  iron deficiency, 203–204
  neonatal causes, 202
  sickle cell, *see* Sickle cell
    anaemia
Andersen's disease (type IV
  glycogenosis), 264
Anencephaly, 67
Angelman syndrome, 23

Anhidrotic ectodermal
  dysplasia, congenital,
  276
Ankylostoma duodenale, 173
Ano–rectal anomaly, 65–66
Anorexia nervosa, 346–347
Anoxic seizures, reflex, 303
Antenatal diagnosis, *see*
  Prenatal diagnosis
Anterior horn cell disorders,
  312–313
Antibiotics
  in congenital heart
    disease, prophylaxis
  in dental treatment,
    155
  meningitis, 306
  osteomyelitis, 284
  rheumatic fever, 156
  tuberculosis, 103–104
  urinary tract infections,
    188, 189
Antibody defects, 108
Anticonvulsants, *see*
  Anti–epileptics
Antidepressant poisoning,
  117–118
Anti–epileptics, 300–301
  dosage/side–effects, 302
  status epilepticus, 302
Anti–inflammatory agents,
  asthma, 133
Anti–oncogenes, 29
Antisocial behaviour, 345
Antituberculous drugs,
  103–104
Anxiety (and fear), 346
  in organic disease, 336
Aorta, coarctation, 147–148
Aortic stenosis, 146–147
Apgar Score, 50
Aplastic anaemia, 204
Apnoeic attacks, 60
Aponeurosis (epicranial),
  bleeding under, 47

Appendicitis, acute, 160
  non–specific abdominal
    pain vs, 160, 161
Arrhythmias, cardiac,
    153–154
Arthritis, 281–283
  juvenile chronic, 282–283
  pyogenic, 281
  tuberculous, 281
  viral, 281
Artificial feeding, 78–80
Aryl sulphatase deficiency,
    266
Ascaris lumbricoides, 173
Ascorbate (vitamin C)
    deficiency, 84–85
Asperger syndrome, 331,
    335–336
Aspiration into lung,
    neonatal, 57–59
Aspirin
  poisoning, 117
  Reye syndrome with, 179,
    308
Asthma, 131–135
  acute exacerbations, 135
Ataxia, 303–304
  acute, 304
  in cerebral palsy, 294, 295,
    303–304
  Friedreich, 304
Ataxia telangiectasia, 304
Athetoid (dystonic) cerebral
    palsy, 294, 295
Atopic eczema, 271–272
Atrial septal defect
  ostium primum, 140–141
  ostium secundum, 139–40
Attention deficit disorder
    with/without
    hyperactivity,
    334–335
Audition, see Hearing
Auscultation,
    cardiopulmonary, 6,
    see also Murmurs;
    Sounds
  neonatal, 44
Autism, 331, 335–336
Autoimmune disease
  liver, chronic, 180
  maternal, 41
  thyroid, 253
Autosomal chromosomes
  numerical/structural
    abnormalities, 14–17
  single gene defects, 19–22
Avascular necrosis of

femoral head, 289

B

Babies, see Infants; Neonates
Bacterial endocarditis, 155
Bacterial gastroenteritis, 165
Bacterial pneumonia, see
    Pneumonia
Bacterial skin infections,
    272–273
Balloon techniques
  transposition of great
    arteries, 153
  valvuloplasty
    aortic stenosis, 147
    pulmonary stenosis, 150
BCG vaccination, 104
Becker muscular dystrophy,
    310
Bedwetting (nocturnal
    enuresis), 331–332,
    343
Behaviour
  illness behaviour, 337
  neonatal, 44
  problems, 326, 341–345
    in cerebral palsy, 295
    factors decreasing
      likelihood, 327
    factors increasing
      likelihood, 327
    management, 348–349
Beta–agonists, asthma, 133
Beta–thalassaemia,
    heterozygous, 209
Beta–thalassaemia major,
    208–209
Biliary atresia, 177–178
Bilirubin excess, see
    Hyperbilirubinaemia
Biochemical screening,
    neonatal, 46
Birth injuries, 46–48
Birth marks, 44–45, 275–276
Birth weight (and size),
    52–57
  low, see Low birth weight
Bladder, exstrophy, 187
Bladder control, 343
Bleeding, see Haemorrhage
Bleeding disorders, 202,
    209–211
Blindness, 316–317
Blisters, see Bullae; Bullous
    impetigo
Block, heart, complete, 154

Blood, exchange transfusion,
    64
Blood disorders, 202–12
Blood group, maternal–fetal
    incompatibility, 35,
    62, 63, 64
Blood pressure
  high, see Hypertension
  measurement, 156
  normal values, 357
Blood tests, renal function
    and, 184, see also
    Haematology
Blue–back pigmented areas,
    45
Body surface area
    calculation, 358–359
Bone, 280
  disorders, 283–292
    neoplastic, 227, 291–292
Bone marrow
  growth factors, with
    cancer chemotherapy,
    216
  transplantation in cancer,
    216
Bordetella pertussis, 99–101,
    128
Bottlefeeding, 78–80
Bow legs, 285
Bowel (intestine)
  in faecal soiling
    bowel control, 333, 343
    empty bowel, 333
  inflammatory bowel
    disease, 162–163
  intussusception, 162–163
  malrotation, 161–162
  neonatal obstruction,
    65–66
  parasites, 173–174
Boys
  growth charts, 233, 234
  incomplete
    masculinisation, 249
  pauciarticular juvenile
    chronic arthritis, 283
  puberty, 244–245
    precocious, 247
Brachial plexus injury, 48
Brain, 293–308
  haemorrhage, preterms,
    55
  hypoxia and its
    consequences
    (perinatal), 51–52, 60
  infections, 307–308
    HSV, 95–6, 307–308

measles, 91, 308
injury, 112–13
non–accidental, 350–351
psychological effects of
    diseases of, 328–329
tumours, 222–223
Breast enlargement
    (thelarche)
normal, 245
premature, 247
neonatal, 45, 247
Breastfeeding, 75–8
advantages, 77
change to bottlefeeding,
    79
choosing not to
    breastfeed, 77
contraindications, 77–8
jaundice with, 177
Breath sounds/noises, 6
Breath–holding attacks, 303,
    342
Brittle–bone disease
    (osteogenesis
    imperfecta), 291, 352
Bronchiectasis, 131
Bronchiolitis, 126–128
Bronchodilators, asthma,
    133
Bronchopulmonary
    dysplasia, 60
Bullae (blisters), 269
    in epidermolysis bullosa,
    276, 277
Bullous impetigo, 273
Burns, 113–114

C

Caecal descent, arrested, 161
Café–au–lait spots, 276, 277
Calcaneovalgus, 290–291
Calculi, renal, 187
Cancer, see Malignancy
Candidiasis
    on nappy rash, 270, 271
    oral (thrush), 72
Capillary haemangioma, 44,
    275
Capillary naevus, 275
Caput succedaneum, 47
Carbon monoxide
    poisoning, 119
Carcinomas, 228
Cardiac problems, see Heart

Cardiovascular
    system,136–158, see
    also Heart
examination, 6
Carditis in rheumatic fever,
    156, see also
    Endocarditis
Caries, 86–87
Carrier detection, 27, 28
    sex–linked recessive
        disorders, 22
Cataracts, 316
Central nervous system
    tumours, 222–223, see
    also Brain
Cephalhaematoma, 47
Cerebral disorders, see Brain
    and specific disorders
Cerebral palsy, 293–296
    ataxic, 294, 295, 303–304
Cerebrospinal fluid
    examination
        encephalitis, 308
        meningitis, 306, 307
        shunts, in hydrocephalus,
        69
Cervical lymphadenopathy,
    93
Chemistry, clinical, normal
    values, 355–356
Chemotherapy (in cancer),
    215–216
    bone marrow growth
        factors in, 216
    specific tumours
        leukaemia, 218, 220
        lymphoma, 221, 222
        neuroblastoma, 224
Chickenpox, see Varicella
Child abuse, 349–354
    physical, 350–353
    sexual, 189, 353
Child health promotion
    programme, 9,
    361–364
Child health service, 9
Child neglect, 353
Children's Coma Scale, 112
Chlamydia trachomatis,
    neonatal, 40, 71–72
Choking, 115
Chondromalacia patellae,
    290
Christmas disease, 210
Chromosomes, 12–19, see
    also Cytogenetics
    abnormalities, 13–19
    learning disability

associated with, 14,
    322
    malignancy associated
        with, 213
Chronic disease
    psychological impact, 336
    short stature, 236
Circumcision, 200, 201
Cirrhosis, 181
Cleft lip/palate, 69–70
Clinical chemistry, normal
    values, 355–356
Clothes, removing, 5
Clumsiness, 330
Coagulation, disseminated
    intravascular, 211–212
Coeliac disease, 169–170
Cold sores, 95
Colic, 3–month, 84
Colitis
    food allergy, 172
    ulcerative, 172
Coma Scales, 112, 113
Complement
    assays, 106
    deficiencies, 108–109
Compulsion, 348
Conception
    folic acid supplements
        around time of, 25
    medicine before, 31
Conduct disorders, 345
Conductive deafness, 319
Congenital disorders
    adrenal hyperplasia, 250
    diaphragmatic hernia,
        64–65
    dislocation of hip, 286–288
    heart disease, see Heart
    hepatic fibrosis, 182
    hypothyroidism, 252
    megacolon
        (Hirschsprung's
        disease), 65, 176
    myopathies, 311
    nephrotic syndrome, 195
    postural deformities, 46
    sacrococcygeal teratoma,
        226
    skin lesions, 275–277
    stridor, 123–124
Conjunctivitis, see also
        Keratoconjunctivitis
    chlamydial, 40, 71–72
    gonococcal, 40, 71–72
Consent, immunisation, 362
Constipation, 174–176, 333
    infant, 84

Constitutional delay in growth and puberty, 235, 246
Consultation, 1–7
Convulsions/seizures, 297–303
    epileptic, 297–300
        types/classification, 297, 298–300
    factitious, 303
    febrile, 302
    neonatal, 72–73
    reflex anoxic, 303
Cori's disease (type III glycogenosis) III, 264
Corynebacterium diphtheriae, 99
Cot death (SIDS), 10
Cough, persistent (infant), differential diagnosis, 132
Cows' milk, 78–79
    protein intolerance, 170
    secondary, 168
Cranial radiotherapy affecting puberty, 248
Craniopharyngioma, 238
Craniosynostosis, 231
Cranium bifidum defects, 67
Cri–du–chat syndrome, 17
Crigler–Najjar syndrome, 177
Crohn disease, 171–172
Cromoglycate, asthma, 133
Croup, 126
Crouzon's syndrome, 70
Crying baby, 84
Cushing syndrome, 251
Cutaneous lesions, *see* Skin lesions
Cyanosis
    in heart disease, 137, 150–153
    in lung disease, 137
Cyst(s)
    bone (simple), 291–292
    oral, neonatal, 45
    renal (simple), 185
Cystic fibrosis, 128–131
    carrier detection, 28
Cystitis, acute haemorrhagic, 191
Cystourethrogram, micturating, 184, 188
Cytogenetics (incl. karyotype), *see also* Chromosomes
    in acute lymphoblastic

leukaemia prognosis, 219
cri–du–chat syndrome, 17
Down syndrome, 15
Edwards syndrome, 15-16
fragile X syndrome, 19
Klinefelter syndrome, 18
Patau syndrome, 17
short stature, 239
Turner syndrome, 18–19
Wilms tumour, 225
Cytomegalovirus, 37–38

D

Day dreams, 303
Deafness, 317, 318–319
    causes, 318
    treatment, 318–319
    types, 318
Deaths, *see* Mortalities
Debranching enzyme deficiency III, 264
Deformity, psychological impact, 337
Dehydration in gastroenteritis, 166–167
Deletion analysis, 28
Dental caries, 86–87
Dental treatment, antibiotic prophylaxis in congenital heart disease, 155
Depression, 347
Deprivation, emotional, 353
Dermatitis/eczema
    atopic, 271–272
    napkin, *see* Nappy rashes
    seborrhoeic, 270
Dermatological disorders, *see* Skin lesions
Dermatomyositis, 311
Development
    delayed, 329–336
        psychological causes, 343
        speech/language, 319–320, 331
    stages in, 3, 4
Diabetes, 255–259
Dialysis, 197
Diaphragmatic hernia, congenital, 64–65
Diarrhoea, 164–168
    chronic, 171–172
    differential diagnosis, 165

infant, 84
Diastolic BP, normal values, 357
Diazepam, status epilepticus, 302
Diet, *see also* Nutrition
    hypercholesterolaemia and, 158
    interventions
        attention deficit disorder with/without hyperactivity, 335
        diabetes, 257
        faecal soiling, 333
        food intolerance, 170, 171
        gluten enteropathy, 170
        migraine, 297
        obesity, 89
Diphtheria, 99
Disability, psychological impact, 337
Dislocation, hip, congenital, 286–288
Disseminated intravascular coagulation, 211–212
Diverticulum, Meckel, 162
Divorce, 339
DNA
    repair defects, malignancy associated with, 213
    Southern blotting, 28
DNA markers, 26, 27
Dominant disorders
    autosomal, 19–20
    X–linked, 2
Doppler ultrasound, fetal, 34
Down syndrome, 13, 14–15
    growth failure, 232
    prenatal screening, 33
Drowning, 114–115
Drug(s), *see also* Poisoning
    in breast milk, 77
    fetus adversely affected by, 36–37
Drug therapy, *see also specific types of drugs*
    arthritis (juvenile chronic), 283
    asthma, 133–134, 135
    cancer, *see* Chemotherapy
    epilepsy, 300–301
    fetal, 35
Dry powder inhalers, 134
Duchenne muscular dystrophy, 28, 309–310

Ductus arteriosus, patent, 143–145
Duodenal atresia, 65
Dyslexia, 320, 330
Dysmorphic syndromes, learning disorder, 323
Dysplasia
  bronchopulmonary, 60
  congenital anhidrotic ectodermal, 276
  hip, developmental, 286–288
  renal, unilateral, 185
  skeletal, 240–241
Dysrhythmias
  cardiac, 153–154
  speech (stammer), 321
Dystonic cerebral palsy, 294, 295
Dystrophin gene, 309, 310

E

Ear infections, middle, 122
Eating disorder, 346–347
Ectodermal dysplasia, congenital anhidrotic, 276
Eczema, see Dermatitis
Education
  child with learning disability, 323, 364
  health (parents), 362, 363, 364
Edwards' syndrome, 15–16
Eisenmenger syndrome, 145
Emesis, see Vomiting
Emotional abuse, 353
Emotional deprivation, 353
Emotional
  problems/psycho-logical problems, 326, 346–348
  factors decreasing likelihood, 327
  factors increasing likelihood, 327
  management, 348–349
Empyema, pleural, 125–126
Encephalitis, 307–308
  HSV, 95–6, 307
  measles, 91, 308
Encephalomyelitis, 307
Encopresis, 332–333
Endocarditis, bacterial, 155
Endocrine disorders, 243–259

with brain tumours, 223
growth disorders in
  excessive height, 242
  short stature, 238
Endotracheal intubation, neonatal, 51
Enterobius vermicularis, 173
Enterocolitis, necrotising, 55
Enuresis, 189–190
  causes, 190
  nocturnal, 331–332, 343
Environmental causes
  accidents, 110, 118–120
  psychological problems, 340–341
  short stature, 235–236
Enzymopathies, 262–267
Epidermolysis bullosa, 276, 277
Epilepsy, 297–302
  assessment, 300
  management, 300–302
  psychological aspects, 328–329
Epiphysis, slipped upper femoral, 289
Epstein pearls, 45
Epstein–Barr virus, 96
Epulis, 45
Equinovarus, 290
Erysipelas, 273
Erythema infectiosum, 38, 97
Erythema multiforme, 278, 279
Erythema nodosum, 278, 279
Erythema toxicum, 270
Erythrocytes, see Red cells
Erythrophagocytic lymphohistiocytosis, familial, 229
Ewing sarcoma, 227
Examination, 5–6, see also specific disorders
  fetal, 32–35
  neonatal (routine), 43–46, 362
Exanthema subitum, 97
Exchange transfusion, 64
Exercise, faecal soiling, 333
Exomphalos, 66
Eye, see also Vision
  migraine related to ocular problems, 297
  neonatal infections, 40, 71–2
  preterm infants, 55–56, 317

tumours, see Retinoblastoma
vitamin A deficiency disorder, 84

F

Face, developmental abnormalities, 70
Facioscapulohumeral muscular dystrophy, 310
Factitious seizures, 303
Factor VIII deficiency, 210
Factor IX deficiency, 210
Faecal soiling, 332–333
  encopresis, 332–333, 343
Failure to thrive, 83
Fainting, 303
Fall(s), 112
Fallot's tetralogy, 150–151
Familial factors
  psychological problems, 326, 338–340
  short stature, 235
Family
  338–340, see Parents
  breakdown, 339
  support in cancer, 214
Family cancer syndromes, 213
Family practice, 8
Fanconi anaemia, 204
Fatalities, see Mortalities
Fathers, bonding, 338–339, see also Family; Parents
Fatty acid oxidation defect, 265
Fear, see Anxiety
Febrile convulsions, 302
Feeding, 74–84
  problems, 80–84
Feet, see Foot
Feminisation, testicular, 22
Femoral head
  avascular necrosis, 289
  slipped epiphysis, 289
Fetus, 31–42
  adult disease and the, 41–42
  examination, 32–35
  therapy, 35–36
  transition to independent life, 48–52
  transplacental infections, 37–40, 92–93

Fibrosis
  cystic, *see* Cystic fibrosis
  hepatic, congenital, 182
Fifth disease, 38, 97
Fistula,
    tracheo–oesophageal,
    64
5p– deletion, 17
Flat feet, 285
Floppy infants, 313
Fluid therapy in diarrhoeal
    illness
  intravenous, 168
  oral, 167
Folic acid supplements,
    periconception, 25
Follicle–stimulating
    hormone (FSH), 245
  abnormal levels, 246
Fontanelles, examination,
    6–7, 45
Food allergy
  colitis, 172
  migraine, 297
Food intolerance, 168, 170,
    171, 264
Foot/feet
  deformities, 290–291
  flat, 285
Foreign body, aerodigestive
    tract, 123
  choking on, 115
Foreskin (prepuce), 200–201
Fragile X syndrome, 19
Friedreich ataxia, 304
Fructose intolerance,
    hereditary, 264
Fungal infections
  cutaneous, 274
  oral, 72

G

Gait
  in–toe, 284–285
  out–toe, 285
Galactosaemia, 264
Galactose–glucose
    malabsorption, 170
Gangliosidosis, GM₂, 266
Gastroenteritis, infective,
    164–168
Gastrointestinal disorders,
    159–182, *see also*
    specific parts
  infections, 160, 164–168,
    173–174

tuberculosis, 103
  neonatal, 64–66
Gastro–oesophageal reflux,
    81–82
Gastroschisis, 66
Gaucher disease, 267
Gender ambiguities,
    248–249
Gene(s), single, defects in,
    19–23
Gene therapy, 29–30
Gene tracking, 26
General practice, 8
Genetic counselling, 30
  autosomal dominant
    disorders, 20
Genetic disorders, 12–30, *see*
    also specific disorders
  blood
    aplastic anaemias, 204
    bleeding disorders,
      210–211
    haemolytic anaemias,
      205–206
  bone/joint, 291
  growth
    excessive height, 241
    short stature, 240
  immune system, 108
  learning disability in, 14,
    322
  metabolic, *see* Metabolic
    disease, inherited
  muscle, 309–311
Genetic factors
  diabetes, 255
  short stature, 235
Genitalia, ambiguous, 249
Genomic imprinting, 23
Genu valgum, 285
Genu varum, 285
Germ cell tumours, 226
German measles, *see* Rubella
Giardia lamblia, 173
Gingivostomatitis, acute, 95,
    273
Girls
  growth charts, 233
  pauciarticular juvenile
    chronic arthritis, 283
  puberty, 244
    early, 246–247
    virilised, 26, 249, 250
Glandular fever, 96
Glasgow Coma Scale, 112, 113
Glomerular filtration rates,
    184
Glomerulonephritis,

poststreptococcal,
    191–2
Glucocerobrosidase
    deficiency, 267
Glucose, blood (glycaemia)
  low, *see* Hypoglycaemia
  monitoring in diabetes,
    257
Glucose–6–phosphatase
    deficiency, 264
Glucose–6–phosphate
    dehydrogenase
    deficiency, 63, 206
α–Glucosidase (acid
    maltase) deficiency,
    267, 311
Glucosuria, 184
Glue ear, 122
Gluten enteropathy, 169–170
Glycaemia, *see* Glucose,
    blood
Glycogen storage diseases
  type I, 264
  type II, 267, 311
  type III, 264
  type IV, 264
Glycosuria, 184
GM₂ gangliosidosis, 266
Goitre, 252–253
  endemic, 252
Graft–versus–host disease,
    216
Granuloma annulare, 277,
    278
Granulomatous disease,
    chronic, 109
Great arteries, transposition,
    152–153
Growth, 230–242
  delay in
    constitutional, 235
    psychological causes,
      343
  disorders, 232–242
  head, 230–231
Growth factors, bone
    marrow, with cancer
    chemotherapy, 216
Growth hormone, 236–237
  deficiency, 236–237, 239
  measurements, 239
  physiology, 236
  treatment using, 239
    in GH deficiency, 237,
      239
    in skeletal dysplasias,
      241
Guillain–Barré syndrome,
    312

Gut, *see* Gastrointestinal
    disorders
Guthrie test, 262, 263
Guttate psoriasis, 277

H

Habits, 343
    habit spasms, 303
Haemangioma
    capillary, 44, 275
    macular, 44
Haematological disorders,
    202–212
Haematology, normal
    values, 184, *see also*
    Blood tests
Haematuria, 183–184,
    190–191
Haemoglobin
    concentration, age–related
        changes, 202, 356
    synthesis disorders,
        206–209
Haemoglobinopathies,
    207–208
Haemolytic anaemia, 202,
    205–206
    in red cell enzyme
        deficiency, 63, 206
Haemolytic disease, 62–63
    rhesus, 35, 62, 63, 64
Haemolytic uraemic
    syndrome, 195–196
Haemophilia A, 210
Haemophilia B, 210
Haemophilus influenzae, 304,
    306
    vaccination, 106, 304
Haemorrhage and bleeding
    anaemia with, 202
    intraventricular, preterms,
        55
    pulmonary, 60
    subaponeurotic, 47
    vitamin K deficiency, 86
Haemorrhagic cystitis,
    acute, 191
Hair loss on scalp, 278
Hand, foot and mouth
    disease, 97
Hashimoto's (autoimmune)
    thyroiditis, 253
Hazards, everyday, 110–120
Head
    growth, 230
        disorders, 230–231

injury, 112–113
    falls, 112
    non–accidental, 350–1
Head lice, 275
Headache, 296–297, *see also*
    Migraine
Health education (parents),
    362, 363, 364
Health promotion
    programme, child, 9,
    361–364
Hearing, 317–319
    assessment, 317–319
    loss, *see* Deafness
Hearing aid, 319
Heart, 136–158
    arrhythmias, 153–154
    congenital disease, 61,
        136–153
        acyanotic, 138–145
        aetiology, 136
        antenatal detection, 136
        antibiotic prophylaxis in
            dental treatment, 155
        cyanotic, 137, 150–153
        obstructive lesions,
            146–150
        presentation, 137
    failure, 137
    murmurs/sounds, *see*
        Murmurs; Sounds
Heat rash, 45
Height, 231–232, *see also*
    Stature
    in body surface area
        calculation, 358–359
    charts, 233, 234
Helicobacter pylori, 163–164
Helminths, intestinal,
    173–174
Henoch–Schönlein purpura,
    192, 281–282
Hepatic problems, *see* Liver
    and below
Hepatitis, chronic, 180
    autoimmune, 180
Hepatitis A, 98, 178–179
Hepatitis B, 98, 179, 180
    neonatal, 41, 98, 179
Hepatitis C, 179, 180
Hepatitis syndrome,
    neonatal, 178
Hepatomegaly, 177
    causes/diagnostic signs,
        182
Heritable disorders, *see*
    Genetic disorders
Hernia

congenital diaphragmatic,
    64–65
    inguinal, 199–200
Herpes simplex infections,
    94–6
    intracranial, 96–97,
        307–308
    neonatal, 40–41, 95
    skin, 273, 274
Herpes varicella zoster, *see*
    Herpes zoster;
    Varicella;
    Varicella–zoster virus
Herpes zoster (shingles), 94,
    273
    maternal, 38
Hexosaminidase complex,
    deficiency, 266
Hip disorders, 286–289
Hirschsprung's disease, 65,
    176
Histiocytosis, 228–289
History–taking, 3–5
HIV disease/AIDS, 105
    infant, 38, 105
Hodgkin disease, 220–221
Home monitoring, diabetes,
    257
Homocystinuria, 241
Hookworm, 173
Hormonal disorders,
    see Endocrine
    disorders
Horseshoe kidney, 186
Hospital service, 8
HPV skin infection (viral
    warts), 273, 274
HSV, *see* Herpes simplex
Human immunodeficiency
    virus, *see* HIV
Human papilloma virus,
    skin infection (viral
    warts), 273, 274
Hunter syndrome, 267
Hurler syndrome, 267
Hyaline membrane disease
    (respiratory distress
    syndrome), 59–60
Hydroceles, 199–200
Hydrocephalus, 68–69, 231
11ß–Hydroxylase deficiency,
    251
21–Hydroxylase deficiency,
    26, 250–251
Hyperactivity, attention
    deficit disorder with,
    334–335
Hyperbetalipoproteinaemia,
    familial, 157–158

Hyperbilirubinaemia, 61–62
  conjugated vs
    unconjugated, causes,
    177
  management, 63–64
Hypercholesterolaemia
  diet and, 158
  familial, 157–158
Hypergonadotrophic
  hypogonadism, 246
Hyperinsulinism, 258, 259
Hyperkinetic syndrome,
  334–335
Hyperlipoproteinaemia,
  157–158
Hyperplasia, congenital
  adrenal, 250
Hypertension (intracranial),
  see Intracranial
    hypertension
Hypertension (vascular),
  156–157
  portal, 181
  pulmonary, see Pulmonary
    hypertension
Hyperthyroidism, 253
Hypertonic dehydration,
  166
Hypochondroplasia,
  240–241
Hypoglycaemia, 258–259
  ketotic, 259
Hypogonadism
  hypergonadotrophic, 246
  hypogonadotrophic, 246
Hypogonadotrophic
  hypogonadism, 246
Hypoparathyroidism,
  253–254
  short stature, 238
  treatment, 254
Hypopituitarism/pituitary
  failure
  GH deficiency in, 237
  tumours causing, 238
Hypoplasia
  left heart, 148–9
  unilateral renal, 185
Hypospadias, 201
Hypothalamic–pituitary
  disorders, 237
  features, 241
Hypothyroidism, 252–3
  congenital, 252
  goitrous, 252–253
  juvenile, 238, 252
Hypotonia, 313

Hypoxaemia, perinatal,
  49–50
Hypoxia, perinatal, 49–50
  neonatal effects, 51–52, 60
Hysterical pseudoseizures,
  303

I

Ichthyosis, 276
Iduronate–2–sulphatase
  deficiency, 267
L–Iduronidase deficiency,
  267
Ileal atresia, 65
Ileus, meconium, see
  Meconium ileus
Illness behaviour, 337
Imaging, renal tract, 184
Immune deficiency, see
  Immunodeficiency
Immune system
  abnormal development,
    107
  investigation, 106
  normal development,
    106–107
Immunisation, see Vaccines
Immunodeficiency, 106–109
  combined, 108
  malignancy associated
    with, 213
Immunoglobulin A
  deficiency, 108
  selective, 107
Immunoglobulins, maternal,
  41–42
Impetigo, 272, 273
Incontinence (urinary), 189,
  see Enuresis
Incontinentia pigmenti, 276,
  277
Infants
  anaemia, causes, 202
  breastfeeding difficulties,
    77–78
  floppy, 313
  health promotion and,
    362–364
  mortality, 10
  newborn, see Neonates
  rashes, 45, 84, 270–271
  spasms, 298–299
  vaccination schedule, 360
Infections, 37–41, 90–109, see
  also specific (types of)
  pathogens and diseases

anaemia in, 202
bone, 283–284
endocardial, 155
gastrointestinal, see
  Gastrointestinal
    disorders
hepatic, see Liver
intracranial, see
  Intracranial infections
joint, 281
neonatal, 57, 70–72, 95, 98,
  179
  acquired in vaginal
    delivery, 40–41
  meningitis, 40, 71,
    306–307
  preterm infants, 54–55
  renal/urinary tract, 163,
    187–189
  respiratory tract, see
    Respiratory infections
  skin, 272–275
  transplacental, 37–40,
    92–93
Infestations, 274–275
Inflammatory bowel
  disease, 171–172
Inguinal hernia, 199–200
Inhalers in asthma, 134
Inherited disorders, see
  Genetic disorders
Injury/trauma, 110, 111–113
  birth, 46–48
  non–accidental, 350–353
  thermal, 113–114
Insulin
  in diabetes therapy, 256,
    257
  high levels
    (hyperinsulinism),
    258, 259
Insulin–dependent diabetes,
  255–259
Intelligence
  measurement, 321
  psychological aspects,
    329, 337
Interview, 1–7
Intestine, see Bowel
In–toe gait, 284–285
Intracranial hypertension
  (raised pressure)
  benign, 297
  brain tumours, 223
Intracranial infections,
  304–308
  herpes simplex, 95–96,
    307–308

measles, 91, 308
Intrauterine growth failure
    persisting into
    childhood, 235
Intravenous fluids,
    diarrhoeal illness, 168
Intraventricular
    haemorrhage,
    preterms, 55
Intubation, neonatal, 51
Intussusception of bowel,
    162–163
Iron deficiency anaemia,
    203–204
Iron poisoning, 117
Irritable hip (transient
    synovitis), 288–289
Isotonic dehydration, 166

J

Jaundice
    infectious, 98
    neonatal, 61–64
        physiological, 61, 177
        prolonged, 61, 63, 177
Joint
    inflammation, *see* Arthritis
    swelling, causes, 281

K

Karyotype, *see*
    Chromosomes;
    Cytogenetics
Kawasaki disease, 96–97
Keratoconjunctivitis, 95
Kernicterus, 62–63
Ketoacidosis, diabetic, 256
Ketotic hypoglycaemia, 259
Kidney, 185, 186, 187
    agenesis, 185
    calculi, 187
    cysts (simple), 185
    failure
        acute, 195–196
        chronic, 196–197
    fetal, examination, 33
    function test, 183–184
    horseshoe, 186
    hypoplasia and dysplasia,
        unilateral, 185
    obstructive abnormalities,
        185, 186
    polycystic, 185
    tumours, 225–256
Klinefelter syndrome, 17–18

Knee, 289–290
    knock, 285
Knock–knees, 285
Kwashiorkor, 87–88

L

Lactation, 75
Lactose intolerance, 170
Langerhans cell
    histiocytosis, 228–229
Language problems,
    319–321
    developmental delay,
        319–320, 331
Large bowel obstruction,
    neonatal, 65–66
Large–for–dates infants,
    52–53
Laryngotracheobronchitis,
    126
Laxatives, 175
    in faecal soiling, 333
Lead poisoning, 119–120
Learning
    disability/disorders
    (mental retardation/
    handicap), 321–324
    assessment, 321
    causes, 321–322
        cerebral palsy, 295, 296
        genetic, 14, 322
    identification, 322–323,
        324
    management, 323–324
        educational, 323, 364
    psychological impact, 329,
        337
Leucocytes (white cells)
    counts, age–related
        changes, 202, 203, 356
    tests in urinary tract
        infection, 184
Leucomalacia,
    periventricular, 55
Leukaemia
    acute, 217–220
    chronic, 220
Leukodystrophy,
    metachromatic, 266
Lice, head, 275
Light, examination using, 7
Limb girdle dystrophy,
    310–311
Lip, cleft, 69–70
Lipid levels, elevated,
    157–158

Lipidoses, 266–7
Listeria monocytogenes, 39
Liver, 177–182
    failure, acute, 179
    fibrosis, congenital, 182
    immaturity in preterms, 54
    infections, 98, 178–179
        neonatal, 41, 98
    tumours, 338
Liver phosphorylase
    deficiency (type IV
    glycogenosis), 264
Louse, head, 275
Low birth weight, 53–57, *see
    also* Failure to thrive
Lumbar puncture, 305
Lung, *see also* Respiratory
    disorders
    cyanotic disease, 137
    fetal, ultrasound, 34
    neonatal
        aspiration into lung,
            57–59
        immaturity, 59–61
Luteinising hormone (LH),
    245
    abnormal levels, 246
Lyell's disease
    (staphylococcal
    scalded skin
    syndrome), 273
Lymphadenopathy, cervical,
    93, *see also* Adenitis;
    Mucocutaneous
    lymph node
    syndrome
Lymphoblastic leukaemia,
    acute, 217, 218–129
Lymphohistiocytosis,
    familial
    erythrophagocytic,
    229
Lymphomas, 220–222
Lysosomal storage
    disorders, 266, 267

M

McCune–Albright
    syndrome, 248
Macrocephaly, 230–231
Macules, 269
    haemangioma, 44
Malabsorption, 168–170
    vomiting and diarrhoea
        in, 165
Malaria, 104
    fetal, 40

Malignancy, 213–29
  management, 214–217
  predisposing conditions, 213
  testicular, 199
Malnutrition, 87–88
Malrotation of bowel, 161–162
Maltreatment, *see* Child abuse
Marasmus, 87
Marble bone disease, 291
Marfan syndrome, 241, 291
Masculinisation/virilisation
  boys, incomplete, 249
  female fetus, 26, 249, 250
Maternal aspects, *see* Mother
Mean corpuscular volume, 356
Measles (rubeola), 90–92
  respiratory problems, 91, 126
Meckel diverticulum, 162
Meconium aspiration, 57–58
Meconium ileus, 65
  in cystic fibrosis, 129
Medium–chain acyl CoA
  dehydrogenase
  deficiency, 265
Megacolon, congenital
  (Hirschsprung's
  disease), 65, 176
Melanocytic naevus, 275–276
Meningitis
  acute purulent, 304–306
  aseptic/viral, 306, 307
  in mumps, 94
  neonatal, 40, 71, 306–307
  tuberculous, 103–104, 306, 307
Meningocele, 67, 68
Meningococcal disease, 304, 305, 306
Meningoencephalitis, HSV, 95–96
Meningomyelocele, *see*
  Myelomeningocele
Mental retardation, *see*
  Learning disability
Mesenteric adenitis, 160
Metabolic acidosis, 60–61
  mechanisms, 261–262
Metabolic disease, inherited, 260–268
  biochemical screening, 46, 261
  clinical and laboratory
  features, 260

management, 268
myopathies in, 311
Metachromatic
  leukodystrophy, 266
Metered dose inhalers, 134
Microcephaly, 230
Microdeletion syndromes, 17
Microscopy, urine, 184
Micturating
  cystourethrogram, 184, 188
Middle ear infections, 122
Migraine, 296–297, 303
  and cyclical vomiting, 163
Milia, 45
Miliaria, 45
Miliary tuberculosis, 103–104
Milk
  aspiration, 58
  cows', *see* Cows' milk
  mammalian, major
  constituents, 74
  humans, 75–76
Miscarriage, chromosomal
  abnormalities, 13
Mitochondrial inheritance, 23
Molecular genetic
  techniques, 25–30
  sex–linked recessive
  disorder detection, 22–23
Molluscum contagiosum, 273, 274
Mongolian blue spots, 45
Mononucleosis, infectious, 96
Morquio syndrome, 267
Mortalities, 10–11, *see also*
  Survival
  neonatal/perinatal, 10
  chromosomal
  abnormalities and, 14
  parental, effect on child, 339
  postneonatal and infant, 10–11
  road traffic accident, 111
Mother, *see also* Family;
  Parents
  blood group
  incompatibility with
  fetus, 35, 62, 63, 64
  bonding with, 338–339
  immunoglobulins, 41
  infections, 37–38, 92–93
Mouth, *see* Oral disorders

Mucocutaneous lymph node
  syndrome, 96–97
Mucopolysaccharidoses, 267
Multifactorial inheritance,
  see Polygenic
  inheritance
Mumps, 93
Münchausen syndrome by
  proxy, 353–354
Murmurs, 137
  aortic coarctation, 148
  aortic stenosis, 146
  atrial septal defect, 139
  Fallot's tetralogy, 152–153
  innocent, 138
  patent ductus arteriosus, 144
  pulmonary hypertension, 145
  pulmonary stenosis, 149
  ventricular septal defect, 142, 143
Muscle disorders
  (myopathies), 309–311
  acquired, 311
  inherited, 309–311
Muscular atrophy, spinal, 312–313
Muscular dystrophy, 309–311
  Becker, 310
  Duchenne, 28, 309–310
  facioscapulohumeral, 310
Mutation analysis
  direct, 27–28
  indirect, 27
Myasthenia gravis, 311–312
Mycobacterium tuberculosis, 102–104
Myelodysplastic disorders, 220
Myeloid leukaemia
  acute, 217, 219–220
  chronic, 220
Myelomeningocele, 67, 68
  spina bifida with, 67
Myoclonic seizures, 298
Myopathies, *see* Muscle
  disorders
Myotonic dystrophy, 311

N

Naevus
  capillary, 275
  pigmented, 275–276
  strawberry, 275, 276

Nappy rashes (napkin dermatitis), 84, 270
candidiasis superimposed on, 270, 271
Nasopharyngeal carcinoma, 228
Near drowning, 114–115
Necrotising enterocolitis, 55
Neglect, 353
Neiserria meningitidis (meningococcus), 304, 305, 306
Neisseria gonorrhoea, conjunctivitis, 40, 71–72
Neonates, 43–73
anaemia, causes, 202
breast enlargement, 45, 247
chromosomal abnormalities, 14
examination (routine), 43–46, 362
hepatitis syndrome, 178
hyperthyroidism, 253
hypoparathyroidism, 253–254
infections, *see* Infections
mortality, *see* Mortalities
screening, *see* Screening
skin lesions, 44–5, 72, 270–271
thrombocytopenia, 211
Neoplasms, *see* Tumours
Nephritic syndrome, acute, 191–192
Nephroblastoma, 225–226
Nephrolithiasis (renal stones), 187
Nephrotic syndrome, 192–193
Nerve fibre disorders, 312
Nesidioblastosis, 259
Neural tube defects, 25, 66–69
AFP levels and, 25, 33
genetic factors, 25
Neuroblastoma, 223–224
Neuroectodermal tumours, peripheral, 224–225
Neuroepithelioma, peripheral, 224–225
Neurological disorders, *see* Brain; Central nervous system; Spine *and specific disorders*
Neurological signs, brain tumours, 223

Neuromuscular junction disorders, 311–12
Newborns, *see* Neonates
Niemann–Pick disease, 267
Night terrors, 303
Nitrite tests, 184
Nocturnal enuresis, 331–332, 343
Nodules, thyroid, isolated, 253
Noises, respiratory, 6
Non–accidental injury, 350–353
Non–Hodgkin lymphoma, 221–222
Nutrition, 74–89, *see also* Diet
deficiencies, 84–86, *see also* Malnutrition
preterm, 56
preterm infant, 54
deficiencies, 56

O

Obesity, 88–89
Observation, 5–6, 6
Obsession, 347, 348
Ocular disorders, *see* Eye
Oedema and nephrotic syndrome, 192–193
Oesophago–tracheal fistula, 64
Oesophagus
atresia, 64
incoordination, 82
reflux into, 81–82
Oligonucleotide probes, point mutations, 27
Omphalocele (exomphalos), 66
Oncogenes, 28–29
Ophthalmopathy, *see* Eye
Oral disorders, neonatal cysts, 45
fungal infections, 72
Oral rehydration therapy, 167
Orchidopexy, 198–199
Organic acidurias, 263
Ornithine transcarbamylase deficiency, 263–264
Ortolani test, 287
Osgood–Schlatter syndrome, 290
Osmolality, urine, 184
Osteogenesis imperfecta

(brittle–bone disease), 291
Osteoid osteoma, 291
Osteomyelitis, 281, 283–284
Osteopetrosis, 291
Osteosarcoma, 227
Ostium primum, 140–141
Ostium secundum, 139–140
Otitis media, 122
with effusion, 122
Out–toe gait, 285

P

Pain, abdominal, *see* Abdominal pain
Palate, cleft, 69–70
Palliative care, cancer, 214
Palpation
abdomen, 6
constipation, 175
fontanelles, 6–7, 45
Pancreatic enzyme supplements, 130
Pancreatitis, chronic recurrent, 164
Panencephalitis, subacute sclerosing, 91, 308
Panhypogammaglobulin-aemia, 108
Papilloma virus, skin infection (viral warts), 273, 274
Papules, 269
Paracetamol poisoning, 117
Paralytic causes of floppiness in infants, 313
Paraphimosis, 201
Parasites
cutaneous, 274–275
intestinal, 173–174
Parathyroid glands, 253–254
insufficiency, *see* Hypoparathyroidism
Parents, *see also* Family; Father; Mother
ability and attitudes, 339–340
health education, 362, 363, 364
at interview, 1–2
Parotitis, epidemic (mumps), 93
Paroxysmal supraventricular tachycardia, 153–154

Paroxysmal vertigo, benign, 303
Partial seizures, 297
    complex, 299
    with secondary generalisation, 300
    simple, 299
Parvovirus B19, 38, 97
Patau syndrome, 16–17
Patellar chondromalacia, 290
Pauciarticular juvenile chronic arthritis, 283
Pediculosis capitis, 275
Pelvi–ureteric junction obstruction, 186
Penicillin in rheumatic fever, 156
Penis, prepuce, 200–201
Peptic ulcers, 163–164
Perinatal period
    hypoxia, see Hypoxia
    learning disability and problems in, 322
    mortality, see Mortalities
Periodic syndrome
    migraine and, 163
    (recurrent episodes of abdominal pain and vomiting), 344
Peripheral neuroepithelioma, 224–225
Peritonitis, primary, 160
Periventricular leucomalacia, 55
Peroxisomal disorders, 268
Perthes disease, 289
Pertussis, 99–101, 128
Pes, see entries under Talipes
pH, urine, 184
Phagocytic function
    defects, 108, 109
    investigation, 106
Phenylketonuria, 262–263
Phimosis, 200
Phobias, 347–348
Pierre Robin syndrome, 70
Pigmented naevus, 275–276
Pituitary failure, see Hypopituitarism
Pityriasis rosea, 277
Placenta, 32
    drugs crossing, 36–37
    infections crossing, 37–40, 92–93
Plants, poisonous, 116
Plaques, 269
Pleural effusions in pneumonia, 125–126

Pneumonia (incl. bacterial pneumonia), 125
    neonatal, 40, 57
    pleural effusions in, 125–126
Pneumothorax, 60
Poisoning, 110, 116–118
Poliomyelitis, 98–9
Polyarthritis (polyarticular arthritis)
    allergic, 282
    juvenile chronic, 282
Polycystic kidneys, 185
Polygenic/multifactorial inheritance, 23–24
    diabetes, 255
    height, 235
Polymerase chain reaction, 28
Polyneuritis, infectious, 312
Pompe disease, 267, 311
Poor families, 340–341
Portal hypertension, 181
Port–wine stain, 275
Poststreptococcal glomerulonephritis, 191–192
Posture
    congenital deformities, 46
    normal variations, 284–285
Poverty, 340–341
Prader–Willi syndrome, 23
Preclinical diagnosis, genetic disorders, 26–27
Preconception medicine, 31
Premature infants, see Preterm infants
Prenatal
    diagnosis/screening
    Down syndrome, 33
    genetic disorders, 26
    heart disease (congenital), 136
    muscular dystrophy, 310
    neural tube defects, 25, 33
    urinary tract malformations, 185
Prepuce, 200–201
Pre–school child
    behavioural problems, 341–342
    vaccination schedule, 360
Preterm infants, 54–56
    perinatal hypoxic damage, 52
    prognosis, 56–57
    retinopathy, 55–6, 316
Processus vaginalis,

persistent patency, 199–200
Proteinuria, 183
Protozoans, intestinal, 173
Prune belly syndrome, 187
Pseudohypoparathyroidism, 254
Pseudopseudohypopara-thyroidism, 254
Pseudoseizures, hysterical, 303
Psoriasis, 277
Psychological problems, see Emotional problems
Pubarche, premature, 247–248
Puberty, 244–8
    cranial radiotherapy affecting, 248
    delay, 246
    constitutional, 235, 246
    height changes, 232
    physiology, 245–246
    precocious, 246–248
Pulmonary flow murmur, 138
Pulmonary hypertension, 145
    in ventricular septal defect, 141
Pulmonary non–vascular disorders, see Lung
Pulmonary valve stenosis, 149–150
Purpura
    Henoch–Schönlein purpura, 192, 281–282
    idiopathic thrombocytopenic, 211
Purulent infections, see Pyogenic infections
Pyloric stenosis, 82–83
Pyogenic/purulent infections
    arthritis, 281
    meningitis, 304–306
Pyruvate kinase deficiency, 206

R

Radiology, renal tract, 184
Radiotherapy
    cancer, 215
    cranial, affecting puberty, 248

Rashes, neonates/early infancy, 45, 84, 270–271
Reading retardation, 330
Recessive disorders
    autosomal, 21–22
    X–linked, 23–4
Rectal agenesis, 66
Red cells
    average volume (MCV), 356
    enzyme deficiency, 63, 206
Reflex(es), primitive, in cerebral palsy, 295
Reflex anoxic seizures, 303
Reflux
    gastro–oesophageal, 81–82
    vesico–ureteric, see Vesico–ureteric reflux
Rehydration therapy, oral, 167
Renal tissue, see Kidney
Renal tract, see Urinary tract
Respiratory disorders, 121–135, see also Lung
    examination, 6
    infections, see Respiratory infections
    neonatal, 57–61
        preterm infants, 54
Respiratory distress syndrome, 59–60
Respiratory infections
    lower, 102–103, 124–128
        in cystic fibrosis, 130–131
        measles, 91, 126
        neonatal, 40, 57
    upper, 121–123
Responsiveness, neonatal, 44
Restriction site, mutations altering, 27
Resuscitation, neonatal, 50–51
    reasons for failing to respond, 51
Reticulocyte count, 356
Retinoblastoma, 228
    preclinical diagnosis, 26
Retinopathy of prematurity, 55–56, 316
Retroviruses in gene therapy, 29
Reye syndrome, 179, 308
Rhabdomyosarcoma, 225
Rhesus incompatibility, 35, 62, 63, 64
Rheumatic fever, 155–156

Rhythmic behaviour, 343
Rickets, 85–86
    secondary, 85–86
Ringworm (tinea), 274
Ritter's disease, 273
Road traffic accidents, 111
Robertsonian translocation, 15
Roseola infantum, 97
Roundworm, 173
Rubella (German measles), 92–93
    maternal, 37, 92–93
Rubeola, see Measles
Russell–Silver syndrome, 236

S

Sacral dimples, 45
Sacrococcygeal teratoma, congenital, 226
Salmon patch, 44
Sarcomas
    bone, 227
    soft tissue, 225
Sarcoptes scabiei (scabies), 274
Scabies, 274
Scalded skin syndrome, staphylococcal, 273
Scales, 269
Scarlet fever, 101
School
    health
        promotion/services in, 364–365
    needs in learning disability, 323, 364
    problems at, 341
    refusal to go/truancy, 344–345
School–age children
    recurrent abdominal pain, 343–344
    vaccination schedules, 360
Sclerosing panencephalitis, subacute, 91, 308
Scoliosis, 285–286
Screening
    deafness, 317
    neonatal, 44
        biochemical, 46, 261
        congenital hip dysplasia, 287–288
        cystic fibrosis, 129
        prenatal, see Prenatal diagnosis

urinary tract infections, 189
Scurvy, 84–85
Seborrhoeic dermatitis, 270
Seeing, see Vision
Seizures, see Convulsions
Sensorineural deafness, 318
    audiograms, 319
    therapy, 319
Separation, 338, 339
Septic arthritis, 281
Septic spots, 72
Severe combined immunodeficiency, 108
Sex chromosomes (X and Y)
    numerical/structural abnormalities, 13, 17–19
    single gene defects, 22–23
Sexual abuse, 189, 353
Sexual characteristics, secondary, staging system, 245
Sexual differentiation disorders, 248–249
Sexually–transmitted diseases, neonatal, 40, 71–72
Shaken baby, 350, 351
Shingles, see Herpes zoster
Short stature, 232–241
    disproportionate, 240–241
    investigation, 239–240
Shunts
    cardiac, left–to–right, 138–415
    CSF, in hydrocephalus treatment, 69
Sickle cell anaemia/disease, 21, 207–208
    mutation detection, 27
SIDS, 10
Sight, see Vision
Skeletal dysplasias, 240–241
Skin lesions, 269–279
    neonatal/infant, 44–45, 72, 84, 270–271
Skin tags, accessory, 45
Skull, growth abnormalities, 230–231
Slapped cheek syndrome, 38, 97
Sleep disorders, 303, 342
Slipped upper femoral epiphysis, 289Small bowel obstruction, neonatal, 65
Small–for–dates infants, 53, 235

Smoking, 119
Social factors (class etc.), 9
  emotional/behavioural
    problems, 326,
    340–341
  short stature, 236
Social misbehaviour, 345
Sodium cromoglycate,
  asthma, 133
Soft tissue sarcomas, 225
Soiling, see Faecal soiling
Sounds
  heart
    aortic stenosis, 146
    Fallot's tetralogy, 152
    neonatal, 44
    pulmonary
      hypertension, 145
    transposition of great
      arteries, 152
    ventricular septal
      defect, 142, 143
  respiratory, 6
Southern blotting, 28
Spasms
  habit, 303
  infantile, 298–299
Spastic cerebral palsy, 294
Speaking, see Speech
Special educational needs
  (in learning
  disability), 323, 364
Speech
  assessment, 320–321
  problems, 319–321
    developmental delay,
    319–320, 331
Spherocytosis, hereditary,
  205–206
Spina bifida cystica, 67–8
Spina bifida occulta, 68
Spinal muscular atrophy,
  312–313
Spine
  scoliosis, 285–286
  tumours, 222, 223
Spitz naevus, 275–276
Squint, 315
Stammering, 321
Staphylococcal scalded skin
  syndrome, 273
Stature, see also Height
  excessive, 241–242
  short, see Short stature
Status epilepticus, 301–302
Stem cell rescue, 216
Steroids
  adrenal

insufficiency/failure, 238,
    251
  arthritis (juvenile chronic),
    283
  asthma
    inhaled, 133, 134
    oral, 134
    prophylactic, 238
  atopic eczema, 272
Stevens–Johnson syndrome,
    278, 279
Still's disease, 282
Stones, renal, 187
Stork bites, 44
Strabismus (squint), 315
Strawberry naevus, 275, 276
Streptococcal infection
  group A haemolytic, 101,
    122
    glomerulonephritis
      following, 191–192
    rheumatic fever and,
      155–156
  group B, neonatal
    meningeal, 40, 71
    respiratory, 40, 57
Stridor, 123–124
Sturge–Weber syndrome,
    275, 276
Subaponeurotic
    haemorrhage, 47
Sucrase–isomaltase
    deficiency, 170
Sudden infant death
    syndrome, 10
Suffocation, 115
Sugar intolerance, 170, 264
Support, family/child, in
    cancer, 214
Supraventricular
    tachycardia,
    paroxysmal, 153–154
Surface area calculation,
    358–359
Surgery
  biliary atresia, 178
  cancer, 214–215
  cleft lip/palate, 70
  fetal, 36
  heart
    aortic coarctation, 148
    aortic stenosis, 147
    atrial septal defect, 140,
      141
    Fallot's tetralogy, 153
    hypoplastic left heart,
      149
    patent ductus
      arteriosus, 144, 145

pulmonary stenosis, 150
    transposition of great
      arteries, 153
    ventricular septal
      defect, 143
  Hirschsprung's disease,
    176
  inguinal
    hernia/hydroceles,
      200
  myelomeningocele, 68
  prepuce, 200, 201
  testicular
    ectopia/maldescent,
      198–9
  urinary tract, 189
Survival, see also Mortalities
  cancer, 217
  preterm infants, 54, 56, 57
Sweat test, 129
Symptom management,
    cancer, 214
Syncope, 303
Synovitis, transient (hip),
    288–289
Systemic juvenile chronic
    arthritis, 282
Systolic BP, normal values,
    357

T

T–cell deficiencies, 107–108
Tachycardia, paroxysmal
    supraventricular,
    153–154
Tachypnoea, transient, 48,
    58–59
Taenia spp., 174
Talipes (pes) calcaneovalgus,
    290–291
Talipes (pes) equinovarus,
    290
Talipes (pes) planus, 285
Tallness, excessive, 241–242
Tay–Sachs disease, 266
Telangiectasia, ataxia, 304
Temper tantrums, 326
Temperament, 337–338
Temporal lobe epilepsy,
    psychological aspects,
    329
Teratoma, congenital
    sacrococcygeal, 226
Testicle/testis, 197–200
  ectopic, 198–199
  maldescent, 198, 198–199
  retractile, 196

torsion, 199
undescent, 197–198, 198
Testicular feminisation, 22
Tetralogy of Fallot, 150–151
Thalassaemia, 208–209
Thelarche, *see* Breast
enlargement
Thermal injuries, 113–14
Thermoregulation, preterm
infant, 54
Threadworm, 173
Thrombocytopenias, 211
Thrombocytopenic purpura,
idiopathic, 211
Thrush, 72
Thyroid, 251–253
carcinoma, 228
overactivity, 253
underactivity, *see*
Hypothyroidism
Thyroiditis, autoimmune,
253
Tibia valga (genu valgum),
285
Tibia vara (genu varum),
285
Tics, 303
Tinea, 274
Toilet training, 333, 343
Tonic–clonic seizures, 299
Tonsillitis, 102, 122–3
Toxic agents, ingested
(poisoning), 110,
116–118
Toxocara canis and *catis*, 174
Toxoplasmosis, 39–40
Toys, 2–3
Tracheal intubation,
neonatal, 51
Tracheomalacia, 124
Tracheo–oesophageal fistula,
64
Transfusion, exchange, 64
Transplantation, bone
marrow, in cancer,
216
Transposition of great
arteries, 152–3
Trauma, *see* Injury
Treacher Collins syndrome,
70
Tricyclic antidepressant
poisoning, 117–118
Trisomies
trisomy–13, 16–17
trisomy–18, 15–16
trisomy–21, *see* Down
syndrome

Truancy, 344–345
Tuberculosis, 102–104
arthritis, 281
meningitis, 103–104, 306,
307
Tumour(s)
bone, 227, 291–292
hypopituitarism caused
by, 238
malignant, *see* Malignancy
Tumour suppressor genes
(anti–oncogenes), 29
Turner (45,X) syndrome,
18–19
short stature, 239

U

Ulcer(s)
peptic, 163–164
skin, 269
Ulcerative colitis, 172
Ultrasound, fetal, 33–35
Umbilical infections, 72
Undressing, 5
Urachal remnants, 187
Urea cycle defects, 263
Ureteric duplication, 186
Ureterocele, 186
Ureteropelvic junction
obstruction, 186
Ureterovesical junction
obstruction, 186
Urethral syndrome, 189
Urethral valves, posterior,
186–187
Urinary tract, *see also specific
parts*
infections, 163, 187–189
malformations, 185–187
Urine, analysis, 183–184
Urolithiasis, 187
Urticaria, neonatal, 45

V

Vaccines (active
immunisation),
105–106
consent, 362
diphtheria, 99
Haemophilus influenzae,
106, 304
hepatitis B, 98
measles, 92
mumps, 93
national schedule, 360

pertussis, 100–101, 128
poliomyelitis, 99
rubella, 37, 92–3
tuberculosis, 104
varicella (chickenpox), 94
Vaginal delivery, infection
risk, 40–41
Valvuloplasty, balloon, *see*
Balloon techniques
Varicella (chickenpox), 39,
94
encephalitis, 308
Varicella–zoster virus,
38–39, *see also* Herpes
zoster
Varicoceles, 199
Venous hum, 138
Ventilation, neonatal, 50–51
Ventricular haemorrhage,
preterms, 55
Ventricular septal defect,
141–143
Vertigo, benign paroxysmal,
303
Vesicles, 269
Vesico–ureteric junction
obstruction, 186
Vesico–ureteric reflux
investigation, 188
management, 189
Vibratory murmur, 138
Viral arthritis, 281
Viral gastroenteritis, 165–166
Viral meningitis, 306, 307
Viral skin infections,
273–274
Viral vectors for genes (in
gene therapy), 29
Virilisation, *see*
Masculinisation
Vision, 314–317
assessment, 314–315
development, 314
loss, 316–317
Vitamin A deficiency, 84
Vitamin C deficiency, 84–85
Vitamin D
deficiency, 85
therapy, in
hypoparathyroidism/
pseudohypoparathy-
roidism, 254
Vitamin K deficiency
bleeding, 86
Vomiting
abdominal pain and,
recurrent episodes,
see Periodic
syndrome

differential diagnosis, 165
von Gierke's disease
(glycogenosis type I),
264
von Willebrand disease,
210–211

W

Warts, viral, 273, 274
Weight, 231–232
at birth, *see* Birth weight
in body surface area
calculation, 358–359
charts
child, 233
fetal, 52

excess, 88–89
infant, regular
assessment, 363
Werdnig–Hoffman
syndrome, 313
Wetting, *see* Enuresis
Wheals, 269
Wheeze, persistent (infant),
differential diagnosis,
132
White cells, *see* Leucocytes
White pimples, 45
Whooping cough, 99–101,
128
Williams syndrome, 17
Wilms tumour, 225–226
Wilson disease, 180–181

Wiskott–Aldrich syndrome,
211

X

X–linked disorders, 22–23
45,X, *see* Turner (45,X)
syndrome
45,X/46,XY, 19
Xeroderma pigmentosum,
276
Xerophthalmia, 84
47,XXY, 17–18

Y

Y chromosomes, *see* Sex
chromosomes